How to Run Your Nurse Practitioner Business

A Guide for Success

How to Run Your Nurse Practitioner Business
A Guide for Success

Sheila Grossman, PhD, FNP-BC, APRN
Martha Burke O'Brien, MS, ANP-BC, APRN

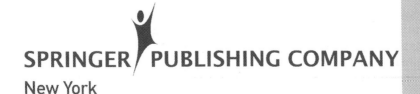

SPRINGER PUBLISHING COMPANY
New York

Springer Publishing Company, LLC
11 West 42nd Street
New York, NY 10036
www.springerpub.com

Acquisitions Editor: Allan Graubard
Project Manager: Barbara A. Chernow
Cover Design: David Levy
Composition: Agnew's, Inc.

E-book ISBN: 978-0-8261-1763-2

09 10 11 12/ 5 4 3 2 1

Library of Congress Cataloging-in-Publication Data

Grossman, Sheila.
    How to run your nurse practitioner business : a guide for success / Sheila Grossman, Martha Burke O'Brien.
        p. ; cm.
    Includes bibliographical references and index.
    ISBN 978-0-8261-1762-5
    1. Nursing—Practice. 2. Nurse practitioners. I. O'Brien, Martha Burke. II. Title.
    [DNLM: 1. Nurse Practitioners—organization & administration. 2. Entrepreneurship—organization & administration. 3. Professional Practice—organization & administration. WY 16 G878h 2010]
    RT86.7.G76 2010
    610.73068—dc22

                                                                    2010012108

Printed in the United States of America by Hamilton Printing Company

The author and the publisher of this Work have made every effort to use sources believed to be reliable to provide information that is accurate and compatible with the standards generally accepted at the time of publication. Because medical science is continually advancing, our knowledge base continues to expand. Therefore, as new information becomes available, changes in procedures become necessary. We recommend that the reader always consult current research and specific institutional policies before performing any clinical procedure. The author and publisher shall not be liable for any special, consequential, or exemplary damages resulting, in whole or in part, from the readers' use of, or reliance on, the information contained in this book. The publisher has no responsibility for the persistence or accuracy of URLs for external or third-party Internet Web sites referred to in this publication and does not guarantee that any content on such Web sites is, or will remain, accurate or appropriate.

This book is dedicated to the many nurse practitioners and nurse practitioner students with whom I have collaborated and worked over the years. I especially want to mention my colleagues, Patricia Poli, PhD, CPA, Associate Professor School of Business, Fairfield University, for her insightful comments regarding business management, Kathleen Wheeler, PhD, APRN-BC, FAAN, who initially inspired me to become a nurse practitioner and always encouraged me, along with Anne Manton, PhD, APRN-BC, FAAN, to be the best I could be. I am privileged to work with the most collegial and knowledgeable nurse practitioners (Maria Banevicius, Martha Burke O'Brien, Lynda Tagliavini, Stephanie Taylor, Kathleen Hayes, and Danielle Morgan) and staff (Jeannette Gomez and Lori Clapis) at Trinity College Health Center, where the mantra is R. E. S. P. E. C. T. for patients and each other.

I also dedicate this book to my sister, Ellen C. Bernstein, who role models the "art of possibility" to perfection and assisted in proofreading this manuscript, to my husband, Bob, for his great humor, sarcasm, and patience, and to our daughters, Lisa and Beth, who have always been motivational forces for me to follow my heart and do things right.

Sheila C. Grossman

This book is dedicated to my husband Kevin for his love and support, for his unequivocal acceptance of my style and practice of nursing, his acceptance of "I'll be late again tonight," his thoughtful and intelligent demeanor that challenges me to be always mindful, and his unfettered encouragement to be and become the only type of clinician and nurse I could respect being.

I also dedicate this book to my professional mentors and clinical role models with whom I have been so blessed to practice: Dr. Elaine Yordan and Dr. Sharon Herzberger. You inspired my creativity, laid the foundation for my high standards, and encouraged me always to practice for the patient.

Lastly, I dedicate this to my current clinical staff, whose members show me the essence of caring, competence, and compassion, and who demonstrate the true meaning of being an independent nurse practitioner each day we work side by side.

Martha Burke O'Brien

Contents

Section I Regulatory Implications for Nurse Practitioner Practice

Section II Essentials of Developing and Managing the Nurse Practitioner Practice

Section III   Templates, Documents, Policy, Procedures, and Plans

About the Authors

Sheila Grossman, PhD, FNP-BC, APRN, is a Professor of Nursing and Coordinator of the Family Nurse Practitioner Track at Fairfield University School of Nursing. She received a BS in nursing from the University of Connecticut, her MS as a Respiratory Clinical Nurse Specialist from the University of Massachusetts/Amherst, a postmasters degree as a Family Nurse Practitioner from Fairfield University, and her PhD from the University of Connecticut. She has worked many years as a clinician on a variety of medical, surgical, and critical care units and presently practices as a Family Nurse Practitioner in a primary care clinic. She is the coauthor of *The New Leadership Challenge: Creating A Preferred Future for Nursing,* which is in its third edition (2009) and received an AJN book of the Year Award. She has also received an AJN Book of the Year Award for *Mentoring in Nursing: A Dynamic and Collaborative Process* (2007), and coauthored *Gerontological Nurse Certification Review* in 2008. She is the author of multiple chapters and journal articles on leadership, mentoring, gerontology, adult health, and palliative care. Her research interests focus on symptom management in palliative care, leadership, pedagogy, cultural competence, and adult patient outcome studies. She is active in Sigma Theta Tau International Honor Society, American Association of Critical Care Nurses, National Organization of Nurse Practitioner Faculty, American College of Nurse Practitioners, and is a certified End of Life Nursing Education Consortium Educator and a Commission on Collegiate Nursing Education Accreditation Site Visitor. She is the winner of the 2009 Josephine Dolan Award for Outstanding Contributions to Nursing Education sponsored by the CT Nurses Association.

Martha Burke O'Brien, MS, ANP-BC, APRN, has been the Director of the Trinity College Health Center (TCHC) in Hartford for 11 years. Early in her tenure, she received a commendation from the American College Health Association for her creative practice model of an all Advanced Practice Nurse staff, using physician collaboration in the "true" sense of collaboration. She received her BSN from Northeastern University and worked at the John Dempsey Hospital of the University of Connecticut Health Center after graduation. She received her MS from Boston College in Adult Primary Care. Before becoming the Director of the TCHC, she worked as a Primary Care Nurse Practitioner in the Adolescent Clinic at St. Francis Hospital and Medical Center for several years. She was involved in the Connecticut Nurse Practitioner Group, Inc., now known as Advanced Practice Registered Nurse Society, serving as President and Membership Chairperson for years. In addition, she has received multiple awards, including The

Nurse Practitioner of the Year Award in 2001. As a member of the American College Health Associations' Consulting Services Program Advisory, she has also consulted with several college health clinics throughout the northeast about setting up nurse practitioner run clinics. She has done several presentations on Adolescent Health, Sexually Transmitted Diseases, and Reproductive Health, and has published in Nurse Practitioner journals.

Foreword

This is a most stimulating time for the expanding number of nurse practitioners (NPs), who are seeking challenges and opportunities that will also be financially profitable. But how does the NP take advantage of these opportunities? Grossman and O'Brien have written *How to Run Your Nurse Practitioner Business: A Guide for Success* for the NP of the twenty-first century.

The authors have threaded their model, "Elements of the Nurse Practitioner Role," throughout the book and given realistic examples to explain the four elements of the NP role: Clinician, Leader, Manager, and Professional. The authors have combined their collective knowledge and experience to illustrate how these four elements can prepare an NP to start a business.

Section III contains templates that the NP can individualize for his or her own practice setting. In addition, examples show how to develop many essential documents, including:

- Letter of intent for applying for a grant
- Résumé and biographical sketch
- Patient satisfaction tool
- Collaborative practice agreement

Everything needed to develop one's own practice is generously shared, along with an explanation of the regulatory statutes for starting a business, managing a practice setting, budgeting and planning for financial stability, obtaining practice accreditation, evaluating staff, and generating high-quality patient outcomes.

In addition, the authors have woven reflective practice into their recommendations as a way for NPs to acquire further insight and skills. The book's purpose, to generate excitement for learning a new way of thinking reflectively, of seeing things more holistically as opposed to in a detail-specific environment, and of collaborating with networks of people on a continuous basis to establish partnerships, comes through clearly and offers the reader a path to gain confidence and growth in each element of the NP role.

Resilience is one of the characteristics NPs embody, as they have the innate ability to persist and succeed in the face of adversity. In *How to Run Your Nurse Practitioner Business: A Guide for Success,* the authors reflect on how NPs need to practice the "art of possibility" (Zander & Zander, 2000), so that they are always prepared to answer the next question about management, address a clinical concern, or resolve a reimbursement issue with a creative plan. Grossman and O'Brien also recommend collaborative networking and partnering as opposed to the mentality that says "everyone for themselves" or "the fittest survive and the others lose." NPs need to learn through collaboration. In this way, NPs will ultimately improve their leadership, management, professional, and practice skills.

Many healthcare work settings are led by managers who have been educated clinically, but often lack proactive leadership skills. Grossman and O'Brien advocate for change that will result in a win-win workplace that is led by NPs who are true leaders, not simply managers. They agree with Bennis and Nannus (1985), who remind us that "managers are people who do things right and leaders are people who do the right things" (p. 21). This is not one of those "Okay, I read that new NP book" that you will put on a bookshelf, but rather a book that you will use time and again.

This is what NPs have been waiting for – a book that inspires them to energize their practices, provide a framework and reference to make their practices more rewarding, and to create work places where all can strive for best practice. Nurse practitioners must take the opportunities that come with these expanded practice and leadership responsibilities and be prepared to fulfill the exciting and challenging role of the twenty-first century NP.

Margaret Fitzgerald, DNP, FNP-BC, NP-C, FAANP, CSP
President, Fitzgerald Health Education Associates, Inc., North Andover, MA
Family Nurse Practitioner, Adjunct Faculty, Family Practice Residency
Greater Lawrence (MA) Family Health Center

References

Bennis, W., & Nanus, B. (1985). *Leaders: The strategies for taking charge.* New York: Harper & Row.

Zander & Zander, (2000). *Using the art of possibility: Transforming professional and personal life.* Cambridge: Harvard Business Book Press.

Preface

How to Run Your Nurse Practitioner Business: A Guide for Success was written as a reference book for nurse practitioners (NPs), masters and doctoral level students, and administrators interested in developing and managing high-quality, cost-effective, and patient-accessible healthcare in NP settings. The Doctor of Nursing Practice (DNP) Essentials are described and implications of the practice doctorate are integrated into this special and comprehensive text designed to assist the reader in learning the principles of business management, including:

- Setting up primary care and other NP specialty practices.
- Collaborating and networking with partners.
- Choosing a business structure.
- Setting up a governing board.
- Creating business plans.
- Developing budgets.
- Writing letters of intent for grants.
- Evaluating patient outcomes.
- Providing ongoing quality improvement.
- Integrating appropriate accreditation regulations.
- Managing compliance, risk, and reimbursement issues.
- Developing policies and procedures to manage a business.

The book was developed with the idea of the NP role as autonomous, but operating within the practice guide parameters determined by local and state legislation. The purpose is to identify the professional, clinical, leadership, and management qualities necessary for a successful patient-centered practice in healthcare settings employing and run by NPs.

The book is divided into three sections. Section I, Regulatory Implications for the Nurse Practitioner Practice, includes the scope and role of the NP, the changing vision of healthcare delivery and its impact on NPs, and an analysis of the impact of statutes and legislation on NP-run practices. Section II, Essentials of Developing and Managing a Nurse Practitioner Practice, offers information about patient safety, evidence-based practice, working with business consultants to develop a practice, financial management of a practice, explanations of the roles of the director/owner and other providers, and collaboration and consultation, as well as a review of entrepreneurial models of NP delivery settings. Section III, Templates, Documents, Policy, Procedures, and Plans, provides templates of policies, procedures, and documents that readers can adapt for their own settings regarding referral, release of healthcare information, on-call correspondence, chart audits, and mission statements. Information regarding all aspects of running a clinic, such as on-call scheduling, job descriptions, staff evaluation, managing patient records, marketing services, collaborative practice agreements, business plans, sample budgets, and specimen processing are shared.

Many entrepreneurial ideas are presented, including delivering health care in creative, innovative, and effective ways in private practice, community health centers, hospital clinics, healthcare homes, homecare, occupational health, juvenile detention centers, prisons, college health, homeless centers, long-term care facilities, and specialty settings. Interviews with experienced NPs representing provider-driven practices are included, as are interviews with new practicing NPs about recommendations for preparing for an NP position.

The major points emphasized throughout this book are: (1) the necessity of knowing local and state legislation and principles of business management as a guide for setting practice parameters; (2) the importance of engaging in reflective practice to enhance creative thinking; and (3) the specific contributions NPs make to health care that result in high patient satisfaction and cost-effective outcomes in providing holistic care as a clinician, leader, manager, and professional.

Key features of the text enhance the readers understanding, including:

- Exploring potential career paths while understanding the breadth of opportunities available to NPs.
- Developing a fundamental framework for establishing an autonomous practice with business management strategies that also take into account the necessary background work needed to start a cost-effective practice.
- Analyzing statutes and legislation affecting the feasibility of developing an NP business.
- Planning for the operational success of an NP practice.
- Implementing changes after evaluation of successes and planning opportunities for continued improvement.
- Providing the business structure necessary to deliver safe and high-quality patient care in an NP clinic.
- Evaluating outcomes, such as patient and provider satisfaction, institutional perception of the healthcare delivery system, and cost effectiveness.
- Examining the structure and functioning of different settings as examples for creating NP practices.
- Integrating the knowledge required to prepare for acquiring and transitioning into the NP role.

Nurse practitioners are encouraged to follow Siegal's (2007) framework on mindfulness to increase their ability to think and learn. Learning through instruction or experience enables NPs to acquire new knowledge and skills by reorganizing neural pathways in the brain. Reflective learning increases the brain's neuroplastic ability, which causes new neurons to be recruited, facilitates different neuronal pathways, and changes the levels of the neurotransmitters. These mechanisms actually have the potential to change the way one thinks. Generally this will improve one's ability to think creatively. By rewiring our brains, reflective thinking enhances our learning ability and passion for our work.

Nurse practitioners need to be aware of how the mind affects who we are, our state of mind, and what information means to us. By practicing active learning strategies, we can improve our clinical, leader, professional, and manager skills. Each chapter includes "Reflective Thinking Exercises" that will assist you in developing the professional leadership, managerial, and clinical aspects of the NP role. Power point slides are available for each chapter.

How to Run Your Nurse Practitioner Business: A Guide for Success is intended to help practicing and student NPs students realize that they must not become the "physician extender" in the physician practice medical model and thereby convert our complex teachings to a 6- to 10-minute meet, treat, and street mentality. Nurse practitioners must resist the temptation to be so cost conscious that they create a health business instead of a healthcare practice. At the same time, NPs must learn to manage a practice like a business.

Many practicing NPs ask: "Why should I go back to get a doctoral degree?" Because, as this text illustrates, the advanced practice role has evolved into one that offers so much more than just excellent care. To be effective as a provider, NPs need to develop skills in the areas of business, policy, statistics, evidence-based practice, billing/coding, and compliance. NPs require additional education in these areas, over and above their education in clinical care, to succeed and to have advanced practice nursing evolve even further.

Acknowledgments

The authors thank Allan Graubard, Senior Acquisitions Editor at Springer Publishing Company, for his creative and exciting ideas for this book, and Barbara Chernow for her editing assistance. For her business expertise, we thank Patricia Poli, PhD, CPA, Associate Professor School of Business, Fairfield University, who is a contributing author in the area of business management. We also thank Dr. Margaret Fitzgerald for her thought-provoking foreword to this book.

We extend our deepest gratitude to the nurse practitioners who expressed their personal thoughts about becoming and being an NP in the interviews cited in Chapters 1 and 8: Jen Cooper, MSN, APRN-BC, Patricia Dunn, MSN, APRN-BC, Michelle Leonard, MSN, APRN-BC, Lesle Spain, MSN, APRN-BC, Mary Tuttle, MSN, APRN-BC, Melinda Wellington, MSN, APRN-BC, Cheryl Anderson, Ed. D, APRN-BC, Christine Berte, MSN, APRN-BC, Jaclyn Conelius, MSN, APRN-BC, Vanessa Pomarico–Denino, MSN, APRN-BC, Louise Moon Rosales, MSN, APRN-BC, Tracy Shamas, MSN, APRN-BC, Corin Shenuski, MSN, APRN-BC, Jacqueline Spano, MSN, APRN-BC, and Kathleen Wheeler, PhD, ARPN-BC.

Regulatory Implications for Nurse Practitioner Practice

Scope and Role of the Nurse Practitioner

1

Learning Objectives

1. Examine the evolving role of the nurse practitioner as a clinician, leader, manager, and professional.

2. Identify the many role opportunities for a nurse practitioner in primary, secondary, and tertiary care.

3. Describe the scope of practice for nurse practitioners.

4. Outline how the Consensus Model for APRN Regulation: Licensure, Accreditation, Certification, and Education will impact the role of the nurse practitioner.

5. Emphasize the value of developing leadership skills to assist nurse practitioners in seeing things from a new perspective and making creative changes.

6. Use self-reflection techniques to create a personal vision of the role of a nurse practitioner.

Key Words: scope of practice, nurse practitioner roles, leadership, Consensus Model for APRN Regulation

This chapter describes how the role of the nurse practitioner (NP) has evolved since the 1960s and teaches advanced and novice practice NPs to create and expand their own roles through self-reflection. Existing employment opportunities are explored, as are ideas for creating new roles consistent with those of advanced nursing practice. As a result of weaknesses and inefficiencies in the delivery of primary and subspecialty health care, NPs now have many more opportunities to expand their scopes of practice by:

- Obtaining new advanced practice skills.
- Acquiring more depth and confidence in their decision making abilities.

▓ Appreciating the resilience of people rather than focusing on the disease model.

▓ Increasing expertise in managing individual patients and populations.

▓ Participating in health policy development.

The Consensus Model for APRN Regulation: Licensure, Accreditation, Certification, and Education (2008) standardizes the NP's preparation, licensure, and maintenance of competency. Nurse practitioners can examine their own visions and goals for developing individualized practice models. They can also mold their practice framework as an advanced practice nurse (APN), rather than as a "physician extender" or "midlevel provider."

The factors affecting the healthcare system—technology, electronic record maintenance, high costs, inefficient payment systems, lack of access to health care, and other variables affecting health maintenance, health promotion, and illness prevention—have created new and exciting opportunities for NPs. In fact, the National Salary and Workplace Survey of Nurse Practitioners, conducted by *ADVANCE for Nurse Practitioners* in 2007, found that 89% of practicing NPs were satisfied with their careers and more than half of these (49%) were very satisfied (http://nurse-practitioners.advanceweb.com/Editorial/Content/Editorial.aspx?CC=200814).

Still, not all NPs are content with their positions. Among the barriers to role fulfillment are issues related to the work setting, including organization, legal problems, and environmental constraints (Plager & Conger, 2007). For example, NPs working at the same location as MDs are often expected to perform RN duties for the physician's patients, as well as for their own. These responsibilities include obtaining laboratory specimens, setting the patient up for a pelvic exam or procedure, and/or teaching a patient about the need for a Coumadin clinic biweekly. Legal and/or organizational problems facing NPs include policies that prevent them from administering desensitization shots without a physician present. Another occurs when the organization's administrators insist that a physician must be the "Medical Director," as opposed to a "Collaborating Physician," even though the physician is not on site. The NP who actually manages the clinic on a 24/7 basis should have the title of Medical Director.

Nurse Practitioner Education

Loretta Ford, PhD, RN, and Henry Silver, MD, started the first NP program, which focused on well child care, at the University of Colorado (Ford, 1979). The four-month program of didactic classes was followed by a 21-month clinical internship, during which NP students worked with experienced NPs in a preceptor format.

As the need for NPs grew, many postbaccalaureate programs emerged, requiring varying amounts of class time and clinical hours. Some of these programs were not college based. Rather, they were continuing education courses with timeframes ranging from a few days to 24 months. In addition, some nurse educators did not want NPs to be graduates of a formal nursing education program. They felt that these nurses had left the nursing profession to become medical professionals or physician extenders.

Since the 1960s, NP programs have grown to include Nurse Practitioner tracks in Family, Adult, Pediatrics, Psychiatric, Neonatal, Geriatric, Acute Care, and Women's Health. In addition, the role of the APN now includes some degree of autonomy, ranging from an autonomous practice with full prescriptive authority without a collaborating physician contract in some states to NPs working under the direct supervision of a physician in other states. Buppert (2008) delineates how each state defines the role in terms of an NP's ability to manage care and prescribe medications independently. Most NPs have two or more years of postbaccalaureate education, certification by a credentialing body in their specialty, the ability to make medical diagnoses, and some degree of prescriptive authority. For further clarification of the legal implications for NPs related to scope of practice, see The American Association of Nurse Attorneys' Web site (http://www.taana.org) (2005).

The American Nurses Association (ANA) defines an APN as a postbaccalaureate educated nurse who is engaged in *practice,* thereby excluding master's-prepared nurses specializing in education, administration, or research. In 2004, the ANA published *Nursing's Social Public Policy Statement* and *Nursing: Scope and Standards of Practice,* which standardized certification, licensure, and educational preparation for the four types of APNs. According to this document, APNs are prepared for "specialization, expansion, and advancement of practice." The policy further describes specialization as a specific area of practice; expansion as the ability to expand one's knowledge and skills duplicating those of the medical profession; and advancement as the integration of research-based evidence. Some functions overlap with the duties of the medical profession, including the ability to diagnose; make differential diagnoses; order and interpret diagnostic and laboratory tests; and prescribe pharmacologic treatments in the direct management of acute and chronic illness. Furthermore, the policy distinguishes APNs from other medical professionals by listing the additional duties of the NP role as comprehensive assessments, health promotion, and the prevention of disease and injury.

Multiple Role Opportunities to Practice as a Nurse Practitioner

Nurse practitioners provide patient-centered health care in acute, primary, and long-term settings. They also serve in various clinical settings as researchers, consultants, and patient advocates for families, individuals, groups, and communities. During the last fifty years, the NP's role has become more complex and autonomous. Ford (2008) emphasizes the continuing evolvement of the NP scope of practice to include all patient populations and multiple medical specialties/subspecialties. She highlights the independence that many NPs in rural areas have enjoyed when compared with NPs working in private practices, who may serve more as physician extenders than autonomous providers. The NP role is truly visible in almost every care setting, but the scope of practice differs depending on the organization's policies and culture, the environment, and even the NP's perception of the role. As NPs continue to expand their skill sets and launch their own practice sites, their scope of practice will further broaden. In today's world, NPs should take the lead in changing healthcare policy, managing care effectively, representing the profession in interdisciplinary initiatives, setting up advocacy programs for patient populations, and practicing as excellent clinicians. Figure 1.1 illustrates the multifaceted and expanding NP role, including clinician, leader, manager, and professional functions. NPs need to incorporate all four of these functions into their daily practices.

One variable that differentiates the NP from the physician is the NP's use of a holistic approach in determining patient care management. This means that an NP who sees a patient presenting with pharyngitis would identify both the need for health advice and pharyngitis as problems, according to the International Classification of Diseases (ICD) codes. In contrast, a physician would generally identify only pharyngitis as the patient's problem. The NP's holistic approach includes assessing the patients' ability to use personal characteristics—such as hardiness, courage, resilience, will to live, basic beliefs, value systems, and literacy level—to create a mutually agreeable plan of care. Primary care providers cannot focus only on the patient's specific complaint(s), such as shortness of breath or fatigue; they must function in an all-encompassing way with each patient encounter.

Clinician

The clinician role encompasses the holistic care NPs render to patients and communities (see Table 1.1). Although the majority of NPs have provided pri-

1.1

Elements of the Ever-Developing Role of the Nurse Practitioner

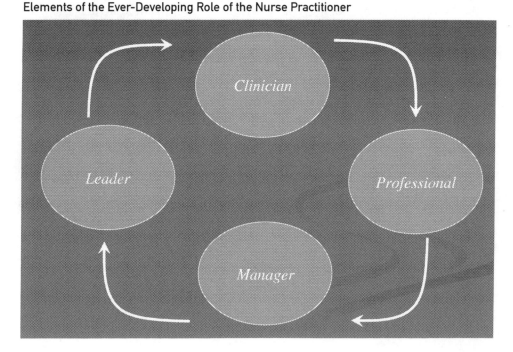

1.1 Levels of Care: Implications for Nurse Practitioners

Level of Prevention	Definition of Level	Examples of NP-Run Activities
Primary	Prevention of disease or injury	Immunizations, good hygiene, smoking cessation, fluoride supplementation, exercise classes
Secondary	Screening of disease or injury in order to diagnose early to decrease further problems	Pregnancy testing, mammography, testicular self assessment, hearing and vision screening
Tertiary	Prevention of complications and rehabilitation to promote health after an injury or disease	Lifestyle changes, diet, exercise regimen, stress management, support groups, psychotherapy

mary care, more NPs are now specializing in specific areas, such as cardiology and dermatology, or working in the community health arena. For example, NPs are often providers of health protection strategies that are related to regulatory or environmental measures needed by large groups of people. Population-based care is receiving more attention, as the focus on health promotion and initiatives increases (see Table 1.2).

Because of the holistic nature of the NP's practice, complementary and alternative techniques are frequently combined with integrative medicine and health teaching. NPs must think about the whole person and not just focus on the episodic nature of the patient's visit.

1.2 Healthy People 2010* Topics

- Exercise and Activity
- Obesity
- Cigarette and Tobacco
- Substance Abuse
- Sexually Transmitted Disease

- Mental Health
- Violence
- Environment
- Prevention of Disease—Immunizations
- Healthcare Access

*U. S. Department of Health and Human Services. *Healthy People 2010.Online Documents.*
http://www.healthypeople.gov/Document/

Leader

The transformational model of leadership provides direction to the NP who wants to make a change. An example is an NP who wants to make a difference for the patient and, therefore, spends extra time teaching patients how to be more responsible for their health. Patients who better understand their health and potential medical problems should see the importance of exercise, reducing caloric intake, and compliance with a health management program. They should, in brief, assume greater responsibility for themselves. Shanta and Kalanek (2008) describe strategic leadership as a way of formulating and implementing a vision. These authors offer a process by which leaders can be successful agents of change. Gardner (1989) also explains how to implement change and includes the following nine tasks in the leadership role:

- Envisioning goals—developing a goal and influencing others to work toward a common goal.
- Affirming values—encouraging people to rethink and change old visions or beliefs.
- Motivating—providing the impetus for the group to make a change and embrace a new way of thinking.
- Managing—moving the group toward the new goals and implementing the new vision.
- Achieving a workable unity—gaining the trust and loyalty of all involved in creating the new vision.
- Explaining—continuously increasing awareness about changes and new beliefs, which will grow as the new vision is achieved.
- Serving as a symbol—being the champion for the new vision and instilling hope in the group as the vision unfolds.
- Representing the group—advocating for the group and its new vision.
- Renewing—reinforcing hope and encouraging others to believe in the new beliefs and vision.

Nurse practitioners often find themselves in situations that demand new ways of thinking. As the challenges arise, a good framework, such as the *Tasks of Leadership* discussed above, will guide the NP in problem solving and reaching the best possible decisions. For example, a colleague tells an NP that their practice, composed of five physicians and three NPs, needs to improve patient management benchmarks. To achieve that mandate, all walk-ins will be assigned to NPs. The rationale is that the physicians will then have more time to achieve benchmarks with their regularly scheduled patients. This approach will significantly improve benchmark goals for the overall practice, as walk-ins generally present with multiple comorbidities, some degree of acuity, and no recent care. As a result, it is more difficult and time consuming to bring these patients to goal and to meet benchmarks. Instead of arguing or complaining about this change in assignment, the NPs decide to accept the challenge and demonstrate that they can succeed in achieving benchmarks even with walk-ins. Using the above framework one NP, Marion, led her group to success by:

Identifying the goal—NP patients will achieve similar, if not increased, benchmarks as compared with the physicians' patients.

Affirming values—Marion holds a dinner meeting at her house for the other two NPs to discuss plans for scheduling/assigning the patients.

Motivating—Marion suggests that each month one of the NPs take all the walk-ins. The other two will cover their own case loads and share the load of the NP doing the walk-ins. As a result, they will have more time to set up achievable plans for the walk-ins, while giving these patients continuity with their first few visits and possibly increased motivation to comply with treatment.

Managing—Marion volunteers to take the walk-ins first and plans weekly lunch meetings to discuss how the new patient assignment is going and to evaluate the benchmarks. The group determines progress has been made and invites the physicians to a meeting to share the results.

Achieving a workable unit—Marion and the other two NPs share their findings via e-mail on a daily basis and strategize on how to best assist each other so that benchmarks can be improved. Two of the physicians volunteer to take a month of walk-ins because they see the NPs new work assignment approach is successful.

Explaining—Marion and the other NPs agree to meet with the remaining physicians to share their progress, and they find these physicians open to participating in the new approach to managing walk-ins.

Serving as a symbol—Marion sets up a schedule and works with the office staff on programming the new method of patient assignment. Lunches are scheduled for all providers to share their concerns and ideas.

Representing the group—Marion analyzes the achieved benchmark data for the patients in the practice and shares positive news with the group as well as the practice group administration.

Renewing—Group meetings reinforce this creative scheduling as a way of improving effective patient management, and increased bonuses are realized for each provider. Marion and one of the physicians present their "Collaborative Scheduling Model" at a primary care conference and receive positive feedback. The group publishes its findings in a family practice journal. Using Gardner's leadership framework, the NP has a method by which to organize strategies to implement a change.

Wheatley (2006) explains how important it is for leaders to capture a holistic view of an organization and examine all aspects of relationships among members of the workforce. By conducting such an in-depth analysis, leaders can more effectively influence how people act and how they interact with others to develop more effective organizations. Wheatley suggests a constant state of change is a good way for organizations and individuals to grow and become more effective. So, to solve the challenges of the chaotic healthcare delivery system currently practiced in the United States, NPs need to lead in creating new methods of healthcare delivery by embracing new ideas and ways of thinking.

Manager

Nurse practitioners must be savvy managers, who are aware of the mission, goals, vision, and strategic plan of the organization with which they are affiliated, as well as those of their own clinic/unit/office. Not only are NPs responsible for managing their patient case loads, but they often also participate in the business aspect of their delivery system. With the changing paradigm of physician-owned to NP-owned primary care practices, understanding financial management has become a necessity. As Gawande (2007) wrote in *Better: A Surgeon's Notes on Performance*, going into a healthcare profession is all about "diagnosis, technical prowess, and some ability to empathize with people," but soon one learns the need to "grapple with systems, resources, circumstances, people—and our own shortcomings" (p. 8). Certainly, this is true for the NP in any healthcare system, including one that is self-owned.

Professional

Because of the complex nature of the illness and health continuum and ever-evolving medical technology, NPs need to be lifelong learners. This involves:

- Continuously learning new information.
- Reviewing research-based studies to assess best practices.
- Being aware of new guidelines of care management.
- Gaining more knowledge regarding variables that impact health, such as the rationale for the regulation of genes so better pharmacological and nonpharmacological treatments can be given to specific patients.

And, the list continues to grow, as there is always something new to learn. For example, NPs need to know about the neuroplasticity of the brain, which allows certain neurons to regenerate and retool certain brain tissue. As a result, patients can relearn function lost because of injury. Another example is a new bio-modulator drug therapy that stops further pathology from developing in specific autoimmune diseases. Continuous learning, knowledge sharing, and networking with other healthcare professionals is crucial for NPs to provide the best care for patients and to know when to refer patients to specialists. Maintaining and gaining new information is certainly part of the professional responsibility of a NP. Such knowledge increases the NPs confidence and depth in clinical decision making.

NPs must learn to manage the care of populations—and not just of individual patients. Some examples include administering influenza vaccines each fall or screening for sexually transmitted infections at a booth at a community health fair. In the first case, the NP-owned practice should consider partnering with a pharmaceutical company so the vaccine can be offered at a reduced cost. In the latter case, an NP-owned practice and a diagnostic laboratory might collaborate to possibly reduce diagnostic testing costs and generate a higher number of participants. To successfully manage an NP-owned business, NPs must be competent and professional. Each time the NP or a designated staff member partners with another agency or company, the potential for positive networking can ultimately improve the quality and outcomes of the business.

In addition, NPs should become involved with national and local professional organizations. Often, the professional agency serves as a vehicle for participation in discussions about regulatory and health policy issues, in developing legislation regarding health care, and in obtaining access to continuing education programs. For example, the American College of Nurse Practitioners (ACNP) offers members access to current legislation on its Legislative Tracking Chart, which is available at www.acnpweb.org. This invaluable forum enables NPs to be involved in the evolving healthcare delivery issues facing the country—who better to assist with developing health policy than NPs who are in the trenches of patient care management? Most policy change seems to focus on quality of services, costs, and access in three areas:

- Public policy—policy developed by local, state, or federal governments.
- Organizational policy—policy formulated by an institution or organization.
- Professional policy—policy set forth by professional organizations, such as the American Academy of Nurse Practitioners or American College of Nurse Practitioners.

Fawcette (2008) also explains that each policy has three components: personnel, services rendered, and costs of services. Nurse practitioners can impact any of the three types of policy depending on their networking interests and abilities.

Scope of Practice for Nurse Practitioners

The scope of practice for APNs is regulated by the State Nurse Practice Act and Board of Nursing. Each state has its own regulations that specify the limits for nursing practice and the sanctions for violation of any nursing regulations. Advanced practice nurses include nurse practitioners, nurse anesthetists, nurse midwives, and clinical nurse specialists. Advanced practice nurses do not include nurses with an advanced education in administration, education, or research. The advanced nursing practice concept focuses on the specialty clinical *practice* of these APNs, although NPs are also involved with fiscal management, education, and research in daily practice.

Nurse practitioners are also responsible for knowing the state Medical Practice Act and Board of Medicine rules that give physicians the authority to delegate certain medical acts to other healthcare professionals. The NP is obliged by law to follow the state's defined scope of practice. An NP who practices beyond the agreed-upon scope may be considered to be practicing medicine without a license. In addition, NPs must be aware of the state Pharmacy Practice Act and Pharmacy Board regulations that may impact prescriptive authority.

Depending on the state where the NP is practicing, a collaborative agreement with a physician may be necessary to comply with an NP's scope of practice. By reviewing the *Pearson Report, the Annual Legislative Update,* by Linda Pearson, who writes the Annual State-by-State National Compilation of Nurse Practitioner Legislation and Healthcare Issues in the *American Journal for Nurse Practitioners* (2009), the reader can determine the scope of the NP's role in every state. This report describes state-specific practice issues, barriers, and legislation affecting NPs and is available at http://www.webnp.net.

At present, the United States has 147,295 licensed NPs (Pearson, 2009), who have a greater opportunity than previously to practice autonomously. Not only do NPs work in traditional settings, such as community health centers, urgent care clinics, and private practices, but also in specialty areas, such as dermatology, infertility, long-term care, pain management, and pediatric psychiatry.

Nurse practitioners also serve as hospitalists in Emergency Departments and intensive care units in hospitals; as palliative care directors; and as owners of primary care and home care practices. They perform a variety of surgical and other invasive procedures and are directly reimbursed for their skill and expertise.

One important variable driving direct reimbursement for NPs is the legal ramifications of the expanded scope of the NP role. Regulatory bodies and insurance companies routinely dictate how health care is delivered. In additional, regulatory and institutional requirements must be met prior to practice. As such, NPs are mandated to have specific curricula, clinical hours, and time with specific patient types to develop certain expertise and certification in their specialty area before they can apply for licensure as an APN.

The Consensus Model for APRN Regulation— Licensure, Accreditation, Certification, and Education: Implications for the Role of the Nurse Practitioner

The National Council of State Boards of Nursing (NCSBN) (2009), which oversees the APN title and scope of practice, endorsed the Consensus Model for APRN Regulation in September 2008. As of 2007, the NCSBN states that "45 out of a total of 50 State Boards of Nursing use APRN certification as one of the requirements of advanced practice licensure for NPs" (Chornick, 2008, p. 90). A distinct difference exists between licensure and certification for APRNs.

The Consensus Model for APRN Regulation: Licensure, Accreditation, Certification, and Education

The Consensus Model for APRN Regulation: Licensure, Accreditation, Certification, and Education (2008) is the product of four years of meetings between members of the country's leading national professional organizations and boards of nursing to develop APN regulation. Licensure, accreditation, certification, and education (LACE) were examined regarding the four advanced practice nurse categories (i.e., nurse practitioners, nurse midwives, nurse anesthetists, and clinical nurse specialists), with the purpose of standardizing criteria. Under this model, NPs "will be educated in one of these four roles in addition to one of six population foci" (Stanley, 2009, p. 101):

- Individual across the lifespan/family
- Adult—gerontology
- Pediatrics
- Neonatal
- Women's health/gender related
- Psychiatric/mental health

Nurse practitioners will only be licensed as APRN, CNP, which represents Advanced Practice Registered Nurse, Certified Nurse Practitioner. Education must include a graduate degree in one of the population-focused NP areas, and the training must include "educational preparation to assume responsibility and accountability for health promotion, assessment, diagnosis, and management of patient problems, including the use and prescription of pharmacologic and non-pharmacologic interventions, and successful passing of the national certification test" (Stanley, p. 101). The Consensus Model, scheduled for implementation in 2015, allows specific grandfathering for NPs practicing in the state that granted their license.

The Consensus Model also defines standards of practice from well care to acute care. Nurse practitioners who are certified as a Family Nurse Practitioner or Pediatric Nurse Practitioner, for example, can be also certified in a specialty area, such as Palliative Care or Oncology. A copy of this Consensus Model can be accessed at http://www.aacn.nche.edu/Education/pdf/APRNReport.pdf.

Licensure

Once the Consensus Model is implemented, all of the standards for licensure, accreditation of educational programs, certification, and education will be universal. Thus, an NP will have less difficulty in obtaining license reciprocity to practice in other states. Until the Consensus Model is implemented, NPs must apply for new APRN licenses when moving to another state. An NP should continue to maintain their RN license as well as their APRN license.

Accreditation

Two bodies provide consistency by accrediting graduate NP programs. The Commission on Collegiate Nursing Education (CCNE) bases its accreditation on the American Association of Collegiate Nursing's (AACN) *Essentials of Master's Education for Advanced Practice Nursing* (1996) and the *Criteria for the Evaluation of NP Programs* (2002) developed by the National Task Force on Quality Nurse Practitioner Education. The National League for Nursing Accrediting Commission (NLNAC) also accredits master's programs using the NLNAC Standards and Criteria for Masters and Pos Master's Certificate accessible at http://www.nlnac.org/manuals/SC2008.htm.

Certification

Certification, under the Consensus Proposal, is earned after an individual completes a Master's Degree NP program, submits an application to the Certification Board, and passes the specialty certification exam. Certification is necessary to apply for licensure in most states. Currently the American Nurses Credentialing Center (ANCC) is the largest certification board and certifies nurse practitioners in eight areas. Once the Consensus Model is in place, all new graduates of NP programs will take a "certification exam recognized by all state licensing bodies" (Stanley, p. 101). These certification exams will evaluate "the nationally recognized competencies of the APRN core, role, and at least one population-focus area of practice" (Stanley, p. 101).

Education

Education is the last component of the Consensus Model. The National Organization of Nurse Practitioner Faculties (NONPF) and the American Association of Colleges of Nursing have worked with the American Nurses Association to further standardize master's program guidelines and NP competencies. The American Association of Colleges of Nursing developed the *Essentials of Master's Education for Advanced Practice Nursing* (1996—in revision, 2009), which specifies the core courses all NPs must take before starting their specialty track courses. These core courses include:

- Advanced Physiology and Pathophysiology
- Advanced Assessment
- Advanced Pharmacology
- Advanced Practice Role
- Epidemiology and Health Promotion
- Advanced Nursing Science and Research
- Advanced Health Care Policy

The NONPF Guidelines for Competencies in each track guide the curriculum development of the didactic specialty courses and list the number of clinical practicum hours mandated for all students.

The Doctorate of Nursing Practice (DNP), which was passed as a resolution by AACN in October 2004, is the goal for NPs graduating after 2015, and educators have worked to prepare curricula to provide the added information NPs need to succeed in the future. AACN and NONPF have standardized the criteria for curricula across programs and also for accrediting bodies, such as the CCNE, to assure all NP graduates are competent in providing safe and high-quality care. See Chapter 2 for a discussion of the DNP Essentials.

Adapting to the Nurse Practitioner Role as a New Graduate NP or NP Considering a Change of Position

In Zander and Zander's *Using the Art of Possibility: Transforming Professional and Personal Life (2002),* the authors provide techniques for a new way of thinking. These techniques can help strengthen self-confidence and decrease the need for ongoing professional reassurance in daily care management. NPs need to imagine a different frame around difficult situations and identify new ways of managing problems. Most NPs know others who have triumphed despite personal difficulties in the workplace. What made those NPs stay and reframe the situation so they could succeed? The Zanders suggest that the world needs to transform itself. We need to shift our very core of "posture, perceptions, beliefs, and thought process" (p. 4), rather than engaging in yet another round of self-improvement exercises. We are all weary of hearing top administrators lament budget cuts, the lack of funding for travel to conferences, and the placing of new initiatives on "hold." NPs must not accept the status quo but try to create new ways of working with new methods of practice. Perhaps, some activities thought to be essential for high-quality care are not necessary. In the end, NPs should work differently and conduct business so practices can remain cost effective while achieving high rates of good-patient outcomes.

These ideas came from interviews with NPs who have 1 to 3 years experience in the role. The demographic was all women, aged 29 to 50 years, and experienced as an RN from 8 to 30 years. None had been in another profession before becoming an NP, and all seemed to respond similarly regardless of age.

Questions and Answers

Question #1—*Approximately how long did it take after you graduated to get a position? When did you begin looking for a position? When did you actually start to apply for a position?*

Answer:

All had started e-mailing, phoning, and interviewing in their final semester of the NP program. All passed the Certification Board before beginning an NP position, except for one who said, "if I could have started after the Boards that would have been good."

Others offered the following advice. "Don't let prospective employers scare you into thinking you will not get the position unless you start when they say." If you are assertive and have good rationales, the employer will demonstrate more respect. Set the right tone from the beginning of the relationship, so the employer will understand the NP will not "cave to their every request," but rather negotiate so both will be satisfied with outcomes. Review local medical practices as any available positions are often listed on Web sites. Word of mouth from colleagues, list-serves, NP journals, newspapers, alumni, and preceptors involved with NP program are all good sources for obtaining information about available positions.

Three NPs obtained positions in practices where they had a practicum during their NP program. And all but one chose a position in a similar setting to their last practice practicum area. All of the NPs said to take a review course, study for four to six weeks while working in the RN position, and then take the certification board exam. All agreed on the importance of looking for a position during the final semester to become familiar with what is available. This early effort often results in first chance at many positions, as many NP graduates wait until they pass the certification board to begin looking. All stressed not rushing into a position; always research the practice thoroughly. All had checked out the practice site with experienced NPs and, if there had been a previous NP in the practice, they investigated why the NP was leaving. During the investigation, check if the practice site is financially solid and if there is a "window on the salary." In other words, can your salary increase as you can gain experience at the practice site. All NPs interviewed stressed the need to have confidence in your abilities to be successful in obtaining a position and salary equal to your competencies. They advised "Never settle for a position—be sure it is what you worked so hard to obtain." You also need to come off as a flexible team player, but not to get "real close" to the registered nurses (if registered nurses work in the setting) or the doctors. Many were the sole NP in the practice and found it best to be professional with everyone. Be careful not to act like a doctor or let patients and staff think you are a doctor; be very clear that you are an NP and just keep sharing your role and practice scope. Unfortunately, RNs are often the most difficult to educate to the NP role. If the NP role is not clear, the RN will let the NP do the RN work for their own patients, as well as provide the NP level care. Once they had been at the site for six to nine months, the majority of the nurses became trusted allies of other staff members.

Question #2—*If you could share anything with someone starting a first NP position or contemplating a change in NP position, what would it be? Did you have a mentor? Have you tried reflective practice and/or meeting with other NPs to share experiences? Do you have any suggestions for the new NP?*

Answer:
Keep in touch with the other providers in your practice. as well as the staff, on a regular basis and get to know them. Be sure they are aware of your experience and, maybe, areas in which you could use more experience. When appropriate, ask them to share knowledge and experiences. Read so you are knowledgeable about the patient types most often seen at your practice site.

Get an iPhone so you can look up information immediately on PubMed or access other Internet resources. Be sure that everyone at the practice site knows the scope of practice for an NP. This is especially crucial when you are the first NP in the practice or, even more so, if you are following an NP who was not well received and left. All recommended having several mentors with whom you can dialogue, plan for the future, and share patient experiences.

All were adamant that the NP role needs to be respected by everyone in the practice. If this does not occur, the NP needs to remedy this by talking with those who do not respect the role and/or enlisting assistance from the supervisor/director.

The only thing I wish was stressed more in my NP program was how big of a change this was going to be—going from RN to APRN. I was one of the senior staff members on my floor at the hospital—most questions about procedure or patient care were directed to me. It was a very big adjustment becoming an APRN. Starting back at the bottom of the totem pole with the feeling of not knowing what you are doing was hard. I was the one asking questions about procedures and patient care again.

So the issue of role needs some attention. Remember when starting the position that most NPs had these same feelings, as most are starting in a whole new type of practice.

I kept a notebook in my pocket in which I wrote anything that was new to me, such as Rx for hidradenitis, pharyngitis, UTI, the usual suspects, un-

til I could remember them without looking them up. I had to learn to say, "I'll be right back with your prescriptions" if I had to look something up online or consult with someone.

I do think it helps to keep a notebook. I carry it to work every day because it gives me security and confidence. Some of the things I put on a page that I add to about once a week I label as "clinical pearls." I then review the notebook and think about how I came up with the patient's differential diagnosis. I also like to reflect on what if . . . meaning what if I had not seen this or the patient had not told me this. I learn a good amount by just reviewing my clinical days. I try to do it on my way home from work.

I save the e-mails from the medical director. Every Sunday I review a "to do" sheet for work. I created a paper that I use for monitoring lab work and Coumadin dosages. I have another sheet that I labeled biological modifiers, where I list the people for whom I need to remember to check labs because they are on Procrit, Aranesp, etc. I review these and feel more prepared. I also have computer access from home to the hospital and the lab. It is not required but I like having the access. Sometimes it is just too noisy at the facility to concentrate.

I did keep a notebook during clinical practica and continue it to this day. Anytime I learn something that is very significant to practice, I write it down. I used this book frequently when I first started, and I still find myself referring to it now. I guess it increased confidence because it helped me build my knowledge base. I have found that I am one of the youngest NPs in the group, so my experiences are a little different than some of the others. That has been one of my frustrations—not knowing any NPs my age. I have one NP with whom I keep in touch from school, but all the other NPs I know are older and at different stages of their lives. Still, it is helpful to dialogue with other NPs.

Question #3—*Kramer's classic work,* Reality Shock *(2004), has been used as a framework to assess new RNs and their adaptation to the role of RN. Given the following framework stages, could you share how you have transitioned through the stages as an NP?*

Answer:

Sometimes, one regresses back a stage before progressing, and it is common to stay in one stage for a long time. All of the participants agreed that knowing the Kramer Framework was helpful in explaining some of the rationales for what they were and are experiencing.

Kramer's *Framework of Reality Shock* (1994) includes the following stages:

- Compliance—The RN [NP] is trying to gain respect from colleagues.
- Identification—Respect is felt and the RN [NP] wants to earn recognition for being good with certain skills, diagnosing certain problem areas, and working with certain age groups, etc.

▨ Internalization—The RN [NP] is responsible and able to manage an "average assignment" of patients independently.

Stage 1, Compliance—One NP had worked as an RN and done some practicum work at her place of employment. As a result, she felt she had already gained respect and went directly to Stage 2. Others asked a lot of questions and often confirmed the information they received on the Internet, particularly as they gained confidence in themselves and also "got a handle on their colleagues' levels of knowledge" and did not just accept their opinions. Because most work was in a primary care settings, few emergencies were presented, so the NPs took the time to be sure patients were managed correctly. Many soon learned they knew more than they had realized and that they had excellent backgrounds from their years of experience as RNs. After a while, most started to share information with colleagues, and this assisted them in garnering respect and improving their confidence.

Many also felt it was important to treat the staff well and thank them for their work. For example, preface requests with, "I know you're really busy, but. . . ." and engage in conversations with them as well as with the providers. One NP felt it took about two weeks before she felt respected; she also believed that she was lucky because her agency had multiple NPs and was aware of the scope of NP practice. Another NP said it took about three months to earn respect. During her formal orientation time, she took her own patients, but had to present each case to a physician before letting the patient leave. (She was the only NP in the practice.) She felt this was a good time for the physicians to get to know her and learn to trust her work. Many felt it was important to teach RNs about laboratory work, how to assess patients for certain problems, such as pneumonia, more critically, and just, in general, to make them feel "valuable" too.

Stage 2, Identification—One NP said her relationship with the Medical Director has been excellent, as he always gets back to her and he is available 24/7 for questions. His motto is, "nothing is a stupid question." After three months, this NP feels more comfortable and shares the following example of avoiding hospitalization of a patient who became acutely ill.

> *I am, as of today, feeling more comfortable managing my residents with certain problems. I had a resident today with dementia, aphasia, and diabetes, who presented with a blood sugar of 482. Her blood sugars are never that high. I noticed that she was also tachycardic at 120, tachypnic, and warm. She had congestion in her chest and was feverish. The tachycardia and tachypnea in the first month I was there would have sent her to the ER. Today I did a stat chest film, had a UA and C&S sent to the laboratory, and started the antibiotic, Avelox. I ordered O_2 and eight units of regular insulin. If she worsens they will send her to the hospital tonight but hopefully I can keep her out of the hospital.*

Another NP said she felt more independent and confident after nine months or so, but still had experiences that "threw her."

I do want the physicians to know that I am doing a good job. There have been occasions where I have noticed something like a lab abnormality that one of my colleagues missed, and I do feel respected when the physician recognizes that I picked it up and followed through on it.

Another NP shared:

I have been sought after by the female patients for sexuality issues while they are undergoing cancer treatments and/or first receiving their diagnoses of cancer. I did not seek this identification, but if I can be helpful to them I am pleased. I am the only female provider. I have chosen to focus on hematological cancers and multiple myeloma, and this has assisted me in gaining some expertise, although I certainly still feel inexperienced with most oncology problems. I am also working on gaining competency with the inpatients so I round daily, cover on-call issues, and make it a point to connect with the hospital staff.

All felt it was important to focus on specific areas and learn as much as one can. Become somewhat of an "expert" in those areas, and then gradually add on more and more diagnostic areas. It is overwhelming to learn everything about everything, so try to focus initially on specific areas.

Stage 3. Internalization—The type of practice determines how one reaches this stage. Here are some of the NPs' ideas:

At eight months into the job I started feeling pretty comfortable and felt I could carry out a day independently. However, some days I have very complicated patients, and I require a lot more collaboration. I have been told this is true with oncology practice for most providers.

It's taken me about six months to get to a 14-day patient load that I could handle. I've seen as many as 25 patients some days. It takes a while to learn to sort through all the information that a patient is bombarding you with and focus on the priority issue of the visit. I was trying to do too much in a visit when I started.

Internalization happened after about three months at the practice. Once I was off orientation, I was expected to handle an average assignment on my own. However, the physicians were always willing to answer questions or consult on a patient. I was much slower in the beginning. I would run behind because they didn't give me any extra time to see patients. In the first two weeks of the job, they scheduled my patients every 30 minutes, after that it was every 15 minutes—the normal time allotted in this office.

Question #4—*What were your five biggest areas of need as you embarked on your NP career and how could they have been less problematic if you had had more of "something" in your program?*

Answer:
Mentoring is the biggest MUST HAVE when you first start out. You have got to have someone who is smart and available to teach you and answer your questions.

The need for a really good physical assessment course cannot be ignored. It's really true when you work in a place where there are no diagnostics (chest X-ray, laboratory, MRI, etc.) available and you have to wait for all of your results. You've got to be really good at physical diagnosis.

My five biggest areas of need were EKG interpretation, physical assessment, billing, support during role transition, and time management. Since I never worked with telemetry patients or ICU/ER patients, I do not have that baseline knowledge or experience and am taking a continuing education course on 12-lead EKG interpretation. I find my physical exam techniques and time management improving as I gain more experience. The practice should have a staff person manage the billing and reimbursement exclusively since this area takes up too much of my time. I am lucky that I belong to an NP Group that meets monthly for dinner and class. This affords me time to network with other NPs and see if they have advice for any issues I am experiencing.

I would have liked to have had to present more patients to my peers and instructors—it seems that is a lot of what I do in an oncology practice. I am learning to be more comprehensive and succinct. I also carry my iPhone so I can be ready with answers during the case rounds. It seems imperative to have knowledge accessible, and the PDA is not as good as the iPhone with instant information access.

Question #5—*List 10 words that describe how you felt during the transition from novice/advanced beginner NP to competent NP this last year?*

Answer:
Benner, Tanner, and Chesla (2009) describe the process of going from advanced beginner to competent to proficient to expert stages in clinical practice for RNs. Each of the interviewees were aware of this framework, because most had used it for their clinical ladder promotion in their hospitals.

They answered this question similarly. As novice NPs, they felt stupid, incompetent, scared, nervous, and unsure, but when they gained self-confidence and competency, these feelings changed to conscientious, good, caring, helpful, smart, like "advanced beginners," and then "competent." No one called themselves expert; they classified themselves as in between the "competent" and "proficient" stages.

Brykczynski (1989) and Brown and Olshansky (1998) studied specifically the transition role of nurse practitioners and developed the following framework of four stages:

▓ Stage 1—Laying the Foundation—This occurs just after graduation, when the new NP is looking for a position, studying for the certification board exam, and working in an RN position.

▓ Stage 2—Launching—Approximately the first 3 months of the first position.

▓ Stage 3—Meeting the Challenge—As one starts feeling more comfortable, the new NP gains competence and believes that he or she is not going to harm or kill a patient.

▓ Stage 4—Broadening the Perspective—When the new NP holds his or her own, feels confident, and does not have to ask as many questions or get approval from another provider as frequently. The individual realizes he or she is a safe and competent provider, but one who could always learn more.

Question #6—*How did you see yourself going through each phase and what feelings are you presently experiencing? If you had had this kind of information about how other new NPs have felt, would it have helped before beginning your position?*

Answer:

Stage 1—Laying the Foundation—Most had secured their positions during the final semester of school, but they had anxiety about taking the certification board. They all took a Board Preparation Course that helped them focus on their weak areas and took the exam 4 to 8 weeks after the Board Review. (They were also working full time in their RN positions). Three took the Board Preparation Course in the beginning of their final semester and thought it helped them feel more confident at graduation. Each NP found it crucial to set aside a certain number of hours to study for the certification board and be serious about completing the hours.

Stage 2—Launching—Here are some ideas the NPs shared about this stage:

The first few weeks, you'd never have known I had been an ER nurse for 25 years. It's like the blackboard in my head had been erased. I didn't know anything. My confidence had totally vanished.

This stage was very difficult. I was very stressed at my new position. I felt like an idiot—like I had learned nothing in school. The "real world" was so different than being in school. Even different than clinical rotations—because I was on my own and nobody was watching my every move. Applying the text book knowledge to real life situations wasn't always easy. The patients didn't fit the text book description. It was also stressful to lose my support system of nurses at the hospital that I had in my RN position. I was out of my comfort zone and thought for a long time that I had made a mistake in changing to an NP career.

*I felt like I knew nothing and was afraid to make a decision at first. How-
ever I was also excited to build "my practice" and often "took" patients from
the physicians. I know I am very fortunate to work with MDs who are very
collaborative focused.*

Stage 3 Meeting the Challenge—Most shared similar findings to the following narratives.

*I've learned that fortunately, people are resilient. I still have daily anxi-
ety, but more about maiming than killing at this point.*

*This is a cool feeling. I am feeling a little overprotective of some of my res-
idents at times. You realize, hey I recognize these symptoms, this is what
I did the last time. Let's try it again.*

*I never thought it would happen but I did reach a point when I felt more
comfortable at my NP job. I really do think it took about a year to start
feeling more confident. There were moments of confidence before a year—
but they came more frequently after the one-year mark. I have to say that
almost two years into this I still have days where I worry that I might kill
someone! I have a feeling that takes a long time to go away. And maybe it
never goes away completely. It is a huge responsibility.*

*It was around eight months that I felt conscious of the fact that I proba-
bly would not kill someone. I am now [about 1.5 years] much more comfortable and enjoy my position for the most part.*

Stage 4—Broadening the Perspective

*This took about ten months. I've gone from 20 questions a day to one or
two and sometimes none. I have worn out the Primary Care Book though.
I always know that I'll never know enough. But I do feel I know something.*

*I think I am somewhere between these last two stages. I am now more reg-
ularly utilizing certain people with important roles. For example, I am not
an expert on wound care. I have a wound care certified RN with whom I
collaborate with regularly. Last week I had a resident diagnosed with
three fractures of the right transverse processes of L2, 3, and 4. My or-
thopedic background told me not to worry about the spine but why did this
72-year-old man have fractures with no trauma? So I called one of the
collaborating MDs but I also spoke with the head of our physical therapy
department and worked it out similar to what the physician had thought.
This was a good growth for me and instilled confidence.*

Conclusions

The background of the registered nurse, along with additional NP education, helps produce an NP who cares holistically for patients, families, and communities. Nurse practitioners are not miniphysicians or extenders of medical care for patients unwanted by physicians. Nurse practitioners evolve from exposure to an integrative approach to medicine that is taught and practiced in nursing undergraduate programs. They need to be successful clinicians, managers, professionals, and leaders at an advanced level. In addition, physical assessment, diagnostic reasoning, and prescriptive authority, as well as other advanced competencies NPs acquire from their education, prepare them to become board certified. The Consensus Model for APRN Regulation is a landmark document describing the titles, defining the specialties, and identifying the new roles and population foci for the NP and three other APN categories in the United States. This regulatory model will direct NPs in forming practice strategies for improved healthcare delivery, role expansion, and standardization of licensure, accreditation, certification, and education.

Reflective Thinking Exercises

1. The American College of Nurse Practitioners (ACNP) has a Legislative Tracking Chart available that lists current legislation affecting NPs. Members can access this invaluable resource at www.acnpweb.org.
2. Use the Pearson Report (2009) to determine the scope of practice for nurse practitioners in your state.
3. Develop an advertisement to market your skills as an NP for a professional nurse practitioner journal. Review your state's Nurse Practice Act regarding the role and scope of practice for an APN.
4. Nurse Practitioners have a Medicare Learning Network Web site that can be accessed at http://www.cms.hhs.gov/MLNProducts/70_APNPA .asp. If an NP provides care to Medicare beneficiaries, this Web site will be an invaluable resource for answering questions regarding policy. It also provides operational updates specific to Medicare Fee-for-Service reimbursement issues. Review the Frequently Asked Questions Section and list the five most frequently asked questions that NPs have regarding Medicare and how it impacts their scope of practice.
5. Review the NP interviews with special attention to the role and feelings of recently graduated NPs. Develop goals and a timeline for seeking NP employment. The Web site from Advance Nurse Practitioners may also be helpful (http://nurse-practitioners.advanceweb.com/Editorial/Content/ Editorial.aspx?CC=200814).

References

ADVANCE. (2009). Your first nurse practitioner position: Advice from those who've been there. *ADVANCE for Nurse Practitioners*. Retrieved June 8, 2009 from http://nurse-practitioners .advanceweb.com/Editorial/Content/Editorial.aspx?CC=200814.

ADVANCE. (2007). National salary workplace survey of NPs ADVANCE for Nurse Practitioners. Retrieved June 9, 2009 from http://nurse-practitioners.Advanceweb.com.

American Association of Colleges of Nursing (1996). *The essentials of master's education for advanced practice nursing.* Washington, D. C: Author.

American Association of Colleges of Nursing. (2008). Consensus Model for APR Regulation. Retrieved April 12, 2009 from http://www.aacn.nche.edu/Education/pdf/APRNReport.pdf.

American Association of Nurse Attorneys (2005). *Business and legal guidebook for nurse practitioners.* Columbus, OH: Author.

American Nurses Association (ANA). (2004a). *Nursing's social policy statement.* Washington, D.C: Author.

American Nurses Association (ANA). (2004b). *Nursing: Scope and standards of practice.* Washington, D.C: Author.

Benner,P., Tanner, C. & Chesla, C. (2009). *Expertise in nursing practice: Caring, clinical judgment, and ethics.* 2nd ed., New York, NY: Springer Publishing Co.

Brown M.& Olshansky, E.(1998). Becoming a primary care nurse practitioner: Challenges of the initial year of practice. *The Nurse Practitioner, 23*(7):46;53–56, 58, 61–62, 64, 66.

Brykczynski, K. (1989) Role delineation studies in advanced practice nursing. An interpretive study describing the clinical judgment of nurse practitioners. *Scholarly Inquiry for Nursing Practice: An International Journal, 3*(2), 75–111.

Buppert, C. (2008). *Nurse Practitioner's Business Practice and Legal Guide.* Sudbury: Jones and Bartlett Publishers.

Chornick, N. (2008). NCSBN Focus-APRN licensure versus APRN certification: What is the difference? *JONA's Healthcare Law, Ethics, and Regulation, 10*(4), 90–93.

Commission on Collegiate Nursing Education. (2009). Procedures on Accreditation. Retrieved April 12, 2009 from http://www.aacn.nche.edu/Accreditation

Fawcette, J. (2008). A comment on integrating nursing and health policy—AAN News & Opinion. *Nursing Outlook, 56*(1), 43.

Ford, J. (2008). 2008 in review: More growing pains, *ADVANCE for Nurse Practitioners 12,* 57.

Ford, L. (1979). A nurse for all settings: The nurse practitioner. *Nursing Outlook, 27,* 516–521.

Gardner, J. (1989). The tasks of leadership. In W. E. Rosenbach & R. L. Taylor (Eds.), *Contemporary issues in leadership* (2nd. Ed.) p. 24–33. Boulder: Westview Press.

Gawande, A. (2007). *Better: A Surgeon's Notes on Performance.* New York: Metropolitan Books.

Kramer, M. (1974). *Reality shock.* St. Louis: C. V. Mosby.

National Council of State Boards of Nursing (NCSBN) (2009). *Advanced Practice Nurses.* www .ncsbn.org

National League for Nursing Accrediting Commission. (2008). Retrieved April 12, 2009 from http://www.nlnac.org/manuals/Manual2008.htm.

National Organization of Nurse Practitioner Faculties. (2002). *Criteria for the Evaluation of NP Programs* developed by the National Task Force on Quality Nurse Practitioner Education. Retrieved June 3, 2009 from www.nonpf.org.

Pearson, L. (2009). Annual state-by-state national compilation of nurse practitioner legislation and healthcare issues. The Pearson Report, the Annual Legislative Update. *American Journal for Nurse Practitioners. 13*(2), 8–82.

Plager, K. & Conger, M. (2007). Advanced practice nursing. *Internet Journal of Advanced Nursing Practice, 9*(1), 13p.

Shanta, L. & Kalanek, C. (2008). Perspectives on nursing leadership in regulation. *JONA's Healthcare Law, Ethics, and Recognition. 10*(4), 106–111.

Stanley, J. (2009). Reaching consensus on a regulatory model: what does this mean for APRNs? *The Journal for Nurse Practitioners. 5*(2), 99–104.

U. S. Department of Health and Human Services. *Healthy People 2010.Online Documents.* Retrieved June 12, 2009 from http://www.healthypeople.gov/Document

Wheatley, M. (2006). *Leadership and the new science: Discovering order in a chaotic world* (3rd ed.). San Francisco: Berrett-Koehler Publishers.

Zander, R., & Zander, B. (2000). *Using the art of possibility: Transforming professional and personal life.* Cambridge: Harvard Business Book Press.

Changing Vision of Healthcare Delivery: Implications for Nurse Practitioners

2

Learning Objectives

1. Describe how changes in healthcare delivery impact the role of nurse practitioners (NPs).

2. Describe how the *Doctorate of Nursing Practice Essentials* will expand the ability of the NP to practice autonomously.

3. Define reflective practice as it influences one's practice.

4. Explain the methods and processes for developing reflective practice as one engages in creative change and translational research.

5. Examine the advantages of increased consulting and collaboration opportunities for NPs.

6. Analyze principles of change management and their application on NP practice.

7. Analyze new healthcare delivery sites for NPs, such as subspecialties, retail health or convenient care, hospitalist, aesthetics, concierge/boutique health care, rural health, and nurse practitioner-owned primary care practices.

Key Words: consultant, collaboration, change, healthcare delivery, nurse practitioner, practice doctorate, primary care, reflective practice, translational research

The healthcare system needs to become more effective and cost efficient. As a result, the NP role has expanded in both inpatient and outpatient settings to include leader, manager, professional, and, of course, clinician. As the system changes, more interprofessional collaboration and networking opportunities have occurred. These opportunities have positively influenced the marketing and expansion of the NP role.

Using reflective practice, the NP's scope is expanding, and new advanced practice roles in consulting, collaborating, partnering, and managing healthcare agencies are being created. As NPs purchase primary care practices or become coowners in multispecialty groups, they need experience in developing and managing a business.

This chapter discusses these changes in terms of the NP role and explains the Doctorate of Nursing Practice (DNP) essentials. Current discussion focuses on how the practice doctorate will influence the paradigm that has NPs assuming more autonomy as they increase their scope of practice.

Healthcare Delivery in the United States

As healthcare prices soar and managed care practice guidelines are continuously revised to cut costs, more NPs are finding employment in primary care, family practice, and "niche" healthcare delivery settings. The financing of health care in the United States is "broken," as costs have become insurmountable. It is hard to disagree with Porter and Teisberg (2006) and others (Knope, 2008; Isaacs, Jellinek, & Walker, 2009), who say that health care has gone from a source of national pride to one of America's preeminent concerns. In fact, the U.S. healthcare system is in need of major change. When compared to other Westernized countries, U.S. patients have the highest risk of receiving poor health care as a result of cost, disorganized care, and errors (Schoen, Osborn, How, Doty, & Peugh, 2008).

Thus far, the healthcare industry has reacted to high costs in two ways: restricting choices of providers and services to patients and increasing the cost share of insurance to members. These changes have had mixed results. Some people are happy just to have any benefits at all and are satisfied with their healthcare costs; some people are angry (since they cannot keep consistency with their providers when their insurance changes); others refuse to go for any uncovered preventive health care because they are unemployed or have no insurance to cover their care; and still others are unhappy their copay and prescription costs have doubled. For many, the extremely high costs of health care have resulted in negotiations between health insurance carriers and employers that lead to reduced coverage for employees with higher premiums and deductibles. For example, many people with employer-driven insurance no longer have coverage for preventive health care, forcing patients to seek treatment only when an emergency occurs. The result is an increase in chronic illness, which prompts more complications and ultimately causes more patients to seek emergency care. The result is higher healthcare costs for everyone.

Kenney (2008) reminds us it has been ten years since the Institute of Medicine (1999) published *To Err is Human: Building a Safer Health System*, yet almost 100,000 preventable patient deaths occur annually in the United States. The United States continues to spend more on health care than any other nation, yet it ranks poorly on every measure of health status. Schroeder (2007) reiterates that there is a chasm, not just a gap, between what our health care is and what it could be. Certainly health promotion and prevention needs more emphasis, and NPs are, and will continue to be, in a position to make a difference by filling this "chasm" with safe and high-quality care.

Reviewing the Ecological Model of Health, it becomes apparent that peoples' behavior toward their health is influenced by more than genes, diet, and exercise patterns (Cohen, Scribner, & Farley, 1998). Hofrichter (2003) agrees that political, environmental, and social factors have more influence on the health status of populations than genetics, personal choices, and access to treatment services. For this reason, the medical community must focus energy at the population level to curb chronic illness. Obesity is just one problem where NPs can make a significant difference if they were more population focused. The community health aspect of health care offers a huge potential for change. In such a practice setting, NPs can be more involved by supporting individual and community choices and by serving as advocates for social justice. All healthcare systems need to foster the idea that everyone is self-accountable and all systems should support these basic human rights:

- The right to access health care,
- The right to dignity and respect, and
- The right to be well and earn a decent wage (Manthey & Disch, 2008).

One innovative healthcare delivery model that provides primary care by NPs to vulnerable populations is the Maryland Governor's Wellmobile (Heller & Goldwater, 2004). Managed by the University of Maryland's School of Nursing faculty, the model describes strategies that prompted the development of similar initiatives on college campuses and in schools, malls, long-term care agencies, churches, Senior Centers, prisons, and anywhere people congregate.

It is general knowledge that sound primary care is more cost effective for the individual and the country than emergency treatment. Nurse practitioners are furthering this goal by providing care and follow-up in all types of settings, including supermarkets, health buses, health fairs, schools, churches, and other storefronts, and by teaching patients to be accountable for their health. Primary care providers effect cost savings when they manage people with chronic illnesses to prevent further complications, which generally result in long hospitalizations, loss of workdays, and decreased quality of life.

Issues Impacting Primary Care and Family Practice

Current issues affecting primary care and family practice for NPs focus on the move from private to collaborative practice. In fact, many private practice physicians and NPs have merged to form larger primary and specialty care practices that have more cost effective outcomes. Most physicians and NPs feel that the advantages of being a part of a larger multigroup practice outweigh the disadvantages. As a result, they have changed the way they run their practices and, more importantly, how they deliver care. They also face decreased financial compensation, specifically in primary care/family practice. The annual salary of most primary care/family practice physicians is approximately $150,000; one-third of what physicians in subspecialty areas earn (Bodenheimer, 2006). Some argue this is only fair, as specialist physicians have studied longer and have more experience in their areas of clinical specialty. However, the multigroup practices are learning to change the delivery of care to maximize efficiency and "fit" the new group model. For example, each provider needs to see a specified numbers of patients every day. This translates into less time with each patient, longer waiting times experienced by patients, and more involved processes to obtain referrals to specialists. The changes in the economy have pressured all businesses to change the way they operate. In some cases, this means not doing some things special for patients, charging patients for time spent reordering medications, and not copying medical records or fulfilling specific requests patients may have.

Insurance reimbursement is based on the insurance companies' determination of a reasonable charge for each procedure. The employer then negotiates with the insurance carriers exactly what they can offer their employees for a specific amount of money. In most cases, the amount of healthcare costs being covered by insurance has decreased, while the healthcare costs have increased exponentially.

Changes in Healthcare Delivery Influence the Role of Nurse Practitioners

With more physicians selecting specialty practices over primary care, multiple opportunities for experienced and new NPs exist. However, similar to physicians, NPs are moving into specialty practices with higher reimbursement than primary care. Table 2.1 lists reasons why the primary care settings may look attractive to NPs.

Nurse practitioners are learning to maximize their education and experience to achieve compensation relative to their market value and their ability to contribute to health care. They should realize that great opportunities exist to start their own businesses and provide consultancies. Often, NPs bring in more revenue than their counterpart physicians, yet the NP salary is much lower than the physician, ranging from $70,000 to $85,000 depending on geographic region. The more experienced NP, who also may have purchased a share in a practice, usually earns a higher salary and bonus payments.

2.1	Factors Influencing NPs to Choose Primary Care

- NPs do not have education loans to pay back [or at least not loans as high as those of a physician], so they may not strive for a pie-in-the-sky salary.
- NPs can start working and earning a salary approximately five years sooner than the physician, who must complete a low-paying residency.
- NPs can have better schedules (e.g. weekends and evenings off) than when they were RNs.
- NPs can generally work close to home and in their community.
- NPs may value the respect and autonomy of their position and feel salary is less important.

With the growing trend for NPs to provide the bulk of primary care, more of them are partnering with physicians or business professionals to learn the skills to practice independently. The ultimate goal is to manage an NP-run clinic. In addition, more NPs are earning the Doctorate of Nursing Practice degree to gain the requisite knowledge and skills to open their own practice or business.

The NP, who is used to practicing with a family-centered model of care, is thus able to deliver holistic care to patients and fit the comprehensive-care-clinician role that is so needed. Nurse practitioners should prepare for lucrative career opportunities by developing their skill sets and confidence, as continued physician attrition in primary care/family practice will yield a greater need for NPs. But the NPs will need the business acumen to market their practices, manage their practices efficiently and effectively, and negotiate for direct insurance reimbursement.

Nurse practitioners also have experience in 24/7 healthcare delivery and will be able to create flexible scheduling to see patients at nontraditional times. Perhaps the use of an NP, an RN, and a medical assistant with different skills will create an efficient work group. All members of the healthcare community and staff must work collaboratively and cooperatively with advanced practice nurses to positively impact patient care and population health outcomes (Mundinger, 2002; Schmalenberg, Kramer, King, Krugman, Lund, Poduska, et al, 2005).

With the increasing burden of chronic illnesses, such as diabetes and cardiovascular disease, the need for interdisciplinary collaboration is even greater. The Group Health Cooperative of Puget Sound, Washington, shows how an interdisciplinary team redesigned the system and developed the Chronic Care Model of Healthcare Delivery. This is a collaborative initiative among primary care physicians, NPs, and specialty physicians to work with patients who had chronic diseases and were not reaching clinical goals. The success of this group effort demonstrates the ability to increase patient clinical goal achievement, increase patient and provider satisfaction, and decrease healthcare costs. They (Boville, Saran, Salem, Clough, Jones, Radwany & Sweet, 2007) recommend the following elements as essential for a successful healthcare practice:

- Delivery system redesign
- Self-management support
- Decision support
- Clinical information systems
- Community resources and policies
- Health care organization mission supportive of patient comorbidities

Nurse practitioners must also be prepared for patients who are Internet savvy and/or listen to direct-to-consumer (DTC) marketing. Many of these patients want to use specific pharmaceuticals or equipment. The NP, as well as the physician, must be knowledgeable about all of these products to recommend evidence-based treatment and avoid market hype. Certainly, one does not want a reputation for satisfying all patients who come to a practice and, compelled by promotional content, ask for a product. Documentation should detail the reason/need for any item prescribed. To decrease the time spent on record keeping, the NP should consider using electronic documentation software, which has many advantages:

- Increased workflow efficiency
- Decreased charting time and error
- Quick access to assignments
- Decreased legal liability
- Increased time spent with patients

Patient-centered medical homes, also called healthcare homes, are another way to improve healthcare. This concept evolved from the need to manage chronic illness more effectively. The Medicare and Medicaid payment systems, which were formerly directed only to physicians in most states, have also recently begun allocating direct reimbursement to NPs in some states. Is this a trend? Only time will tell. Some states have also changed the term, medical home, to healthcare home, but this is not universal.

The Rittenhouse, Casalino, Gillies, et al. study (2008) described findings from 291 medical practices involving twenty or more physicians from the Study of Physician Organizations and the Management of Chronic Illness. They focused on four elements of the Patient-Centered Medical Home (PCMH) model:

- Physician-directed medical practice
- Care coordination and integration
- Quality and safety
- Enhanced access

Essentially Rittenhouse et al. believe this model will not be successful unless physicians make serious changes in how they deliver care, invest in using electronic records, and increase medical staff.

Primary care in 2009 is in need of a total overhaul, including the way primary care physicians are paid. Paulus, Davis, and Steele (2008) describe the experience of the Geisinger Health System in Pennsylvania: Its redesign of health care delivery, installation and use of electronic health information systems, development of an integrated team approach, and a restructured financial incentive program. Findings of this study are far more positive and support the Rittenhouse study group regarding primary care. Ideas generated from this study for the healthcare home can be used in any primary care setting. For its part, the American College of Physicians (ACP) has a three-part series on the medical home, which may be helpful in explaining how the ACP believes primary care should be delivered. It is available at http://www.acponline.org/running _practice/pcmh/resources_tools/abstracts.htm.

O'Grady (2009) suggests our current 9:00 AM to 5:00 PM primary care model needs to be restructured to provide 24 hour access seven days a week to medical care. This change involves availability, such as a patient-centered health care home or practice setting with NPs and physicians working collaboratively. O'Grady also describes a reformed reimbursement program that gives incentives to increase provider consistency, integrate health care, and provide a healthcare home model that pays for successful outcomes, not just procedures. In other words, O'Grady recommends NPs abandon the outdated fee-for-service payment system and think more about payment for success. Perhaps having patient outcomes determine reimbursement will link patient outcomes with incentive. This is an example of a healthcare pay-for-performance strategy versus a new innovative business strategy. Many organizations are building this incentive into the pay structure since it offers a merit or bonus award for excellent patient outcomes.

The American Academy of Pediatrics supports the medical home concept since it provides all children with services and support for full community inclusion. This organization introduced the medical home concept in 1967 and initially referred to it as a centralized location for the child's medical record. Since then, the concept has continued to evolve and, in 2002, was expanded to include the following qualities of care:

- Accessible
- Continuous
- Comprehensive
- Family-centered
- Coordinated
- Compassionate
- Culturally effective

More information is accessible at http://www.medicalhomeinfo.org. The Academy of Pediatrics sees the medical home as a method of providing primary care with an underlying family-centered partnership, community-based system that provides healthcare services as the child transitions from infant to young adult. The efficiency of this method generates high-quality care and patient/family satisfaction. It was developed further by the American Academy of Family Physicians (2004) and the American College of Physicians (2006) and can be accessed at their Web sites. The National Association of Pediatric Nurse Practitioners also supports the medical home for children concept and believes that Pediatric Nurse Practitioners have the training to provide and manage children's care in such a setting (Duderstadt, 2008).

Studies comparing NPs and physicians in primary care show outcomes that are favorable for nurse practitioners (Spitzer, Sackett, Sibley, Roberts, Kergin, Hackett, & Olynich, 1974; Sakr, Angus, Perrin, Nixon, Nicholl, & Wardrope, 1999; Kinnersley, Anderson, Parry, Clement, Archard, Turton, Stainhorpe, Fraser, Butler, & Rogers, 2000). The seminal study by Mundinger, Kane, Lenz, et al. (2000) involved a randomized trial of patient outcomes (patient satisfaction with care, health status, physiological test results, and service use by physicians and NPs) and found the outcomes are similar for both providers. The follow-up study of this trial confirmed sustained equal management outcomes for both NPs and physicians (Lenz, Mundinger, Kane, et al, 2004). Diers (2004) found experienced NPs can manage 70 to 90% of primary care ambulatory care visits effectively autonomously. Several studies indicate that NP outcomes are not statistically significantly different from those of physicians in primary care. In some cases, NP outcomes are actually better (Wilson, Landon, Hirschorn, McInnes, Ding, Marsden, & Cleary, 2005; Laurant, Reeves, & Hermens, et al, 2006; Horrocks, Anderson, & Salisbury, 2002). The implications of these studies for NPs are extraordinary. However, the same problems facing physicians in primary care also face NPs. Still, creative thinking can overcome barriers.

One solution for many primary care providers is to integrate mental health specialists or psychiatric NPs with primary care NPs. Roberts, Robinson, Stewart, and Wright (2008) developed an Integrated Mental Health Practice Model that combines mental health specialists with primary care providers. This acknowledges that most primary care providers are not prepared to meet patients' mental health needs and that many problems seen in primary care have a mental health etiology. Therefore, such integration is an excellent arrangement for clinics that serve multiple walk-ins and vulnerable populations. Certainly, no one needs to be reminded there is an increased number of patients categorized as vulnerable. Thus, the Integrated Mental Health Practice Model is an effective, efficient, and high-quality one-stop process for patients with mental health needs. Westheimer Steinley-Bumgarner, and Brown (2008) share similar findings from their study of the integration of primary care and mental health providers in a university health center. This integration of practitioners is especially desirable in a college setting because this is often the time when individuals first experience mental health issues. Lastly, Baumann (2004) relates how the integration of mental health services with primary care in a not-for-profit site was successful.

Nurse practitioners in all settings also need to use cost-efficient treatments for patients, especially those without insurance prescription plans (Luthy, Peterson, & Wilkinson, 2008). One solution is sending patients to a pharmacy that generally charges a copayment of $4 per prescription or to grocery stores that offer specials, such as free antibiotics. Approximately 360 different generic medications are in the $4/per prescription price bracket, and they tend to be for the most common health problems. A sample listing can be accessed at www.walmart.com/pharmacy. Another possibility is to refer the patient to a patient assistance program that provides the medication at a lower cost or sometimes free to patients with financial need (Chauncey, Mullins, Tran, McNally, & McEwan, 2006). For individuals who do not speak English, use the translation Web site, http://translate.google.com/translate_t#, to assist with communication. Practice settings using teams is another cost-efficient method to provide care. Table 2.2 provides practical considerations.

A large group of " baby boomers" is starting to flood the healthcare market. Some are demanding health promotion and disease prevention strategies to maintain their health as they age. This group has been satisfied with the care they receive from NPs. But more initiatives to promote self-responsibility for health and cost-efficient care need to be generated for this market.

Grossman and Burke (2002) determined that some of their patients were making appointments without really needing them, so they developed a model

2.2 Strategies for Success With Team-Run Practices

- Have NP students do a practicum in an underserved area to maximize their primary care experience.
- Educate each team member to his or her roles and responsibilities.
- Assure mentors are available for NPs.
- Provide time for staff to share experiences and concerns.
- Be a role model by showing respect for all staff and patients.
- Provide constructive feedback daily to staff and suggest they do the same.

for self-management of the common cold. A checklist was created containing questions regarding the presence of a fever, sore throat, or ear discomfort and the duration of the illness. This was available in the waiting room with over-the-counter remedies for the common cold. Directions to make an appointment if they experienced certain symptoms were also provided. This helped patients determine whether they could manage their symptoms independently or whether they needed to be seen by an NP. The self-management model was considered satisfactory by the individuals, saved appointment time for people who really need to be seen, was cost effective, and instilled a degree of self-responsibility for one's health.

Having a one-stop practice setting for multiple healthcare needs, such as dental, health, vision, hearing, diagnostic laboratory, and pharmacy is another good marketing method. This family-centered approach is helpful for both the patient and healthcare professionals. Huer (2007), in the *Journal for Specialists in Pediatric Nursing,* offers an example where dental and healthcare offered at the same location demonstrate effective patient outcomes—another model of care to increase access to individuals who may not otherwise obtain health care.

DNP Essentials

In 2004, the American Association of Colleges of Nursing (AACN) developed a position paper, *Position Statement on the Practice Doctorate in Nursing,* regarding a change in the terminal degree for advanced practice nurses (nurse practitioners, nurse anesthetists, nurse midwives, and clinical nurse specialists) from a master's degree to a doctoral degree by the year 2015. This paper can be accessed at http://www.aacn.nche.edu/DNP/pdf/DNP.pdf. Between 2004 and 2006, multiple meetings of stakeholders discussed the Doctorate of Nursing Practice. Then, in 2006, the AACN, in cooperation with multiple professional organizations, introduced *The Essentials of Doctoral Education for Advanced Practice Nurses* (http://www.aacn.nche.edu/DNP/pdf/Essentials.pdf). The *DNP Roadmap Task Force Report* is accessible at http://www.aacn.nche.edu/DNP/pdf/DNProadmapreport.pdf. Also in 2006, the National Organization of Nurse Practitioner Faculties (NONPF) introduced the *Practice Doctorate Nurse Practitioner Entry-level Competencies* (http://nonpf.com/NONPF-2005/PracticeDoctorate ResourceCenter/CompetencyDraftFinalApril2006.pdf).

This change is in response to requests from the Institute of Medicine, Joint Commission, and National Academy of Science Report, *Advancing the Nation's Health Needs: NIH Research Training Programs (2005),* to educate nurses at a level consistent with role expectations and on a par with other health professions. For example, the fields of pharmacy, psychology, medicine, dentistry, physical therapy, and occupational therapy require doctoral degrees for entry into practice, and each has a practice doctoral degree.

Never has the healthcare system demanded so much from nurses, and never has there been such a shortage of nurses, nurse educators, and nurse executives. At the same time, nurses need to acquire more skills in management, organizational behavior and systems, and business. In addition, it is time for the nursing profession to negotiate a place at the podium rather than in a front row seat. Nursing professionals must become a direct part of the complex healthcare system and not remain as those to whom other healthcare professionals delegate their plans.

According to O'Sullivan, Carter, Marion, Pohl, and Werner (2005), APNs need more in-depth knowledge in practice management, health policy, informatics, risk management, evaluation of symptoms, and advanced diagnosis and care management. Each of these areas should be part of the practice doctorate curriculum. Other background information is also worth noting. The DNP Essentials were developed primarily for future APNs (i.e., for graduates of baccalaureate nursing programs who wish to become advanced practice nurses as of 2015). The year 2015 is the year when graduates of advanced practice nursing programs will be required to have a DNP to be certified to practice as an NP or other advanced practice role. The remaining certified master's prepared NPs will be grandfathered.

The doctoral degree will provide nurses with a terminal degree earlier in their careers. They will have the credentials to propel themselves to leadership positions faster than if only prepared at the master's level. Graduates of most advance practice nursing master's programs have completed the same number of courses and clinical hours as many graduates of doctoral programs in other disciplines. The question for many is: What about the MSN-prepared NP who wants to pursue the DNP? And what about those who don't? Those who don't will be grandfathered. As for those who do, some Schools of Nursing have established MSN-DNP completion programs. Generally these programs include a two-year, part-time program averaging approximately 35 to 45 credits and 400 immersion clinical hours. Most programs use the following formula to determine how many clinical hours the student needs: take the student's clinical hours from the MSN program and subtract it from 1000; the remaining hours are completed in the DNP completion program. This usually equals about 400 immersion clinical hours.

Many NP clinicians have not had the inclination or time to learn the business aspect of their practice because each day is spent seeing patients every 15 minutes. Nurse practitioners who want to become educators will need to pursue a doctoral degree, learn more research skills, and maintain their clinical competency. To maintain their academic positions, the nurse educators teach, conduct research, publish, and do university/community/professional service. The practice doctoral degree will augment a nurse's ability to focus on clinically based research.

Table 2.3 can help almost every NP enhance what he or she has learned in master's preparation. The DNP Curriculum includes foundational and specialty competencies for APNs. Of the eight essentials, the first seven delineate the foundational competencies and the eighth deals with the competencies, content, and practice experiences delineated by the National Specialty Organizations of nurse practitioners, nurse anesthetists, nurse midwives, and clinical nurse specialists. Each essential delineates the student competencies.

Many issues are still under discussion as APNs and members of the nursing profession do not agree on solutions. One of the most important issues is the certification process for DNP graduates. Carter and Apold (2009) present their differing viewpoints on whether graduates from a DNP program should be required to pass the National Board of Medical Examiners (NBME) exam. This exam is similar to the Step 3, U.S. Medical Licensing Examination (USMLE).

2.3 The AACN-DNP Essentials

http://www.aacn.nche.edu/DNP/pdf/Essentials.pdf

1. *Scientific Underpinnings for Practice*
   includes a focus on both the natural and social sciences such as the traditional physiology, pathophysiology, microbiology, pharmacology, chemistry, physics, psychology, sociology, nutrition, and the less traditional genomics, advances in immunology and inflammation, and the science of organizational structures. Most significantly there is nursing science including reflective practice theory which has expanded greatly and will guide practice.

2. *Organizational and Systems Leadership for Quality Improvement and Systems Thinking*
   involves quality improvement, organizational & systems leadership theory, quality indicators, patient safety, management, organizational behavior, organizational culture, ob design, health care delivery environment, leadership, practice models for patient panels and populations, micro, meso, macrosystems, peer review, practice guidelines, and standards of care, power, budgeting, fiscal management, economics, outcome management, patient centered care, patient advocacy, ethics, corporate compliance, and risk management.

3. *Clinical Scholarship and Analytical Methods for Evidence-Based Practice*
   includes critiquing skills, knowledge development pathways, patterns of knowing, reflective practice, nature of science, use of data bases, knowledge synthesis, research—theory practice links, evidence based practice, levels of evidence, practice problems, middle range theories, research designs, sampling strategies, ethical principles, measurement errors, qualitative and quantitative research methods and analysis, data collection strategies, use of human subjects, evaluating evidence, descriptive and inferential statistics, multivariate statistics, instrument resources, use of research methods for outcome improvement, Boyer's Model, translational research, information technology, research dissemination and publication, and application of research to practice.

4. *Information Systems/Technology and Patient Care Technology for the Improvement of Transformation of Health Care*
   includes evaluation & use of information systems and technology, macro and meso-system levels, information system design, outcome evaluation, patient web-based learning tools, productivity tools, quality improvement, communication networks, patient care technology, Informatics Models, informatics, theories, ergonomics, telemedicine, practice applications, consumer health information, utilization, data sets, legal and ethical issues.

5. *Health Care Policy for Advocacy in Healthcare*
   includes lobbying, building coalitions, health policy initiative impacting healthcare, healthcare financing , role expansion, policy makers, policy development, economics,

(continued)

regulation, role, scope of practice, licensure, accreditation, certification, education, political activism, resource allocation, communication skills, advanced practice role, legislation, business ethics, advocacy, workforce issues, and healthcare reform.

6. *Clinical Prevention and Population Health for Improving the Nation's Health*
   includes models of health promotion & disease prevention, prevention interventions, health disparities, at-risk populations, community partnerships, wellness and self-care, Healthy People 2010/2020, adherence, resiliency, social determinants, population–based care, chronic illness, cultural diversity, lifestyle modifications, motivational interviewing, change, pain relief, trauma treatment, advanced communication techniques, biostatistics, epidemiology, genomics, population genetics, clinical trials, outbreak management, public health, program planning, models of disease transmission, and practice guidelines

7. *Inter-professional Collaboration for Improving Patient and Population Health Outcomes*
   includes communication, politics, collaboration, partnerships, advance practice role, reflective practice, consultation, coaching, mentoring, leadership models and theories, vision development, strategic planning, career development, group dynamics, healthcare teams, change and chaos theory.

8. *Advanced Nursing Practice*
   is the specialty competencies for the NP, nurse anesthetist, nurse midwife, or CNS along with the advanced practice role.

Carter suggests graduates of DNP programs take the exam. The Consensus Model states only APNs (nurse midwives, nurse practitioners, nurse anesthetists, and clinical nurse specialists) can graduate from a DNP program, but the DNP will become the entry level for advanced practice in 2015, which would prepare the DNP graduate to take the APN certification exam. Dr. Apold believes it is the role not the credential being certified. She believes the current established certification bodies have psychometrically sound tests measuring NP clinical competency. Dr. Aphold suggests these tests constitute what a nurse practitioner needs to know to pass and become certified. Further, she points out that if DNP graduates take this exam and MSN-prepared NPs do not, a gap between the two types of APNs (those who are certified by the medical profession's NBME exam and those who are credentialed by nursing's APRN exam) will exist. "Leveling" of NPs would not be favorable for anyone.

The classic article from the *Wall Street Journal*, "Making Room for Dr. Nurse," dated April 2, 2008, speaks to whether the APN should take the medical profession's NBME exam. It can be accessed at http://online.wsj.com/article/SBI20710036831882059.html. In response, the American Association of Colleges of Nursing sent a letter to the *New York Times* stressing that DNPs are not being prepared to be physicians or hybrid practitioners. For further information regarding the NBME exam or Comprehensive Care Certification exam, access http://www.abcc.dnpcert.org/pdf/AACN_Statement_on_CC%20Exam_3-6-091.pdf.

Reflective Practice Influences the NP Role

Reflective practice involves learning from one's experiences to improve one's practice. However, when one realizes the potential of this process regarding one's way of thinking, it becomes more multidimensional. Johns and Freshwater (2004), Bulman and Schutz, (2008) and Freshwater, Taylor, and Sherwood (2008) offer various definitions of reflection and suggest it is a way of learning to see the world in a different manner. Using reflective practice can change one's perceptions about experiences, learning, and one's way of thinking. To develop autonomy, accountability, competency, knowledge, and creativity, it is necessary to allow reflection time for the NP. Obtaining improved skills will assist the NP to make better clinical decisions, since practitioners, as a rule, make decisions based on experience and not on technical rationality (Schon, 1983). Most important, self-reflection and inquiry will assist the NP to gain confidence and, subsequently, improve patient outcomes.

Hardy, Titchen, and Manley (2007) suggest NPs can evaluate the effectiveness of their practices with research and, with self-reflection, can improve both professionally and personally. Reflection is a means of collecting data regarding one's practice. One can continue to learn by reflecting in, reflecting on, and critically thinking about the patient encounter. "Reflecting-in-action" is being able to relate to the intuitive process of "thinking on one's feet," and "reflecting-on-action" is a retrospective process that occurs when one reflects on what happened after an experience occurs (Schon, 1983). Consistent use of reflective practice should assist NPs in identifying how their actions impact their patients so that outcomes can be maximized.

Advanced practice nurses need to reflect more on their experiences so they will gain more knowledge, develop intuitive thinking for the future, and just "know" how to respond better to their patients. It is kind of a *déjà vu,* as one thinks about the process of becoming an RN and how one currently learns in everyday advanced practice or practica about patient management. Initially, one learns the skills and is task oriented. Then, as more theory is integrated, one assesses and analyzes a situation. Finally, one integrates all of the nuances gained in advanced preparation classes and, if one is interested in continuing to improve performance, she or he should use reflection. One gains insight, learns to inquire more, uses the evidence, and applies what one successfully did in the past regarding a specific situation. This new way of practicing is forever evolving with critical reflection. Freshwater, Taylor, and Sherwood (2008) present helpful reasons why individuals use reflection in everyday practice:

- Development of nursing theory
- Integration of theory and practice
- Encouragement of a holistic and flexible approach to practice
- Enhancement of self-esteem
- Improvement of image of the advanced practice nurse
- Creation of teams, partnerships
- Development of new practice models

Reflective practice is based on neurophysiology. Daniel Siegel (2007) in his book, *The Mindful Brain,* explains that being "fully present" in the "here and now" allows for mindful awareness, which has been researched and proven to:

- Enhance physical, social, and mental being
- Create an attunement or resonance with oneself that promotes improved neural circuitry—which, in turn, fosters physiological benefits
- Expand specific social and emotional circuits in brain and develop the prefrontal cortex

Siegel further says continued mindfulness or critical thinking:

- Improves resilience, flexibility, and emotional balance
- Increases immune and cardiac function
- Enhances a sense of empathy and self-understanding

By expanding our neural circuits with reflective learning, our brain reorganizes neural pathways based on new experiences, called neuroplasticity. This is a lifelong ability. Learning, through instruction or experience, allows us to acquire new knowledge and skills (Zull, 2002; Facione & Facione, 2008; Brookfield, 1995). Increased mindfulness enhances our ability to think and learn. Changing the prefrontal cortex by using reflective learning increases the brain's neuroplastic ability. NPs need to create awareness that the mind matters—who we are, our state of mind, and what information means to us. More reflective thinking will rewire our brains and enhance our learning ability and passion about our work (Siegal, 2007). Using more active learning strategies to teach and learn knowledge will assist NPs in improving their neuroplastic ability. This, in turn, will increase clinical reasoning ability and clinical and case management skills, as well as expand critical thinking.

NPs Are Involved in Evidence-Based Practice and Translational Research

APNs and other care providers use practice guidelines from evidence-based practice to manage patients. Many NPs have acquired new knowledge about advanced practice, but they never have the time to disseminate it. Nurse practitioners need to gain the skills to evaluate evidence they collect and share the outcomes they generate. At times, NPs may become too disease focused. However, NPs generally have holistic techniques for practice that could (and should) be shared and incorporated into practice guidelines along with the medical practice hints. The Agency for Healthcare Research and Quality (AHRQ) presents guidelines that focus on the problems or responses of patients versus just the disease as the focus and can be accessed at www.ahcpr.gov. The National Guideline Clearinghouse is another source of interest regarding practice (http://www.guideline.gov/).

Advanced practice nurses also incorporate midrange theories into their management plans. If more information was disseminated from practice, NPs would be able to improve their management of various patient responses, including patient uncertainty, pain, discomfort, anxiety, and fear. Most NPs plan their care using one or a combination of the grand theories, such as self-care, adaptation, crisis, or caring and are guided by national practice and agency guidelines.

The literature describes many translational research studies regarding creative strategies of patient management and examples of small research studies which have generated cost-effective outcomes and patient satisfaction. The term, translational research, is research intended to enhance the adoption of best practices in the community. Koeniger–Donahue (2007) shared results of a qualitative study regarding NP-client interactions in two women's health settings, where types of exchange relationships between patients and NPs were identified. The results are helpful for other NPs to apply to clinical practice and serve as an excellent example of how to apply reflective thinking to practice. Alexander (2004) identified problems discovered in her study of ethnically diverse groups of women regarding system delivery issues and one-to-one interactions with providers. NPs can apply the findings of these two examples of translational research in other delivery settings to improve patient care.

NPs Use Principles of Change Management to Expand Role

Certainly our society has experienced great changes; this is particularly true with approaches to health care. Change is a dynamic process that generally causes conflict for an individual or among people but ultimately results in positive growth. Although not everyone may perceive the outcome(s) of change as positive, unbiased outsiders usually do. Ultimately, the change that constantly occurs in most organizations as a result of some type of chaos leads to continued evolution and growth.

For example, everyone is discussing needed reform and change in the U.S. healthcare system. In doing so, people tend to blame others for the problems. The insurance companies blame the healthcare providers for ordering too many diagnostic tests. The providers blame the lawyers because the diagnostics are ordered to protect them from liability in case patients do not respond to a treatment or experience errors or omissions by a healthcare provider. This vicious cycle is compounded by healthcare organizations that do not operate efficiently, technology not working properly, and the human error that occurs because healthcare providers are working under too much stress with too many complex patients. One must also consider political forces and the politics of health care in our chaotic delivery system. Unending problems cause the costs of health care to increase.

Each NP can teach patients techniques they can use to adapt to change. Nurse practitioners can also become leaders of change in their practice or community. Individuals can probably improve their skills in managing change by reviewing Lewin's and Prochaska, DiClemente, and Norcross's frameworks. Lewin's (1951) theory of change discusses three stages:

▨ **Unfreezing** is the assessment period when a need for change arises. Sometimes, only a few people realize change is required, and they have to lead others to understand that change could improve the situation. Change proponents need to allow time for those who do not readily see this need to conclude for themselves that change is necessary. Allowing a majority to decide in favor of change results in a greater likelihood of success. During this time, the proponents of the change can prepare others for the change and its impact on them. A time should be set aside for meetings to discuss the change. Providing a timeframe for the actual change is also helpful. If the NP is working with a patient to change some behavior, a contract with the patient can be developed. This will provide a method of communication between the patient and healthcare provider known as coaching. A good resource for different methods of coaching is found in Kilburg's *Executive Wisdom: Coaching and the Emergence of Virtuous Leaders* (2006).

- **Moving** occurs when people have accepted the need for change and begin to implement it. During this stage, proponents function as coaches. It is also helpful to have established communication so everyone can share ideas about the change and make recommendations for adapting to it. Once again, coaching and mentoring of others by the change proponents are important parts of the process. Sometimes, during this stage, the change may need to be modified; it is crucial everyone involved is part of the decision-making process for these adjustments. This stage can vary in terms of time and, in some cases, can last forever. It is a good time to "get the kinks out of the new change" and obtain acceptance from the majority involved. Of course, some will never support the change. They may be "up-front" about sharing their objections to the change or they may try to sabotage the change. The "passive-aggressive" individual working against the change is the real challenge, and it will require some ingenuity to either win them over or proceed without them. Everyone reading this book has probably experienced this challenge and will agree there is no one easy way to solve it. Another approach is to attempt a compromise with those not willing to participate in the change. If compromising with the participants is unsuccessful, the nonchangers will need to come to terms with the change.
- **Refreezing** is the time when the new change is integrated into the system and becomes part of the culture. Naysayers who still complain and try to sabotage the change will have to accept that the change has been made and all need to adapt.

Another framework NPs can use to assist people with change is the *Change Framework* by Prochaska, DiClemente, and Norcross (1992). This method is appropriate for working with patients who are attempting to change unhealthy behaviors. It is always difficult to change habits, such as substance abuse or overeating. As previously discussed, a "contract" can be developed with the patient describing the specifics of the required change, methods of communication to be used between themselves and the provider, and development of a list of the consequences that may result if the change process is not followed. Patients often make mistakes and encounter negative reaction from others when they choose to abandon the behavior modification process. The NP can be an invaluable support in this situation.

NPs Involved in Intra- and Interprofessional Collaborating and Consulting: Implications for Further Role Expansion

Collaboration is a process of working together to meet each individual's needs. Jenerette, Funk, Ruff, Grey, Adderley-Kelly, and McCorkle (2008) recommend that everyone involved in the decision-making process be a part of the collaborative initiative. However, an NP who works with other NPs is not necessarily "collaborating." Nurse practitioners have been invisible for too long and need to become more transparent by collaborating more with physicians. They need to explain their role and market their services to physicians and other interprofessional healthcare team members. Keith and Askin (2008) recommend more interprofessional education between medical and nursing schools to increase understanding of roles. This understanding may increase interprofessional consultation and collaboration. Intraprofessional collaboration is also important and involves other NPs and nursing teams cooperating with each other.

Effective collaboration includes clear communication, honest dialogue, active listening, awareness of each person's different role, and the ability to negotiate responsibilities (Keleher, 1998). Common knowledge accepts that one can learn more from a group project than working alone. It is beneficial to see things through other people's eyes; this generally widens everyone's perspective. So, with a wider knowledge and experiential base, the finished project should result in improved care.

Broome (2007) describes that "magic happens" when each member of a group shares specific knowledge and skills. This collaboration involves two or more individuals acting to maximize outcomes. The team could be a patient and an NP working to attain results with an antihypertensive treatment; a group of healthcare team members discussing the treatment of a morbidly obese patient who needs surgery; or NPs from various states developing a new Guideline for Care who are collaborating via conference calls. Collaboration means genuinely working together to reach a goal.

Collaboration does not mean there is a change in responsibility. For example, there is no change in responsibility if a primary care provider collaborates with a specialist to obtain the specialist's general opinion. However, if the primary care provider feels the need for the specialist to actually see the patient, a referral occurs.

Consulting

There are numerous advantages for the NP who serves as a consultant:

- Increased networking
- Enhanced credibility of the NP and the practice the NP represents
- Greater visibility of the NP role
- Improved knowledge sharing between other NPs, physicians, and members of the interprofessional team

These opportunities will ultimately yield higher quality patient care and improved patient outcomes.

The process of consulting is similar to the nursing process—it includes assessment of the problem or area of need, analysis of the data regarding the problem, development of a plan to manage the problem, completion of the management intervention for eradicating the problem, and evaluation of the intervention(s) performed. Sometimes the consultant is asked to confer on a complex patient situation. Other times, an NP may be hired to develop a care delivery system or an aspect of one, revise a management process not operating the way the agency hoped, or set up staff development regarding a specific topic(s).

A successful consultant needs good communication and conflict management skills. The NP meets first with the person requesting the consultation and then with those who will be affected by the outcome. One will need to develop the plan and obtain feedback from the hiring agency. When the plan is implemented, the actual consultation begins. After completing the assignment, feedback needs to be analyzed and used to market the work with other prospective consultees. If the consultation involved a change process, a follow-up evaluation should occur about four weeks after the change is initiated. This follow-up visit is crucial to determine whether the change is proceeding as planned.

Clinical consultations are conducted with providers who have specific expertise. Nurse practitioners must realize, however, that responsibility for the patient's care remains with them and that they must decide whether to follow the recommendation. The consultant has no liability unless the consultant actually sees and examines the patient. In that case, the consultant can be liable and must be sure the consultee follows up with some type of action for the patient. The consultant should obtain a copy of the consultee's decision and management plan for the patient.

The referral visit is completed by a specialist who manages the specific problem and shares findings with the primary care provider. The primary care provider may not take part in managing the referred problem unless a mutual agreement is reached between the specialist and the primary care provider. Still, the primary care provided must perform a follow-up to ensure the recommended care was completed.

Informal consultations usually occur on the spur of the moment, are not billable, and involve a patient problem the consultee has little or no experience managing. The patient is probably in the examination room, and the consultee has come out to obtain assistance from a more experienced clinician. If the patient's issue is too complex for the consultee, the consultant provider may mentor the consultee in caring for the patient. There may be some schedule or assignment change so the consultant's work schedule is freed up to accommodate the patient.

A formal consultation may involve direct contact with the patient. The consultee maintains responsibility for the patient and should document the consultant's visit and participation in the management plan in the patient's chart. This documents the consultant's involvement if a future liability issue arises. The information in the patient's chart also serves as a reminder to the consultee that follow-up by the consultant may be needed. In addition, a formal consultation takes more time and may be billed by the consultant; this would require the consultee to notify the patient about the extra charge before the consultation.

The United Kingdom Healthcare System has four consultant roles given to experienced nurses, midwives, and allied health professionals that comprise four key functions. These functions, which delineate the consultant's responsibilities, include practice, leadership, education, and research. The role specifies that the consultant must be involved in the direct care of patients to maintain clinical competency (Humphreys, Johnson, Richardson, Stenhouse, & Watkins, 2007). Although consultant roles are not identified in the literature for NPs in the United States, they are doing more consulting, and primary care NPs are requesting assistance with complex patient care issues from other subspecialists who may also be NPs. An example would be consulting a Psychiatric NP to help manage patients with mental health problems.

Healthcare Delivery Settings for Nurse Practitioners

Many practice models for NPs have been studied, and new models are continuously evolving. Nurse practitioners and physicians are providing collaborative care in rural areas of the United States that have fewer than 20,000 people (Brown, Hary, & Burman, 2009). These authors' findings equate NP and physician primary care outcomes. The descriptive study indicates NPs in Wyoming are independently managing simple as well as complex patients with physician collaboration in a variety of rural settings.

Williamson and LeBlanc (2008) share a genetics service practice model that includes an NP, genetics counselor, and collaboration with a geneticist. This model depicts a new NP practice setting. Recommendations for NPs not working in a genetic service are also identified regarding the importance of integrating genomics into practice.

"Concierge medicine" describes a new relationship between healthcare providers and their patients. In this scenario, patients pay an annual fee for the right to seen by the provider as circumstances require. The patient, however, is still required to pay for services rendered. Most concierge providers have smaller caseloads than average and make visits to the patient's home or long-term care facility. The revenue collected from the annual fees offsets the lower number of patients in the practice, so the concierge generates a positive cash flow. Providers are assured continued financial stability and the patients have a sense of being "well cared for," with easier access to their provider.

"Boutique medicine" is a model of practice in which the provider does not accept insurance. Instead, only cash is accepted for payment. This eliminates the large portion of overhead used to manage insurance reimbursement. The patient does not pay an annual fee. Otherwise, this type of practice is similar to any private practice.

Retail medical clinics are successful because they rent space at a low cost from a retail store or pharmacy and see patients on a walk-in basis only. This model is truly patient-centered in terms of access to care. In fact, hospitals and private practices are beginning to open up their hours to walk-ins and also provide weekend and evening hours to recruit some of this business. An example of this care model is the Mayo Clinic in Minneapolis, which has increased revenue since it opened Mayo Express Clinics in shopping centers (2008). The Convenient Care Association (www.ccaclinics.org) represents the retail health industry, such as the Minute Clinics with CVS Drug Stores or the Redi-Clinics with Wal-Mart. The retail clinics' business plan offers high-quality, effective, and convenient care to those with common primary care complaints. The five most frequent complaints seen in retail clinics are sore throat, otitis media, acute sinusitis, conjunctivitis, and urinary tract infection. The cost for a visit is approximately $75, compared to $127 for a private physician's office visit or $356 for Emergency Department care (Hansen-Turton, 2008). Management strategies for all practices can be identified by reviewing retail clinic Web sites (Hansen-Turton, Ryan, Miller, Counts, & Nash; 2007).

The impact of NPs in critical care is not well identified. In a search of literature databases covering the past ten years, only 31 research studies were found describing the role of the NP and/or physician assistant in the care of acute and critically ill patients. Kleinpell, Ely, and Grabenkort (2008) note only two of the 31 studies were randomized control trials, with both highly supportive of the advanced practice role. The authors conclude that more studies are needed to focus on the NP role and its impact on patient outcomes in acute and critical care.

Acute care NPs work in a variety of settings, such as the emergency department, the operating room, post anesthesia care units, and intensive care units. Many NPs also work as hospitalists and with specialty groups in surgical centers and other ambulatory care facilities. Some of these NPs are Acute Care NPs and some may be Family, Pediatric, or Adult NPs. Galicyznski (2006) gives a description of her role as a Trauma Acute Care NP and discusses her impact on patient outcomes.

These are just a few of the settings where NPs are working. The opportunities for NPs in acute, primary, and long-term care are infinite and seem to be growing. The profession would benefit with more descriptions of NP roles in different settings. Chapter 8, *Entrepreneurial Models of Facilitating Best Practice,* presents interviews with NPs in a variety of areas regarding their practices.

Conclusions

It is important for NPs to engage in reflective practice as they continue to grow and expand their roles. Nurse practitioners use a patient-centered focus, rather than a disease focus, in their delivery of care. They are participating in all levels of care in both new and more traditional practice settings. Nurse practitioners have been, and continue to be, a significant part of the health promotion and disease prevention movement. As new challenges surface in care delivery, it is likely the NP will have a major role in healthcare design and provision. Certainly, the DNP offers an opportunity for nurses to enhance skills and knowledge to prepare them for a career in advanced practice nursing as a NP. The DNP can also help showcase the expansion of the nursing profession. It provides areas of instruction to build skills needed for improved business literacy, so NPs can become change agents for future healthcare delivery models.

Reflective Thinking Exercises

1. Gain access to an electronic portfolio or computer program such as Microsoft 2007 One Note and manage your curriculum vita and accomplishments. Keep copies of your papers, abstracts, executive summaries, journals, cases, and anything that describes your abilities.

2. Prepare an advertisement marketing a clinic/office. Use the Online Media Training Tutorial offered by the Kaiser Family foundation (accessible at www.kaieredu.org/tutorials/media/player.html) to help develop an advertisement for radio, television, or print media. This tutorial can also assist NPs when talking with insurance providers, politicians, or other groups in explaining why consumers should come to a specific practice.

3. Using *UpToDate* (either on a PDA device or desktop computer), the NP can have continuing education units tracked. For every hour you participate in *UpToDate,* you can receive 1.0 contact hour through the American Academy of Nurse Practitioners. This program provides current and prompt answers to all clinical questions when the information is needed. Access to this site is www.uptodate.com. Review a clinical concern you recently experienced with a patient using *UpToDate* or some other Internet-based resource site. Evaluate how the information improved your differential diagnosing and expanded your ability to develop other potential differential diagnoses regarding the patient's chief complaint.

4. Create a vision for your role as a nurse practitioner in primary care or a specialty area using reflection and experience. Use the Mindfulness Tool at http://www.springerlink.com/content/g784k7783j4w73j1/ to assess your awareness.

5. Read the *Scholarship of Reflective Practice* Sigma Theta Tau Paper available at http://www.nursingsociety.org/aboutus/Documents/resource_reflective.doc. Develop a definition of reflective practice for yourself. Reflect on your own practice and determine whether your deeper sense of self has assisted you in providing better therapeutic outcomes for your patients.

References

Agency for Healthcare Research & Quality. Retrieved April 3, 2009 from www.ahcpr.gov.

American Academy of Family Physicians. Retrieved April 3, 2009 from http://www.futurefamilymed.org

Alexander, I. (2004). Characteristics of and problems with primary care interactions experienced by an ethnically diverse group of women. *Journal of the American Academy of Nurse Practitioners, 16*(7), 300–310.

American Academy of Pediatrics Retrieved April 3, 2009 from http://aappolicy.aappublications.org/policy_statement/index.dtl#M

American Association of Colleges of Nursing (2004). *AACN position statement on the practice doctorate in nursing.* Retrieved March 12, 2009 from http://www.aacn.nche.edu/DNPpdf/ Essentials.pdf

American Association of Colleges of Nursing. (2006a). *Doctor of nursing practice roadmap task force report.* Retrieved March 12, 2009, from http://www.aacn.nche.edu/DNP/pdf/DNP roadmapreport.pdf.

American Association of College of Nursing. (2006b). *Essentials of doctoral education for advanced nursing practice.* Retrieved March 8, 2009, from http://www.aacn.nche.edu/DNP/ pdf/Essentials.pdf

American Association of Colleges of Nursing. (2009). *DNP program list.* Retrieved March 9, 2009, from http://www.aacn.nche.edu/dnp/DNPProgramList.html.

American Board of Comprehensive Care. Competency Care Certification Exam. Retrieved April 12, 2009 from http://www.abcc.dnpcert.org/.

American College of Physicians. Retrieved April 13, 2009 from http://www.acponline.org/ advocacy/?hp.

American Medical Association. (2004). *Guidelines for integrated practice of physician and nurse practitioner.* (H-160.950). Retrieved April 1, 2009 from http://www.ama.-assn.org/apps/ pf_new

Apold, S. (2008). The doctor of nursing practice: Looking back, moving forward. *The Journal for Nurse Practitioners, 4*(2), 101–107.

Baumann, S. (2004). Integrating psychiatry in inner-city primary care with psychiatric nurse practitioners. *Clinical Excellence for Nurse Practitioners, 8*(3), 103–108.

Bodenheimer, T. (2006). Primary care-Will it survive? *The New England Journal of Medicine. 355,* 861–864.

Boville, D., Saran, M., Salem, J., Clough, L., Jones, R., Radwany, S. & Sweet, D. (2007). An innovative role for nurse practitioners in managing chronic disease. *Nursing Economics, 25*(6), 359–364.

Brookfield, S. (1995). *Becoming a critically reflective teacher.* San Francisco: Jossey-Bass.

Broome, M. (2007). Collaboration: The devil's in the detail. *Nursing Outlook, 55*(1), 1–2.

Brown, J., Hart, A., & Burman, M. (2009). A day in the life of rural advanced practice nurses. *The Journal of Nurse Practitioners, 2,* 108–114.

Brykczynski, K. (1989) Role delineation studies in advanced practice nursing. An interpretive study describing the clinical judgment of nurse practitioners. *Scholarly Inquiry for Nursing Practice: An International Journal, 3*(2), 75–111.

Bulman, C. & Schutz, S. Eds. (2008). *Reflective practice in nursing.* 4th ed., Oxford, UK: Wiley & Sons.

Carter, M. & Apold, S. (2009). Point/Counterpoint: Should DNP graduates take the NBME certification examination? *The Journal of Nurse Practitioners 5*(2), 106–7.

Chauncey, D., Mullins, C., Tran, B., McNally, D., & McEwan, R. (2006). Medication access through patient assistance programs. *American Journal of Health—System Pharmacology. 63,* 1254–9.

Cohen, D., Scribner, R., & Farley, T. (1998). A Structural Model of Health Behavior: A Pragmatic Approach to Explain and Influence Health Behaviors at the Population Level. *Preventive Medicine, 30*(2) 146–154.

Diers, D. (2004). *Speaking of nursing: Narratives of practice, research, and policy, and the profession.* Sudbury: Jones and Bartlett Publishers.

Duderstadt, K. (2008). Medical Home: Nurse practitioners' role in health care delivery to vulnerable populations. *Journal of Pediatric Health Care, 22,* 390–3.

Facione, N. & Facione, P.Eds. (2008). *Critical thinking and clinical reasoning in the health sciences: An international multidisciplinary teaching anthology.* Millbrae: The California Academic Press. http://www.amazon.com/Critical-Thinking-Clinical-Reasoning-Sciences/ dp/1891557602/ref=sr_1_1?ie=UTF8&qid=1244999702&sr=8-1

Freshwater, D., Taylor, B. & Sherwood, G. (2008). *International textbook of reflective practice in nursing.* Oxford: John Wiley & Sons, LTD.

Galicyznski, S. (2006). Top 10 reasons to become a trauma nurse practitioner. *Journal of Trauma Nursing, 13*(3), 107–110.

Grossman, S. & Burke, M. (2002). Providing self-care models for well adults can increase cost-effectiveness. *The International Journal of NPACE, 6,* 2, 1–6.

Hansen-Turton, T. (2008). Editorial: A business model with staying power. *Clinician Reviews. 8*(12) 1.

Hanson-Turton, T., Ryan, S., Miller, K., Counts, M., & Nash, D. (2007). Convenient care clinics: the future of accessible health care. *Disease Management, 10*(2), 61–73.

Hardy, S., Tichen, A., & Manley, K. (2007). Patient narratives in the investigation and development of nursing practice expertise: A potential for transformation. *Nursing Inquiry 14*(1): 80–88.

Heller, B. & Goldwater, M. (2004). The governor's wellmobile: Maryland's mobile primary care clinic. *Journal of Nursing Education, 43*(2), 92–94.

Hofrichter, R. (2003) *Health and Social Justice.* San Francisco: Jossey-Bass Inc Pub.

Horrocks, S. Anderson, E., & Salisbury, C. (2002). Systematic review of whether nurse practitioners working in primary care can provide equivalent care to doctors. *British Medical Journal 324*(7341), 819–23.

Huer, S. (2007). Integrated medical and dental halth in primary care. *Journal for Specialists in Pediatric Nursing. 12*(1), 61–65.

Humphreys, A., Johnson, S., Richardson, J., Stenhouse, E., & Watkins, M. (2007). A systematic review and meta-synthesis: Evaluating the effectiveness of nurse, midwife,/allied health professional consultants. *Journal of Clinical Nursing, 16,* 1792–1808.

Institute of Medicine. (2003). *Health professions educations: A bridge to quality.* Washington, DC: National Academy Press.

Institute of Medicine. (1999). *To err is human: Building a safer health system.* Washington, DC: National Academy Press

Isaacs, S. L., Jellinek, P. S., & Walker, R. L. (2009). The independent physician—Going, going. . . . *The New England Journal of Medicine, 360,* 655–657

Jenerette, C., Funk, M., Ruff, C. Grey, M., Adderley-Kelly, B., & McCorkle, R. (2008). Models of inter-institutional collaboration to build research capacity for reducing health disparities. *Nursing Outlook, 56*(1), 16–24.

Johns, C. & Freshwater, D. Eds. (2004). *Becoming a reflective practitioner: A reflective and holistic approach to clinical nursing, practice development, and clinical supervision.* 2nd ed. London, England: Blackwell Publishers.

Keith, K. & Askin, D. (2008). Effective collaboration: The key to better healthcare. *Canadian Journal of Nursing Leadership. 21*(2), 51–61.

Keleher, K. (1998). Collaborative practice: Characteristics, barriers, benefits, and implications for midwifery. *Journal of Nurse Midwifery, 43,* 8–11.

Kenney, Charles, (2008). *The best practice: How the new quality movement is transforming medicine.* New York, Public Affairs.

Kilburg, R. (2006). *Executive wisdom: Coaching and the emergence of virtuous leaders.* Washington, DC: American Psychological Association.

Kinnersley, P., Anderson, E., Parry, K., Clement, J., Archard, L., Turton, P., Stainhorpe, A., Fraser, A., Butler, C., & Rogers, C.(2000). Randomised control trial of nurse practitioner versus general practitioner care for patients requesting "same day" consultation in primary care. *British Medical Journal, 320,* 1043–1048.

Kleinpell, R., Ely, E., & Grabenkort, R. (2008). Nurse practitioners and physician assistants in the intensive care unit: an evidence-based review. *Critical Care Medicine, 36*(10), 2888–2897.

Knope, S. (2008). *Concierge medicine: A new system to get the best healthcare.* Westport: Prager Pub.

Koeniger-Donahue, R. (2007). Nurse practitioner-client interaction as resource exchange: The nurse's view (NP-client interaction). *Journal of Clinical Nursing, 16,* 1050–1060.

Laurant, M., Reeves, D., Hermens, R., Braspenning, J., Grol, R., & Sibbald, B. (2006). Substitution of doctors by nurses in primary care. Cochrane Database of systematic reviews. Issue 1.

Lenz, E., Mundinger, M., Kane, R., Hopkins, S. & Lin, S. (2004). Primary care outcomes in patients treated by nurse practitioners or physicians: Two-year follow-up. *Medical Care Research and Review, 61*(3), 332–351.

Lewin, K. (1951). *Field theory in social science.* New York: Harper & Row.

Making Room for Dr. Nurse. (4/2/08) Wall Street Journal. Retrieved May 16, 2009 from http://online.wsj.com/article/SBI20710036831882059.html.

Manthey, M. & Disch, J.(2008). Social Justice and Nursing: The Key is Respect. *Creative Nursing, 14*(2), 62–65.

Mundinger, M. (2002). Twenty-first century primary care: New partnerships between doctors and nurses. *Academic Medicine, 77*(8), 776–780.

Mundinger, M., Kane, R., Lenz, E., Tsai, W-Y., Cleary, P., Friedewald, W., Siu, A. & Shelanski, M. (2000).Primary care outcomes in patients treated by nurse practitioners or physicians. *Journal of the American Medical Association. 283*(1) 59–69.

The National Guideline Clearinghouse. Patient Care Guidelines. Retrieved April 3, 2009 from http://www.guideline.gov/.

National Institutes of Health Roadmap. National Institutes of Health. Retrieved on June 1, 2009 from http://www.grants.nih.gov/grants/oer.htm.

National Organization of NP Faculties. (2002). *Domains and competencies of nurse practitioner practice.* Washington, DC: Author.

National Organization of NP Faculties (2006). *Practice doctorate nurse practitioner entry-level competencies.* Retrieved March, 4, 2009, from http://www/nonpf.com/NPNPF2005/PRactice DoctorateResourceCenter/CompetencyDraftFinalApril2006.pdf.

O'Grady, E. (2009). Garbage cans and barking dogs: Health care reform 2009. Nurse *Practitioner World News. 14*(1)/2 8–9.

O'Sullivan, A., Carter, M., Marion, L., Pohl, J.,& Werner, K. (2005). Moving forward together: the practice doctorate in nursing. *Online Journal of Issues in Nursing, 10*(3), 5.

Paulus, R., Davis, K., & Steele, G. (2008).Continuous innovation in health care: Implications of the Geisinger experience. *Health Affairs, 27(5), 1235–45.*

Porter, M. & Teisberg, E. (2006). *Redefining health care: Creating value-based competition on results.* Boston: Harvard Business School Publishing.

Prochaska, J., DiClemente, C. & Norcross, J. (1992). In Search of how people change: Applications to addictive behaviors. *American Psychologist, 47,* 1102–1114.

Rittenhouse, D., Casalino, L., Gillies, R., Shortell, S. & Lau, B.(2008).Measuring the medical home infrastructure in large medical groups *Health Affairs, 27*(5):1246–58.

Roberts, K., Robinson, K., Stewart, C., & Wright, J. (2008). Integrated mental health Practice in a nurse-managed health center. *American Journal for Nurse Practitioners. 12(*10), 33–34, 37–40, 43–44.

Sakr, M., Angus, J., Perrin, J., Nixon, C., Nicholl, J., & Wardrope, J. (1999). Care of minor injuries by emergency nurse practitioners or junior doctors: A randomized controlled trial. *The Lancet, 354,* 1321–1326.

Schoen C., Osborn, R., How, S., Doty, M. & Peugh, J. (2008). In chronic condition: Experiences of patients with complex health care needs, in eight countries. *Health Affairs, 28*(1), w1-w16.

Schroeder, S. (2007). We Can Do Better—Improving the Health of the American People. *New England Journal of Medicine, 357*(12) 1221–1228.

Schmalenberg, C., Kramer, M., King, C., Krugman, M., Lund, C., Poduska, D., & Rapp, D. (2005).Excellence through evidence: Securing collegial/collaborative nurse-physician relationships. *Journal of Nursing Administration, 35*(10), 450–458.

Schon, D. (1983). *The reflective practitioner: How practitioners think in action.* New York: Basic Books.

Siegal, D. (2007). *The Mindful Brain.* New York W. W. Norton & Company.

Spitzer, W., Sackett, D., Sibley, J., Roberts, R., Kergin, D., Hackett, B., & Olynich, A. (1974). The Burlington randomized trial of the nurse practitioner. *New England Journal of Medicine. 290,* 251–256.

Westheimer, J., Steinley-Bumgarner, M. & Brown, C. (2008). Primary care providers' perceptions of and experiences with an integrated healthcare model. *Journal of American College Health, 57*(1), 101–108.

White, J.E., Natvio, D. G., Kobert, S. N., & Engberg, S. J. (1992). Content and process in clinical decision making by nurse practitioners. *Image: Journal of Nursing Scholarship, 24,* 153–158.

Williamson, L. & LeBlanc, D. (2008). A genetic services practice model: Advanced practice nurse and genetic counselor team. *Newborn & Infant Nursing Reviews. 8*(1), 30–35.

Wilson, I., Landon, B., Hirschorn, L., McInnes, K., Ding, L., Marsden, P., & Cleary, P. 2005). Quality of HIV care provided by nurse practitioners, physician assistants, and physicians. *Annals of Internal Medicine, 143,* 729–736.

Yee, C. M. (2008). Mayo Express Clinic. *Minneapolis Star Tribune,* November 12, 2007.

Zallen, D. (2008). *To test or not to test: A guide to genetic screening and risk.* New Brunswick: Rutgers University Press.

Zull, J. (2002). *The Art of Changing the Brain: Enriching the Practice of Teaching by Exploring the Biology of Learning.* Sterling: Stylus Publishing, LLC.

Analysis of Statutes and Legislation: Impact on Nurse Practitioner Practice

3

Learning Objectives

1. Articulate the differences among certification, licensure and credentialing, and accreditation of educational programs and healthcare practices.

2. Identify and describe the national organizations that certify nurse practitioners.

3. Enumerate the available certification specialties and the differences among them.

4. Describe how role, scope, statute, certification, and licensure define the requirements for implementation of standards for clinical practice.

5. Conduct an investigation of state statutes to obtain mandates on practice within a state.

6. Discuss how the scope of practice creates the legal path for all actions executed by the nurse practitioner (NP).

7. Describe the advantage of individual malpractice versus group coverage and the difference in "Occurrence" versus "Claims Made, with tail" coverage.

8. Articulate the difference between licensure of an individual and of a practice.

Key Words: certification, licensure, statute, practice acts, standards of practice, malpractice coverage, scope of practice, credentialing

Advanced Nursing Practice

An effective NP who provides professional and clinical care must understand the nomenclature of advanced practice. The working language of nursing can be confusing to individuals within the profession; to those outside the profession, it can sound like a foreign language.

To begin an advanced nursing practice, one needs to earn a degree, pass certification, obtain licensure, acquire malpractice insurance coverage, understand how legislative and professional scope-of-practice requirements create job limitations, and complete credentialing. An NP needs to understand, articulate, and complete these mandates so professionals, consumers, and appropriate legal bodies recognize his or her competency and readiness to practice. This chapter describes the step-by-step process NPs need to follow to meet all these requirements. Although Advanced Nursing Practice (ANP) is a term encompassing the four separate clinical practice roles available for nurses who obtain advanced education (i.e., nurse practitioner, nurse anesthetist, nurse midwife, and clinical nurse specialist), this text describes only the NP role.

The American Nursing Association (ANA) is a national professional organization that advocates on behalf of the nursing profession. According to the ANA Web site:

> *Nursing is the protection, promotion, and optimization of health and abilities, prevention of illness and injury, alleviation of suffering through the diagnosis and treatment of human response, and advocacy in the care of individuals, families, communities, and populations.*
>
> (American Nursing Association, 2009)

Accreditation: Educational and Practice

To practice as an NP, one needs to graduate from an accredited master's program. Accreditation means that an institution of higher education has been approved by a certifying body, such as the Commission on Collegiate Nursing Education (CCNE) or the National League for Nursing Accrediting Commission (NLNAC). The accreditation process has specific criteria for each program area. Copies of CCNE and NLNAC Accreditation Manuals are accessible on their respective Web sites. Colleges and Schools of Nursing must maintain accreditation standards and be reaccredited in specific time increments. By using established criteria to validate educational requirements, these organizations publically attest that graduates from specific programs have received adequate educational preparation according to the accepted standard.

Accreditation in health care is granted to large organizations, such as hospitals or large group practices, not to independent or individual practices. All hospitals must be accredited by the Joint Commission previously known as the Joint Commission on Accreditation of Health Care Organizations (JCAHO). Each state's public health code specifies the accreditation requirements. In some states, businesses such as surgical centers and medical practices that have received certain licensures may be required to obtain accreditation from organizations such as the Accreditation Association of Ambulatory Health Care (AAAHC), a not-for-profit organization that accredits ambulatory clinics and healthcare provider offices. In doing so, "AAAHC helps to improve the quality of care through the adoption of standards of care and best practices" (Accreditation Association for Ambulatory Health Care, 2009). The Joint Commission publishes a *Compre-*

hensive Manual for Ambulatory Care to guide a practice through the process of accreditation. Additional information for practice accreditation can be accessed at www.jointcommision.org and www.aaahc.org.

Graduate Degree

An NP student who meets all the criteria of an accredited program receives a master's degree, which is the official *credential* awarded for successful completion of the program of study. Because colleges and schools of nursing have different curricula, the credential conferred is not the same for all graduates. The credential varies according to the educational institution attended and the state in which it is earned. For example, one can earn a Master's of Science (MS), Master's of Science in Nursing (MSN), Doctorate of Philosophy in Nursing (PhD), Doctorate of Nursing Science (DNSc), or Doctorate of Nursing Practice (DNP). Although a strong movement exists to require at least a master's degree to become a nurse practitioner (NP), a minority of states still do not require it (Pearson, 2009). In contrast, medical students attend institutions that have similar curricula and are universally granted either a Doctor of Medicine (MD) or Doctor of Osteopathic Medicine (DO). The American Nurses Credentialing Center (ANCC) recommends that the academic credential be listed after a person's name on a signature line as follows: Sarah Connor, DNP (Smolenski, 2008).

For a nurse, a postgraduate/master's certificate is validation of an additional level of specialized education. These certificates indicate educational preparation in a different specialty field than the master's already received. For example, an NP who completed an MSN as an ANP may realize a preference for a broader range of patients and decide to earn a postgraduate Family Nurse Practitioner Certificate. This new certificate requires the NP to pass a Family Nurse Practitioner certification exam before expanding his or her scope of practice.

Although earning an academic credential is the first step in becoming an NP, graduation alone does not grant the ability to practice.

Certification

The second step for the majority of individuals who want to become NPs is certification. Requirements are stipulated by state law or by regulations set by a governing board of professional peers and appointed laypeople. The Nurse Practice Act stipulates whether certification is required to practice as an NP. Most, but not all, states require certification (Pearson, 2009).

A candidate acquires certification by passing a national exam. Several certifying agencies exist; each has different eligibility requirements, renewal requirements, and specializations. The candidate chooses a "specialty track" during the educational process—sometimes on application and sometimes at matriculation. All tracks contain "core" coursework necessary for all NPs, such as advanced physical assessment and pharmacology. Specialty tracks then provide the curriculum specific to the desired area of concentration, such as Adult Nurse Practitioner, Family Nurse Practitioner, Pediatric Nurse Practitioner, Acute Care Nurse Practitioner, and so on.

3.1 List of Agencies and Specializations for Certification

Organization and Web Site Address	Certification Name	Previous Credential (a 2008)	Current Credential
ANCC (American Nurses Credentialing Center) www.nursecredentialing.org/default.aspx	Acute Care NP	APRN-BC	ACNP-BC
	Adult NP	APRN-BC	ANP-BC
	Adult Psychiatric and Mental Health NP	APRN-BC	PMHNP-BC
	Advanced Diabetes Management NP	APRN-BC-ADM	BC-ADM
	Family Psychiatric and Family NP	APRN-BC	FNP-BC
	Mental Health NP	APRN-BC	PMHNP-BC
	Gerontology NP	APRN-BC	GNP-BC
	Pediatric NP	APRN-BC	PNP-BC
	School NP	APRN-BC	SPN-BC
AANP (American Academy of Nurse Practitioners) www.aanp.org	Adult NP		NP-C
	Family NP		NP-C
NAPNAP (National Association of Pediatric Nurse Practitioners)	Pediatric NP		
NCC (National Certification Corporation) www.nccnet.org	Women's Health Care NP		RN-0C
	Neonatal NP		
PNCB (Pediatric Nursing Certification Board) www.PNCB.org	Primary PNP		CPNP-PC
	Acute PNP		CPNP-AC

The National Council of the State Boards of Nursing (NCSBN) (2002) established the criteria that agencies use to create and offer national certification exams. Some specialty tracks have more than one certifying body. For example, a student completing a pediatric concentration can seek certification from:

▓ The National Association of Pediatric Nurse Practitioners (NAPNAP),
▓ The Pediatric Nursing Certification Board (PNCB),
▓ The American Academy of Nurse Practitioners (AANP) or,
▓ The American Nurses' Credentialing Center (ANCC).

When choosing a certification agency, students should consider acceptance by state, federal, and employment agency authorities, recertification requirements, and cost. Licensing and employer authorities detail which certifications are acceptable, as not all certifications are accepted equally in all circumstances. Once the organization for certification is chosen, the candidate submits an application to the certifying body offering the exam (see Table 3.1).

The applicant's eligibility requires corroboration from the academic institution's Specialty Track Coordinator. As a result of technology and the increased creativity of desktop publishing products, copies of degrees are no longer valid proof of graduation as a standalone item of documentation. Corroboration is also required (see Table 3.2).

The national certification granted by passing an exam publicly acknowledges that the NP has the knowledge and competencies to perform clinical care at an advanced level within the tested specialty. Not all states require certification, but those that do require the NP to renew certification on a regular basis, usually every three to eight years. As with advanced degrees, the initials again differ. If certification is obtained through ANCC for an Adult NP, the credential is ANP-BC, which means Adult Nurse Practitioner—Board Certified. If obtained from AANP in the same specialization, Adult NP, the credential RN-C is granted. The certification credential is generally listed after the educational credential in a signature line, as in Sarah Connor, DNP, ANP-BC. Two NPs working side by side doing an identical job can have different academic and certification credentials, as shown by these examples: Sally Smith, MSN, ANP-BC, and Derek Lane, MS, RN-C. No wonder titles and roles are confusing to many in our society (Landro, 2008).

Note, however, an NP with a degree and certification still does not have all the papers needed to begin practice.

Licensure

Once certified, an NP needs a license to practice in the state where employment is anticipated. Each state has its own governing regulations regarding licensure and practice to which healthcare practitioners must comply. Stipulations such as certification, malpractice coverage, and working relationships with other healthcare professionals are delineated in the Nurse Practice Act of each state. Through licensure, each state ensures the safety of its residents.

Licensure applications are obtained from the agency overseeing practice. It may be the State Board of Nursing or another agency, such as the Department of Public Health. The process entails verifying all credentials obtained. Once

3.2   Directions for Applying for APRN Certification, State Licensure

1) Choose the certification agency to apply for exam and contact them for an application
   * Your university must complete a form of verification.
   * You need an official transcript to include with the application.
   * Attach a copy of your RN license.

2) When an authorization-to-test number is received, schedule the exam.
   The exam is computerized, as is the NCLEX. Complete all 175 questions (150 count and 25 are tested for reliability and do not count toward your score. There is no way to determine which are not being counted from those that are counted.) Results are available immediately after the test is completed!

3) Once notified of passing, apply to the state for an APRN license.
   * [See Web site for your state Board of Nursing]. This process has several steps. In addition:
   * A recent passport size photo is needed.
   * The application must be notarized.
   * Your university must complete another form to verify all requirements were completed.

4) You need to provide verification of every RN license you hold. If you hold licenses from several states, contact each state. There is a separate form for this. Depending on the state, it is possible that some verification of RN licenses can be done online.

5) After passing the test, instruct the certifying agency to send the results to the State Nursing Board. The ANCC will not automatically send the results, nor will the state automatically request them. The agency's Web site includes a link for this purpose. Note that the first request is free, but you must do it through regular mail. If the information is needed quickly, pay the $40 fee to do it online.

again the muddy waters of alphabet nonsense in nursing get confusing because each state has its own authority and its own requirements to practice; each state also names the license issued. Again, there is no uniformity is the nomenclature of NP licensure. Licensure variations include: APRN, ARNP, CRNP, CANP, CPNP, RNP, ANP, CNP (Pearson, 2009). The Consensus Model for APRN Licensure, Accreditation, Certification, and Education (2008) is projected to standardize all nomenclature and practice preparation in 2015.

A *Google* search of the term "nurse licensure" and (specific state) should yield results for the state of interest to the reader, and lead to an online application with instructions. Within the search results, look for a Web address with the suffix .gov or state.gov. Pearson (2009) does an extensive review annually of all state legislative mandates and publishes them in *The American Journal for Nurse Practitioners.*

Just as obtaining a driver's license allows one to operate a motor vehicle, obtaining an NP license allows one to "operate" or practice as an NP. Different from a driver's license though, state NP licensure is NOT automatically reciprocated in adjacent states because the steps to obtain licensure are different in each state. That means living and working in Hoboken, New Jersey and volunteering to cover a branch clinic of the same agency in the City (New York) would require licenses in both states, New Jersey and New York. Some work has addressed this boundary issue where practice restriction at a state border isn't convenient. Tristate areas of NJ/NY/MD have started a process of examining licensure acceptance without additional scrutiny known as reciprocity. This process creates a Multi-state Nursing Licensure Compact or "Compacts." Compacts acknowledge that the licensure requirements of the first state were met, so practice in an adjacent state can be granted preliminarily, while awaiting completion of the entire new licensure process to work in the second state. Many states have been able to make progress on Compacts at the Registered Nurse (RN) level of practice, but only two states (Utah and Iowa) are in a compact agreement at the Advanced Nursing Level. The Institute of Medicine (1999) report recommended movement in the NP Compact direction to make Nursing more understandable and consistent (Philipsen & Haynes, 2007; Harbison, 2003).

As Advanced Practice Nursing is, at its foundation, the practice of Nursing, some states require that practicing NPs have both a Registered Nurse (RN) license and an Advanced Practice Nurse license. States differ on which license gives the NP authority to practice. As in Connecticut (see insert of Practice Act next page), where having both the RN and APRN license is required, the RN license is valid for all assessment and care, and prescriptive authority is rendered on the Advanced Nursing license. Some states simply require one license for all care. Knowledge of the law within the state of practice is *imperative*. Licensure is a required component for ANP and all NPs must have one.

Boards of Nursing—Regulation of Nurse Practitioner Practice

Nurse practitioners should be informed about state regulatory practices, as healthcare colleagues, consumers, or insurance companies can bring complaints of illegal practice, practicing without a license, and/or practicing beyond one's scope. Although variations exist, often the state governing board that oversees the issuance of licensure and practice hears the complaint. This may be the Board of Nursing (BON), if it is the supervising body, or the BON may share joint oversight with another Board. Pearson's (2009) annual review includes licensure oversight, state by state, for easy access to up-to-date information. Practitioners and consumers both need to know where a complaint can be filed if wrongdoing is suspected.

Depending on the testimony presented during a complaint, the Board can revoke, suspend, or discipline a nurse by stipulating a probationary period. Only governing bodies can discipline an NP's license. In the case of a malpractice lawsuit, courts cannot revoke or suspend a nursing license, but rather file a report with the BON stating the accusations of substandard care. The BON would then investigate the complaint. It is also customary on annual licensure renewal to be asked, "Have you been convicted of a felony in the last year?" Answering "Yes" will most likely invoke a BON review.

One question that often surfaces is, "Why is the practice of nursing overseen by any profession other than nursing?" Most believe it is an attempt to maintain control over the Scope of Practice of ANP. A general contractor would not allow a plumber to oversee and judge work done if the possibility of losing a license to work was possible. Each professional wants to be judged only by professional peers. It is a common goal among national nursing organizations to have all nursing practice report only to nursing authorities.

Scope of Practice

A Scope of Practice is an in-depth definition of professional expectations and behaviors. They are written by authoritative bodies, mostly legislative, but also by regulatory bodies, such as BONs, with the goal of establishing parameters for the activities of professional practitioners. Every profession engaging in patient care has a Scope of Practice detailing the authority and boundaries of actions while practicing. One enacted into law, these are called Practice Acts. Regulations are invoked through state boards. Different scopes exist for each area of medicine, such as dentistry, medicine, and nursing. Different scopes also exist for levels within each profession, such as Licensed Practice Nurse (LPNs), Registered Nurse (RN), and Advanced Nurse Practice (ANP). Finally, if necessary, different scopes are delineated for roles within a level of practice. For instance, Nurse Practitioner and Nurse Anesthetist are enumerated in the Nurse Practice Act separately. In states where NP practice is governed by laws, legislation dictates the Scope of Practice. The variation does not stop there, as some scopes are very detailed to clarify expectations and some are left purposefully vague in an attempt to alleviate demanding structure. However, this vagueness can lead to an inability to interpret the scope clearly and results in inconsistency among practitioners. This variation adds another level of confusion to the understanding and acceptance of NP practice (Buppert, 2008).

To find the Scope of Practice for a particular state, search the Internet for "nurse practice act" and (the state) of interest. Two examples are given below, one from Connecticut and the other from New Mexico. The example from Connecticut shows the RN scope first. The ANP scope follows in this excerpt. Clearly, the requisites of NP practice in Connecticut include post basic education and collaboration with a physician. In the insert below, allowed NP actions are bolded and defining requirements for the NP role are underlined.

Sec. 20-87a. Definitions. Scope of practice.

(a) The practice of nursing by a registered nurse is defined as the process of diagnosing human responses to actual or potential health problems, providing supportive and restorative care, health counseling and teaching, case finding and referral, collaborating in the implementation of the total health care regimen, and executing the medical regimen under the direction of a licensed physician, dentist or advanced practice registered nurse.

(b) Advanced nursing practice is defined as the performance of advanced level nursing practice activities that, by virtue of <u>postbasic specialized education and experience,</u> are appropriate to and may be performed by an advanced practice registered nurse. The advanced practice registered nurse *performs acts of diagnosis and treatment of alterations in health status,* as described in subsection (a) of this section, and <u>shall collaborate with a physician licensed to practice medicine in this state.</u> If practicing in (1) an institution licensed pursuant to subsection (a) of section 19a-491 as a hospital, residential care home, health care facility for the handicapped, nursing home, rest home, mental health facility, substance abuse treatment facility, infirmary operated by an educational institution for the care of students enrolled in, and faculty and staff of, such institution, or facility operated and maintained by any state agency and *providing services for the prevention, diagnosis and treatment or care of human health conditions,>* or (2) an industrial health facility licensed pursuant to subsection (h) of section 31-374 which serves at least two thousand employees, or (3) a clinic operated by a state agency, municipality, or private nonprofit corporation, or (4) a clinic operated by any educational institution prescribed by regulations adopted pursuant to section 20-99a, the advanced practice registered nurse may, in collaboration with a physician licensed to practice medicine in this state, **prescribe, dispense, and administer medical therapeutics and corrective measures.** In all other settings, the advanced practice registered nurse may, in collaboration with a physician licensed to practice medicine in the state, *prescribe and administer medical therapeutics and corrective measures and may request, sign for, receive and dispense drugs in the form of professional samples* in accordance with sections 20-14c to 20-14e, inclusive, except that an advanced practice registered nurse licensed pursuant to section 20-94a and maintaining current certification from the American Association of Nurse Anesthetists who is prescribing and administrating medical therapeutics during surgery may only do so if the physician who is medically directing the prescriptive activity is physically present in the institution, clinic or other setting where the surgery is being performed. For purposes of this subsection, "collaboration" means a mutually agreed upon relationship between an advanced practice registered nurse and a physician who is educated, trained or has relevant experience that is related to the work of such advanced practice registered nurse. The <u>collaboration shall address a reasonable and appro-</u>

priate level of consultation and referral, coverage for the patient in the absence of the advanced practice registered nurse, a method to review patient outcomes and a method of disclosure of the relationship to the patient. Relative to the exercise of prescriptive authority, the collaboration between an advanced practice registered nurse and a physician shall be in writing and shall address the level of schedule II and III controlled substances that the advanced practice registered nurse may prescribe and provide a method to review patient outcomes, including, but not limited to, the review of medical therapeutics, corrective measures, laboratory tests and other diagnostic procedures that the advanced practice registered nurse may prescribe, dispense and administer. An advanced practice registered nurse licensed under the provisions of this chapter **may make the determination and pronouncement of death of a patient,** provided the advanced practice registered nurse attests to such pronouncement on the certificate of death and signs the certificate of death no later than twenty-four hours after the pronouncement.

Conn. Gen Stat. 20-87 a,b.

Although the legalese is not easy to read or interpret, it is necessary to review the document that grants permissions for practice. Note too, this text makes no mention of malpractice insurance. Those requirements are listed in another subsection of the public statute, as are the requirements for running a business that provides clinical care. To become an NP to the fullest allowable legal extent, review of all areas of the state statute to ascertain the limits and capabilities of the role. To perform legally and avoid BON or trial exposure, a consultation with a healthcare attorney in the state is a valuable exercise.

In contrast to Connecticut's Act, New Mexico's Nurse Practice Act articulates the requirements of practice simply: credential of RN licensure, master's degree, and certification. It articulates the Scope of Practice in New Mexico as independent practice including prescriptive authority.

61-3-23.2. Certified nurse practitioner; qualifications; practice; examination; endorsement. (Repealed effective July 1, 2010)

A. The board may license for advanced practice as a certified nurse practitioner an applicant who furnishes evidence satisfactory to the board that the applicant:

    (1) is a registered nurse;

    (2) has successfully completed a program for the education and preparation of nurse practitioners; provided that if the applicant is initially

licensed by the board or a board in another jurisdiction after January 1, 2001, the program shall be at the master's level or higher;
  (3) has successfully completed the national certifying examination in the applicant's specialty area; and
  (4) is certified by a national nursing organization.
B. Certified nurse practitioners may:
  (1) perform an advanced practice that is beyond the scope of practice of professional registered nursing;
  (2) practice independently and make decisions regarding health care needs of the individual, family or community and carry out health regimens, including the prescription and distribution of dangerous drugs and controlled substances included in Schedules II through V of the Controlled Substances Act [30-31-1 NMSA 1978]; and
  (3) serve as a primary acute, chronic long-term and end of life health care provider and as necessary collaborate with licensed medical doctors, osteopathic physicians or podiatrists.
C. Certified nurse practitioners who have fulfilled requirements for prescriptive authority may prescribe in accordance with rules, regulations, guidelines and formularies for individual certified nurse practitioners promulgated by the board.
D. Certified nurse practitioners who have fulfilled requirements for prescriptive authority may distribute to their patients dangerous drugs and controlled substances included in Schedules II through V of the Controlled Substances Act [30-31-1 NMSA 1978], that have been prepared, packaged or fabricated by a registered pharmacist or doses of drugs that have been prepackaged by a pharmaceutical manufacturer in accordance with the Pharmacy Act [Chapter 61, Article 11 NMSA 1978] and the New Mexico Drug, Device and Cosmetic Act [Chapter 26, Article 1 NMSA 1978].
E. Certified nurse practitioners licensed by the board on and after December 2, 1985 shall successfully complete a national certifying examination and shall maintain national professional certification in their specialty area. Certified nurse practitioners licensed by a board prior to December 2, 1985 are not required to sit for a national certification examination or be certified by a national organization.
N.M.Stat.Ann 61-3-23.2

Because Practice Acts are passed by state legislatures, variations are inevitable. The governing bodies that write and vote on these rules are comprised of average citizens who may not be thoroughly aware of the competencies an NP education provides. In addition, each state acts independently, based on input from constituents and groups and organizations with an interest in the legislation. Some constituents may see advantages to limiting an NP's Scope of Practice, so they maintain an edge in the healthcare business. This is why legislative advocacy is so crucial to NPs.

Most of the progress made in the expansion of the ANP role has happened since the 1970s. These changes have opened up many and varied employment opportunities in ANP. This expansion is the result of changes in Nurse Practice Acts to allow increased responsibility and actions on behalf of patients. One of the most important extracurricular requirements facing nurses today is the role of "practice advocate." This is achieved by educating patients, legislators, and healthcare peers about the potential outcomes and the impact on health outcomes if NPs practice fully to their certified level of preparation.

One stop along the way to improved practice (which would provide considerable momentum) would be to invoke a universal nomenclature and one national Nurse Practice Act—in other words, a National Compact. Proponents agree that simplifying the nomenclature would provide greater understanding, but opponents fear losing professional ground and reimbursement in states where independent practice is already a reality. Because state laws and regulations control Practice Acts, every NP needs to advocate for change on a state-by-state basis.

Laws at the federal level do dictate some care mandates. Federal laws cover implementation of Medicare, the Health Insurance Portability and Accountability Act (HIPAA) confidentiality, and Occupational Safety and Health Administration (OSHA) regulations, but they defer to the state for implementation of other programs, such as Medicaid. Most private and state run reimbursement programs mimic Medicare or look to the federal level for guidance.

Understanding NP practice and lobbying for less restrictive practice will continue to expand the possibilities of entrepreneurship and business opportunities. Supporters of NPs have shown that in the eleven states where NPs currently have independent practice, they offer safe, accessible, and quality health care without regulatory oversight by another profession. What is different between the NPs in these states and nurses in the other thirty-nine? What "magic" helps NPs in New Mexico to provide care, and how can others import it? The magic begins with Nurse Practice Act advocacy.

State medical societies and insurance companies comprise the opposition. They offer dissenting opinions because their goal is to eliminate competition by containing the NP scope. For example, Medicare, which was enacted before the NP role existed, speaks only to the role of the physician in regard to care and reimbursement. As a result of the actual language (i.e, the use of physician instead of provider), sometimes empanelling, which is the acceptance of NPs by insurance companies as care providers, reimbursement, and hospital privileges, are not accessible to NPs. This, however, can change.

All graduating NPs and those in practice should be able to articulate the Scope of Practice that guides and limits their practice. An understanding of these regulations can help generate ideas for improvements and initiate changes.

For example, pharmaceutical companies recently began requiring a physician signature on paperwork to drop off samples for the practice. In most states, physicians are not required to be on-site for NPs to practice, so drug representatives could not leave samples if no physician was present to sign. This presented problems for patients, who needed the unavailable samples, and for the pharmaceutical companies, whose representatives had to make return visits. A pharmaceutical company explained that a single policy company-wide was easier. Therefore, policy was based on the Practice Act from the most restrictive state in which it does business. The pharmaceutical company chose the "lowest common denominator" in terms of Practice Act restrictions. NPs in states with complete legal authority to sign for samples began advocating for their patients who needed samples, and NPs educated the company with a better understanding of their scopes of practice. As a result, new systems were created to meet the needs of the states with lenient Acts.

The NP profession does not as a rule function on the "because it has always been done that way" mentality. Using educational and people skills to bring about change is readily possible. In this example, change was achieved and the pharmaceutical company altered its policies to be broader in states where it legally could be. Change is readily possible, and NPs can become empowered to advocate for it!

During this episode, one NP stated, "Oh, I didn't even know we could have signed for samples before this uprising." This is unacceptable. Familiarity with Practice Acts, Scope of Practice, and Standards of Care is truly essential in becoming the most qualified and effective NP possible.

One common concern regarding broader scope of practice is, "I don't want any more to do than I do right now." Consider an analogy. Interstate 75 in Michigan has a speed limit of 65 miles per hour. Some motorists may drive 62, 57, or 40 miles per hour for various reasons, including safety. Although driving 40 miles per hour is legal, it is not the norm. The same is true of a broader scope of practice. The Practice Act explains the MOST one can do, but an NP can always do less as long as peers are notified and appropriate referrals are executed. If a state law allows for practice without a written agreement, but both the NP and the physician prefer to have one in place, write one and adhere to it. For example, many male pediatricians and male primary care physicians have the authority and knowledge to perform annual gynecology exams, but choose to make arrangements with practice partners or for an appropriate and timely referral to a gynecologist. Other examples of voluntary limitations on the scope is the restricting practice hours on religious holidays or not engaging in some forms of reproductive health care based on personal beliefs. All of these circumstances allow a practitioner to offer a level lower than afforded by statute.

Another point is that legislative regulations can and do change frequently, but those changes are often not communicated to the parties affected. If a change affects the general population, such as laws governing cell phone usage, the local news often provides coverage, thereby informing citizens of the change. The same is not true of legislation affecting professional practices. Therefore, a practitioner has the responsibility to stay informed about changes in the law even without formal notification. And remember that change can be initiated by any party, so it can create a more restrictive environment. Not all change allows for more lenient action. Perhaps NPs should advocate for a change in how they are notified of legislation affecting their practices. Increasing awareness of change is achieved in one of two ways.

- An annual review of the Practice Act can be completed, perhaps at the time of licensure renewal. This method presents some difficulty, as there are multiple areas within statute dictating rules about practice and a thorough review can be time consuming.
- Membership in a state or national professional group is another method of keeping informed of legislative changes affecting NP practice.

State advocacy groups often have a legislative component, a continuing education component, and a social networking component. Membership fees for joining is money well spent, as these groups notify members of important practice changing legislation. They often monitor all proposed legislation impacting ANP practice, even in completely different statutes. For instance, a change in the Physician Assistant Practice Act or Medical Assistant Practice Act might alter the functioning in daily practice by allowing or curtailing duties of other professionals. State advocacy groups may also hire a lobbyist to monitor all proposed legislation, as it can be voluminous.

National professional NP organizations offer resources to practice and provide leadership in advocacy for changes needed on a national level. Specialty organizations vary on focus and philosophy but all have NP advocacy as a motivational passion. These groups include:

- Association of Women's Health, Obstetric and Neonatal Nurses (AWHONN)
- National Association of Pediatric Nurse Practitioners (NAPNAP)
- National Geriatric Nursing Association (NGNA)
- American Nurses Association (ANA)
- American Academy of Nurse Practitioners (AANP)
- American College of Nurse Practitioners (ACNP)

Standards of Practice

Scopes of Practice differ from Standards of Practice. A Scope of Practice legislatively defines the practice of a professional and broadly places requirements and limits on the professional functioning. In comparison, Standards of Practice define the proficiencies, skills, and competencies expected of an individual while working within the normal functioning of the profession.

Standards of Practice are written and published by professional organizations offering certification exams or representing the profession. The ANA defines a standard as "the authoritative statement defined and promoted by the profession by which the quality of practice, service, or education can be evaluated" (ANA, 2004, p.49) and, as the overarching national nursing professional organization, publishes a "Standards" package (http://nursingworld.org/books/pdescr.cfm?cnum=15#PKG). Below is a partial listing of associations that publish NP Standards of Practice and their Web sites:

- Pediatric NPs: www.napnap.org/practice/pnpstandards
  http://www.napnap.org/aboutUs/ourPerspective/ScopeAndStandards.aspx
- Adult NPs: www.ACNP.org or www.AANP.org
- Family NPs: www.ACNP.org or www.AANP.org
- Women's Health:
  http://www.awhonn.org/awhonn/store/productDetail.do?productCode=PSS6

Standards of practice are used primarily in two ways. First, Standards enumerate the skills and proficiencies an NP learns in an educational program and is expected to use in practice. Educational institutions receive accreditation by teaching Standards. Nurse practitioners receive certification when they correctly test their knowledge base against the acceptable Standards of Care. These Standards must guide care rendered in everyday practice. Secondly, Standards answer the question, "What would someone equally educated do?" Standards serve as a guide for expected clinical behavior. If all adult NPs are taught blood pressure assessment and methods of treating hypertension, it is assumed that when encountering a patient with hypertension, NPs will initiate care to the accepted standard. This "reasonable approach" perspective is used in evaluating care in a court or a BON action. Lawyers will investigate whether the care rendered by the NP in question meets the Standard of Care by comparing it with care rendered by an equally prepared NP in the profession. Actions are held accountable to these Standards of Care when a complaint is filed about an NP's practice.

How can care differ so greatly if all practice has care frameworks? First, varied fields of science have nonparallel facts guiding care. Second, care is not based solely in science. ANP care is often referred to both as an art and a science. Standards provide the science of ANP care and nursing practice provides the art. Herein lies the possibility of variance.

To assist the NP in following Standards of Care, Clinical Guideline texts have been written for most specialties to use as reference. Each NP should have at arm's length a current text or electronic reference to assist in the formulation or validation of care. The NP can also consult government up-to-date clinical care guidelines that compare the care generally widely with the results of evidence-based studies. Visit www.AHRQ.gov for examples.

In addition, some employers have written protocols for NP-provided care in daily practice. Protocols can, however, be a help and a hindrance. The ways they are helpful are easily identifiable. Following written protocols ensures consistent care among providers. Uniformity is guaranteed by following "the letter of the protocol."

In fact, some states mandate written protocols for NP practice. The Nurse Practice Act can mandate that an NP provide independent care only as mandated by a physician. The intent is for the physician to sanction and approve all care. No care outside the protocol is to be provided without the direct supervision and approval of the physician authority. Protocols can present other problems as well. Health care is not amenable to a cookie-cutter approach. If written protocols are strict and do not allow variance, an NP's professional hands can be tied. Some physicians are not familiar with the breadth and extent of Standards of Care taught in NP education. As a result, the permitted level of care per protocol may be too narrow. NPs can become increasingly frustrated when a situation in practice calls for intervention learned in an educational program, but practice protocol does not permit the NP to practice to the full extent proven by certification.

In addition, if a protocol is written for practice and not followed, liability can follow. For example, a protocol written for the care of a patient with abdominal pain includes a laundry list of diagnostics. If any one of those diagnostics is omitted, the protocol was not followed. If that omission is not documented adequately, complaints of oversight in care can arise. Protocols not only **LIMIT WHAT CAN BE DONE,** they also articulate what **MUST BE DONE.** The use of the term protocol in practice infers a legal interpretation. When not mandated by authority, the same uniformity and efficiency in practice can be achieved with the use of accepted *guidelines* for care. Using guidelines allows for consistent structure but also for variation and customization as the realities of practice require.

Malpractice Requirements

The Nurse Practice Act also enumerates malpractice requirements. Every NP should have coverage, which can come in three forms. The first is provided by the employer. Some consider this the best coverage because it precludes an NP being named independently in a suit, but this is not true. A lawsuit can name any and all parties as responsible for an injury. Having or not having independent coverage doesn't protect or expose the NP to liability. Many times, it has proved helpful for the NP to be represented by a private attorney, as the larger umbrella policy of the employer might have other parties to protect. If employer umbrella coverage is the option chosen, the NP needs to have written proof from Human Resources or the Medical Staff Director that the NP is named as an individual on the policy. A copy of the policy face sheet, with the NP's name printed on it, should be maintained with other important licenses and documents.

The second form of coverage is "Claims Made" coverage. This coverage is only in effect while the policy is in effect. Thus, if the policy ends because of change of practice or employment and a suit is filed three years later, the individual is no longer covered. If Claims Made coverage is ended, the NP should purchase "Tail Coverage" to ensure protection. The statute of limitations for filing a suit is seven years.

The third form is "Occurrence" coverage, which protects the NP for any occurrence of claim. Most consider Occurrence coverage as comprehensive individual coverage. The amounts and limits of coverage can be set as desired, available, or mandated by the Nurse Practice Act. These limits may be mandated in statute, so examine the statute closely.

Nurse practitioners need to be cognizant of potential malpractice complaints. After sacrificing and completing all the steps necessary to become an NP, the realization that a malpractice suit can quickly take it all away can be overwhelming, especially when first starting out in practice. Steps to protect one's practice require that the NP:

- Be familiar with the state's Scope of Practice and not exceed it.
- Be credentialed and licensed appropriately.
- Have clinical references handy to maintain Standards of Care.
- Maintain complete and thorough patient documentation easier said than done, but worth the effort).
- Know that malpractice claims need to show an NP's actions did not meet those of a reasonable NP and practice accordingly.

Malpractice complaints arise from any number of motivations. Remember that an NP is considered to have committed malpractice when a standard of care is not met and patient injury results (Buppert, 2008).

Prescriptive Privilege

The Nurse Practice Act of each state clearly delineates what documents and training are required to empower the NP to write prescriptions. The writing of prescriptions is inherent in the role of ANPs. An NP has many skills and embracing nonpharmacotherapeutic modalities in treatment plans is a strong talent. The nursing theory chosen as the foundation of practice can guide these modalities, including theories related to patient adaptation, self-care, autonomy, and caring. Handing out the prescription to eradicate invading biological offenders feels powerful, but increasing a patient's self-care efficacy through education, teaching environmental adaptation skills, and self-advocacy has a much longer impact than "twice a day for 10 days."

A small arena of controversy is worth mentioning. In most patient encounters, NPs educate and instruct. Sometimes, the instructions are specific and clear cut. They concern how and when to take a prescription medication, along with information about possible side effects, as in: "Doxycycline is a capsule in a 100 mg dose. Taking it twice a day for 10 days is recommended. It is best when taken with an equal time span between each dose to help keep a therapeutic level in the blood." The experienced NP also adds "this medication can make skin more susceptible to sunburn than usual so please avoid sun exposure while on it, or carefully apply sunscreen." These directions are easy to understand and packed with information. Not so much attention is given when encouraging use of over-the-counter (OTC) medications. The controversy is whether or not OTC medications are prescribed or "recommended." In either case, the *perception* of the patient may be that the OTC medication was "ordered" by the NP to help relieve the complaint. Access to OTC medications is not restricted to prescriptions, but that does not constrain the NP from discussing complete and thorough instructions in the plan of care. If advocating use of OTC medications, such as nonsteroidal anti-inflammatories for symptom relief, always add the phrase "according to package directions" and emphasize if it should be taken with food.

A mention of prescription pads is also prudent. Requirements specify what can and must be printed on them. These regulations are found in either the Nurse Practice Act or in a statute regarding state Drug Enforcement Agency (DEA) protocols. Pads are a necessary tool for practice, as much as stethoscopes and exam tables, but they are even more valuable on the black market. Take care not to leave them unattended in an examination room. DEA numbers should not be printed on the front for everyone to see, as those numbers are as sacred as a social security number. This problem may soon be a nonissue with the increase use of electronic prescription filing, but remember that even with electronic filing, all of the statute requirements must be met. Pearson (2009) reports a comprehensive overview of what an NP can prescribe and how much involvement by another healthcare provider is necessary. In states where a physician's cosignature is required on prescriptions, do not allow "presigning" to occur. For the convenience of all parties—patients, NPs and physicians alike— the act of presigning the physician name on the script has been known to happen. It is mostly a time constraint or physician availability issue, but it is unequivocally against the law. If physicians are not always available for supervision while the NP is practicing or if inconveniencing the patient is not a desired outcome, physicians and NPs can approach the legislature together and request a change in the prescriptive privilege law. Many configurations and levels of prescribing are available to choose from in other states; it need not be an all or nothing proposal. Great changes have happened in all states by taking small steps at a time.

Federal Drug Enforcement Agency License

The state Practice Act gives NPs the authority to write prescriptions for non-scheduled drugs, scheduled drugs, or both. Nonscheduled drugs include those not prone to addiction, such as antibiotics and hypertension therapies. If statute permits scheduled drugs to be prescribed, they are written under the authority of a state license. But, in addition to the state license, the prescriber must have a DEA license at the federal and state levels. In 1973, the federal government created the DEA to provide oversight of substances that have the potential for abuse. This oversight was designed to protect individuals from addiction to these substances and to prevent the mishandling or diversion of these drugs into illegal hands (www.usdoj.gov). The Web site www.usdoj/dea/index.gov has a plethora of information about applying for a license and on the drugs themselves.

Drugs with the potential for abuse and/or addiction were categorized into schedules according to that potential, along with a note of evidence of medical efficacy. With this information, the prescriber can determine much danger a medication may possess for a specific patient. A brief interpretation of each of the five schedules is presented in Table 3.3. A complete definition can be found on the United States Department of Justice Web site.

3.3 Schedules: Intravenous (IV) Drugs

Schedule I: Drugs with high abuse potential and little data to support medical use or safety.

Schedule II: Drugs with high abuse and dependence potential and only some data to support medicinal efficacy

Schedule III: Drugs with some abuse and dependence potential and data to support medicinal use and efficacy.

Schedule IV: Drugs with low abuse and limited dependence potential and data to support medicinal use and efficacy.

Schedule V: Drugs with low abuse potential and minimal dependence and data to support medicinal use and efficacy.

Adapted from the Code of Federal Regulations, Part 1308 of Title 21, U.S Drug Enforcement Agency, retrieved from www.usdoj.gov/dea

An application for DEA licensure can be completed on-line. Licensure is good for three years and currently costs $550. Writing a prescription for a legend or scheduled drug without a DEA license is illegal. A pharmacy cannot dispense a Schedule II or III medication without the original prescriptions; faxes are not acceptable.

All NPs should obtain a DEA license; the application process is outlined at the DEA Web site: http://www.deadiversion.usdoj.gov. Some NPs, who do not prescribe scheduled medications in the course of a normal clinical day, prefer not to spend money for such a license. But, the DEA license is one of the tools to full implementation of the clinical role and practice of the NP. With the license, NPs will receive national recognition of their role as a potential provider of service and be "counted" as a player in the healthcare arena. In addition, drugs are put on and off schedules by way of the DEA. Something currently prescribed may have its classification changed as a result of new information gleaned from additional research or practice use. For example, long-acting amphetamine salts may go off schedule or sleep aids now nonscheduled may be added as increased knowledge of potential side effects is gathered. The best strategy is to be prepared by obtaining DEA licensure.

The use of DEA license number when prescribing may soon be replaced with a National Provider Identifier (NPI) number. In an effort to streamline government, a single identifier number in can effectively track professionals who submit claims for reimbursement to Centers for Medicare and Medicaid Services (CMS) and who write prescriptions for scheduled medications.

State Drug Enforcement Agency License

The federal DEA license defers to states the authority to grant NPs the right to write pharmaceutical prescriptions. States have consumer protection laws and/or DEA departments that oversee the prescribing of healthcare professionals. It is one more licensure requirement needed to function fully in the NP role.

NPI Numbers

The Health Insurance Portability and Accountability Act of 1996 (HIPAA) mandated a numerical identifier for healthcare providers so that claims could be tracked across established insurance, provider, and hospital systems. Since implementation of the act, the National Provider Identifier (NPI) number has become known as the provider's identification number in many electronic transaction and payment systems. Because NPIs are unique to the provider or setting and are used for reimbursement in the Medicare system, their acceptance has been without contention. As a result, NPIs are now used in addition to and, may possibly replace, the DEA number as an authenticity identifier on prescriptions. Because of the widespread acceptance and utilization of the NPI, information on provider practices can be captured. In addition, provider databanks can address multiple subjects. This should yield useful information to promote ANP practice.

Another number, once known as the Medicare Identifier, is the UPIN. Many NPs did not obtain a UPIN because patients utilizing Medicare were not normally in the practice panels of NPs or reimbursement was sought under the name of the physician practicing with the NP.

Now, however, with an increased interest in data gathering and accountability for NP practice, each NP should apply for an NPI. The application is easy to complete, without cost, and available online at http://www.cms.hhs.gov/cmsforms/downloads/CMS10114.pdf

Physician Colleagues in the Nurse Practitioner Scope of Practice

Some physicians prefer physician colleagues to NP colleagues. Although this is neither universal nor endemic across the nation, it is a simple fact. Many physicians do not understand the role of the NP. As a result, their opinions are not based on accurate data. In some cases, the physicians are influenced by cues from national professional organizations or insurance and pharmaceutical businesses that may infer NPs are business competitors in health care and negatively affect a physician's financial potential. In any case, one theme should dominate: patients are plentiful, not well, and need access to care.

State statute will dictate the minimum level of physician involvement mandated in an NP practice. These levels range from no daily involvement, known as independent practice, to having physicians collaborate with the NP on care rendered, to strict on-site supervision of care. These levels are mandated, but nothing precludes additional arrangements with physician colleagues as agreed on by both parties. Note, however, that any addendums to the agreement may voluntarily limit the scope of practice granted by law.

Independent practice is an easily understood concept, but its implementation sometimes invokes concern. Independent practice actualizes into patient assessment, diagnosis, and treatment without oversight, but consultation and referral are and will always be an integral part of an ANP. Standards of Care dictate that management of care MUST include consultations with healthcare colleagues and referrals to specialists, both of whom are often physicians. Nurse Practitioners work in a connected healthcare system that includes all levels of providers, including physical therapists, pharmacists, physicians, and psychologists. Nurse practitioners cannot preclude physicians from care planning if goals remain patient focused. Neither can NPs "steal" business as providers. Idle physicians are just not a common entity; most are overbooked and working feverishly. Nurse practitioners have been shown to provide competent, quality-driven, patient-accepted health care within the approved scope of practice.

Strict supervision is also rather easily understood. In most cases, the physician must be on-site or immediately available to co-manage the care given by the NP. In these cases, the NP is an extender of the physician and has a very limited scope. In these situations, NPs must be careful not to do more than is allowed. The presigned prescription pad is an example. Arrangements skirting the statute requirements are done to provide leeway for implementation, but they are dangerous in terms of liability. Physicians can provide that leeway legally by assisting NPs in their fight to widen statutory scope by allowing greater auton-omy in providing standards of care with the skills and competencies acquired through education.

Collaboration is the "middle ground," as physicians and NPs alike question how to accurately implement the concept. The American College of Physicians (2009) offers a definition of collaboration that emphasizes communication based on interdisciplinary respect for complementary scopes of practice and skills among team members. This communication promotes quality and cost-effective care, which, in this definition, is led by the physician. According to the College, the rigors of medical education are so much higher than those of ANP educa-tion that the role of the ANP can be complementary but not collegial. Further, state variations in education and scopes of practice mean that NP care cannot be substituted for physician-rendered care.

Other regulatory agencies and legislative sources define collaboration as the act of working together for a common goal. Each state Nurse Practice Act em-phasizes the aspects of practice that need to be put in writing. The particulars must be agreed upon by all parties. Examples of points of emphasis per practice site are:

- What type of care can be provided.
- Demographic descriptors of the population of patients.
- When is consultation with the physician required.
- How the physician will evaluate the NP's care.
- What limits or access to pharmacotherapeutics exist.
- Who will cover the NP's patients when the NP is not available.
- How will patients be told the NP works with this physician.

Collaboration agreements must also include dates of effect and the written signatures of both parties (Buppert, 2008). This is a legal document that must be kept along with other licenses, certifications, and degrees.

Employee Credentialing/Hospital Privileges

Credentialing NPs for employment verification or for issuance of privileges has become increasingly commonplace. Employee credentialing is the process that verifies an NP's graduation from an accredited educational program, certifica-tion, licensure, and NPI number. Admitting privileges or hospital affiliations are traditionally for physicians only, and refer to admission, inpatient care, and dis-charging of patients. The move by hospitals to a "hospitalist" model of care means that the facility provides a care team for inpatient management and out-side providers are not required to be on the medical staff to have patients ac-cepted for admission. This helps NPs in primary care who do not have local hospital privileges.

The expansion of inpatient roles for NPs and interest in maximizing fund-ing and reimbursement have propelled the evolution of credentialing for NPs. Klein (2004, 2008) details the process and explains the increased need for un-derstanding NP credentialing. Unfortunately, the process is still quite confusing for a number of reasons. First, the process is relatively new for NPs; only with the passage of the federal Balanced Budget Act of 1997 were NPs allowed the possibility for direct reimbursement for care. Since then, administrations and billing specialists have creatively tried to mimic the physician credentialing process, but that is not easily done because of the lack of uniformity in NP practice. Employees of the hospital business office may not understand the role of the inpatient NP, so billing can be difficult and incomplete. These employees need accurate training on the role, scope, and legal practice of the NP as a new player in the field of hospital reimbursement. More importantly, NPs need a strong understanding of billing rules so they can advocate for accurate billing and easy-to-read financial reporting of profit attributed directly to NP care. Only with such reporting can the true fiscal evaluation of the inpatient NP role occur.

Outside of the hospital setting, financial conundrums abound. Private insurers generally follow Medicare rules (Buppert, 2008; Klein, 2008), which means they require an empanelling process that means the credentialing and acceptance of healthcare professionals before they can to be listed for patient access and for the reimbursement of patient services. Several multistate insurance companies have blocked the empanelling of NPs based on lack of hospital affiliation or lack of credential. For years, NPs in practice have argued against this unfair restriction to empanelling and are now making strides toward direct reimbursement. This will enable patients to access NP care. Still, the issue continues because insurance companies are hesitant to change the healthcare arena by directly reimbursing NPs as primary care providers. Healthcare colleagues who lack awareness and understanding of the NP scope and role need to be educated further. Misunderstanding occurs even with colleagues who support NP care. For example, one physician queried appropriate billing techniques when using the NP in his employment for new (in-home) house-call coverage. In response, Martin (2009) explained Medicare does not allow billing for NPs with new patients or existing patients with new problems for visits at home unless the physician is on-site too. Many colleagues erroneously use "incident to" billing rules from a lack of understanding. More and more colleagues want to expand the use of the NP role, but current reimbursement and practice act barriers prevent that from happening.

The Joint Commission issued a Comprehensive Accreditation Manual for Ambulatory Care (2009) that provides for NPs for be licensed independent providers "LIPs," so that they can bill for services and receive reimbursement. This allows a billing route based on the NPI, but it does not override individual state or BON licensure, scope, or practice limitations. This federal government could adopt this manual, thereby allowing independent NP billing and reimbursement, but NP reimbursement would still remains tied to Scope of Practice and Standards of Care at the state level.

The credentialing process begins with a signed release or "permission to contact" that grants employers the right to investigate an NP—an investigation that is NOT limited to the NP's professional life. The investigation includes:

- Completion of a demographic background check.
- Verification of all education and certifications listed on the curriculum vitae or résumé.
- Examination of any past licenses, including complaints against them.
- Examination of any malpractice claims, pending or resolved.

- Verification of any specialty education or training attested to.
- Completion of a criminal background check.
- Completion of a credit report check, and often.
- Investigation of any *Facebook* account and postings or other electronic social networking pages, driving records, or additional public records.

Credentialing is a thorough task and can take many weeks to complete.

Obtaining Licensure for a Practice

The components discussed so far relate to the licensure of an individual for practice. When starting a business or independent practice, these components apply to all employees and NP clinicians working for the practice. The business itself falls into a different set of regulations that provide for its legal functioning. Regulations in the form of Public Health Codes or Department of Health mandates dictate necessary actions for a practice to open and provide care to patients. The regulations are required and conferred based on the type and level of business opened. Private practices may not be subject to inspection or mandate unless they are considered a surgical center. In addition, if a business has less than 10 employees, it is exempted from the federal paperwork mandate, but it still must comply with federal standards. Those would include Occupational Safety and Health Administration (OSHA) regulations Standard 29 CFR 1910. A succinct overview of OSHA regulations can be found at www.ehso.com/oshareview.php.

If in-office laboratory testing is performed, such as urine dipsticks, rapid streptococcal throat cultures, and so on, regulations are set forth in the Clinical Laboratory Improvement Amendments (CLIA). Centers for Medicare and Medicaid oversee CLIA regulations. Similar to the two-tier DEA system, CLIA has federal and state level regulations. The level of CLIA licensure required is dictated the type of laboratory testing done on-site. These are discussed in detail in later chapters.

Conclusions

The advanced practice nurse faces a number of professional challenges and options. These require inordinate attention to detail, as no two states have the identical requirements, no two educational programs have identical curricula, no two certifications are identical, and few titles of licensure are identical. The process to become an ANP is both exciting and arduous, but the benefits are gratifying and overwhelming. Never has it been truer that "the sky is the limit." An ANP's potential is only limited by the individual's motivation and imagination. In the process of embracing that potential, requisite steps must be followed. For the sake of the evolving NP practice and the expansion of public acceptance of it, every NP must be a leader in advocacy, possess professional credentials, an expert in clinical acumen, and an overseer of the management of the role of the NP.

The components for advanced nursing practice have been highlighted. Clearly, it differs for each state. In addition, federal law sometimes defers to state law. With the variation in state law, confusion abounds about the role of the NP.

It is crucial for an NP to analyze, understand, and implement the laws and regulations that oversee practice. Regular review is also highly recommended to be sure of continued compliance.

Reflective Thinking Exercises

1. Formulate a debate concerning the expansion of the Scope of Practice in a given state to include completely unrestricted independent practice.
2. Prepare a list of points to support independent practice and reimbursement within a given state using the Nursing Practice Act from a state that currently allows independent practice.
3. Complete a legislative search within your state for both registered nurse licensure and advanced practice registered nurse licensure requirements.
4. Complete a legislative search for the Nurse Practice Act within your state. Find the requirements for licensure, requirements for practice, scope of practice parameters, prescribing parameters, and malpractice requirements.
5. Legislative Advocacy is crucial in the expansion of the Scope of Practice of NPs. Locate your local officials, state senators, and congresspeople. Email or call them to let them know you are a constituent and would be happy to share opinions for proposed healthcare legislation.

References

20th annual survey of state boards of nursing and selected national professional certifying boards/associations. (2009). *Journal of Continuing Education in Nursing,* Retrieved June 14, 2009, from CINAHL with Full text database.

Accreditation Association for Ambulatory Health Care. (2009). Retrieved June 6, 2009, from http://www.aaahc.org.

American Association of Colleges of Nursing. (1998). Certification and Regulation of Advanced Practice Nurse. from http://www.aacn.nche.edu/Publications/positions/cerreg.htm

Web site of the American Academy of Nurse Practitioners. Available at http://www.aanpweb.org. Accessed June 2009

Web site of the American College of Nurse Practitioners. Available at http://www.acnpweb.org. Accessed June 2009

American Nurses Association (ANA). (2009). What is Nursing? Abstract: definition of Nursing. Retrieved June 18, 2009, from http://www.nursingworld.org/search.aspx?SearchMode=1&SearchPhrase=definition+of+nursing&SearchWithin=2

American Nurses Association (ANA). (2004). *Nursing: scope and standards of practice.* Silver Spring, Maryland, Author.

American Nurse Credentialing Center (2009). American Nurses Association. Retrieved June 3, 2009, from http://www.nursecredentialing.org

Byrd, D. (2004, September). Recognition of advanced practice nurses. *ASMN Update,* 8(5), 16. Retrieved July 3, 2009, from CINAHL with Full text database.

Buppert, C. (2008). *Nurse Practitioner's Business Practice and Legal Guide, 3rd Ed.* Bethesda: Jones and Bartlett Publishers.

Centers for Medicare & Medicaid Services. Nurse Practitioner (NP) services and clinical nurse specialist services. Pub 100-02, transmittal 75. Available at: http://www.cms.hhs.gov/Transmittals/downloads/R75BP.pdf . Accessed June, 2009.

American College of Physicians. Nurse Practitioners in Primary Care Philadelphia: American College of Physicians; 2009: Policy Monograph. (available from American College of Physicians, 190 N. Independence Mall West, Philadelphia, PA 19106.)

GovTrack.us. H.R. 2015-105th Congress (1997): Balanced Budget Act of 1997 GovTrack.us (database of federal legislation). Available at: www.govtrack.us/congress/bill.xpd?tab=summary &bill=h105-2015. Accessed June 26, 2009.

Harbison, S. (2003, November). Legislation and health policy. APRNs and multi-state licensure compacts. *Journal of Pediatric Healthcare,* 17(6), 321–323. Retrieved June 14, 2009, from CINAHL with Full text database.

Hansen-Turton, T., Ritter, A. Rothman, N., Valdez, B. (2006). Insurer policies create barriers to health care access and consumer choice.*Nursing Economics, 24*(4), 204–11, 175. Retrieved June 12, 2009, from ABI/INFORM Trade & Industry database. (Document ID:1118040371).

Institute of Medicine (1999). *To Err is Human.* Washington, DC: National Academies of Science Press.

Joint Commission on Accreditation of Health Care Organizations. (2009). Retrieved June 6, 2009, from http://www.jointcommission.org.

The Joint Commission (2009). *A Comprehensive Accreditation Manual for Ambulatory Care.* Available at www.JCRinc.com.

Klein T. (2004). Scope of practice and the nurse practitioner: regulation, competency, expansion, and evolution. *Topics in Advanced Practice Nursing eJournal 4*(4), 1–11. Retrieved from MedScape June 28, 2009.

Klein T. (2008, October). Credentialing the nurse practitioner in your workplace: evaluating scope of safe practice. *Nursing Administration Quarterly, 32*(4), 273–278. Retrieved June 14, 2009, from CINAHL with Full Text database.

Landro, L. (2008, April 2) "The Informed Patient: Making Room for Dr. Nurse." *The Wall Street Journal,* New York, Eastern Edition: Wall Street Journal.

Martin, V. (2009, February). Billing for a nurse practitioner. *Medical Economics, 86*(4) 45.

National Council of State Boards of Nursing. Available at: www.ncsbn.org. Accessed June 12, 2009.

National Nursing Centers Consortium (NNCC). (2005). Nurse-managed health centers from http://www.nncc.us/about/nmhc.html

NPFreebies.com. (n.d.). Retrieved June 22, 2009, from NPFreebies.com: http://www.npfreebies .com/Nurse_Practitioner_Download_Forms_and_Resources.htm

Pearson, L. J. (2009). THE PEARSON REPORT, A National Overview of Nurse Practitioner Legislation and Health Care Issues. *The American Journal for Nursing Practitioners,* 8–82.

Philipsen, Nayna, and Haynes, Dorothy (2007). The Multi-State Nursing Licensure Compact: Making Nurses Mobile. *Journal for Nurse Practitioners, 3(1):36–40.* Retrieved June 28, 2009 from Medscape.com.

Requirements for Accrediting Agencies and the Criteria for Certification Programs.pdf retrieved 6/18/09 from https://www.ncsbn.org.

Smolenski, M. (2008, June). *Playing the Credentials Game.* www.nursecredentialing.org.

Website of the United States Department of Health and Human Services. Available at http:// www.hhs.gov/ocr/privacy/index.html HIPAA. Accessed June 10, 2009.

Web site of the CT Nurse Practice Act. Available at http://www.acnpweb.org. Accessed June 12, 2009

Web site of the NM Nurse Practice Act. Available at http://www.acnpweb.org. Accessed June 12, 2009

Website of National Association of Pediatric Nurse Practitioners. Available at http://www .napnap.org/aboutUs/ourPerspective/ScopeAndStandards.aspx. Accessed June, 28 2009.

Website of the United States Department of Justice. Available at http://www.usdoj.gov, accessed June 23, 2009.

BLOG: http://npbusiness.org/nurse-practitioner-sites/

Essentials of Developing and Managing the Nurse Practitioner Practice

Development of a Nurse Practitioner Run Clinic: Variables Affecting a Nurse Practitioner's Business

4

Learning Objectives

1. Differentiate among protocols, standards of care, practice, and disease-focused guidelines.

2. Identify a mechanism for evaluating competency of practicing nurse practitioners (NPs).

3. Develop a professional résumé.

4. Describe the process by which quality of care is monitored in NP practices.

5. Describe the three major components of an individual malpractice policy.

6. Identify ways to augment one's salary and gain experience performing the leader, manager, and professional functions of the NP.

7. Describe the process of grant writing.

8. Develop a letter of intent/interest for applying for start-up funding or expansion of existing healthcare care programs for a private foundation/organization.

Key Words: quality improvement, patient safety, evidence-based practice, individual malpractice, grant writing, peer review, provider competency, standards of care, practice protocols, practice guidelines, résumé

Providing a safe and high-quality, evidence-based practice is essential for NPs. Understanding the various methods for managing appropriate use of practice guidelines and protocols is also important. Thus, this chapter describes how to follow protocols, standards of care, practice, and disease-focused guidelines. As all providers are evaluated by some audit and/or peer review process to determine competency, quality improvement mechanisms are illustrated for evaluating practice and maximizing patient safety. Ideas for partnering with other agencies to maximize resources, increase quality, and reduce costs are also presented. Salaries are identified for NPs in various parts of the country and in different practice settings. Ideas for using the leadership, management, clinical, and professional functions of the NP role are discussed. The difference between a curriculum vitae, résumé, and biosketch are presented, along with an examples of a résumé and biosketch.

Types of funding and ideas for grant writing are described, as are strategies for obtaining funding. This includes advice on how an NP might obtain seed money for a project or even larger funding for further expansion of an initiative. Examples of a letter of interest for applying for start-up funding or expansion of new healthcare programs for private foundations are offered.

Use of Practice Protocols, Standards of Care, Practice, and Disease-Focused Guidelines

Nurse practitioners and physicians must follow a *protocol* step by step. For example, NPs follow specific steps when evaluating a patients' pacemaker, determining a patient's Coumadin level, or perhaps visiting a postoperative patient who has had a hip replacement. Practice *guidelines* tend to be developed by NP experts and have support from NP professional organizations. They offer a framework for patient care, describing recommended interventions based on a diagnosis. Nurse practitioners practice autonomously and provide patient-focused care, using *guidelines* to meet the needs of each patient. Guidelines give more flexibility than rigid protocols. Several published clinical guideline texts are available for purchase in each specialty area and can be used as resources in practice. These texts are a good foundation for clinical care management and can provide consistency among providers. Even if alone in practice, it behooves one to have a clinical guideline named in a Policy and Procedure Manual as the clinic's accepted *Standard of Care*. An example is Uphold and Graham's *Clinical Guidelines in Family Practice* (2003). Online sources and free texts also explain clinical guidelines and sometimes provide additional content concerning the level of research or evidence upon which the guideline is based. These are the foundations of the "Evidenced-Based Practice Model," toward which health care is moving. In addition, specialty organizations have accumulated care-based evidence for more than a single intervention, as well as for the management of an entire disease process. These disease management guidelines are available through the Web sites of the specialty organizations that did the research.

- *Nursing Care and Management of the Second Stage of Labor: Evidence-based Clinical Practice Guidelines* published by the Association of Women's Health, Obstetric and Neonatal Nurses and accessible at www.awhonn.org/store.
- Diabetes Type 2 Update Treatment Recommendations from the American Diabetes Association and the European Association for the Study of Dia-

betes. This is accessible at http://www.diabetes.org/for-media/pr-ada-easd-publish-consensus-algorithm-for-type-2-diabetes-treatment.jsp.

These specific guidelines are not to be confused with the *Standards of Practice for Nurse Practitioners,* such as the set published by the American Academy of Nurse Practitioners and revised frequently to support the NP scope of practice (2007). These standards list:

- Qualifications
- Process of care
- Care priorities
- Interdisciplinary/collaborative responsibilities
- Accurate documentation of patient status and care
- Responsibility as patient advocate
- Quality assurance
- Continued competency
- Roles of NPs
- Research in practice

Best practices are similar to evidence-based guidelines in that research and experience are used to indicate proven ways to do things most effectively. Two agencies house the largest collections of evidence-based guidelines. The Cochrane Collaborating Center, which assesses the literature and makes recommendations for practice (www.cochrane.org/index0.htm), and the Agency for Healthcare Research and Quality (www.ahrq.gov/clinic/epcix.htm).

Do NPs practice only with evidence-based guidelines and protocols or do they use some type of reasoning to frame decisions concerning patient care? How does the culture of the individual being treated or the patient's socioeconomic status impact the NP's plan? Do all factors influence how NPs practice? Is there only one way of practicing? Do NPs practice medicine or should NPs follow the Medical Model? Most NPs fall back on the Nursing Models learned in their baccalaureate program and/or used in their RN practice. Nurses use models such as Orem's Self-Care Theory (1980) or Roy's Adaptation Model (1984) to make decisions about care for each patient, albeit sometimes not consciously. Some NPs use one model exclusively, while others use combinations of models by which they frame their patients' situations and determine the best ways to manage their care.

Others, such as Bourbonniere and Evans (2002), developed their own model of care. These authors conducted a literature review focusing on the functions and skills of advanced practice nurses (APNs) regarding the care of frail older adults. They found the APNs had expertise in managing groups of patients and determined that patient care outcomes evaluating care management were positive. The evaluation of care management occurred along with the evaluation of the entire interprofessional team's care. It centered on cost effectiveness, patient and family satisfaction with services, and the clinician's use of consultants. Patient health included input from the APN, physician, and social worker and consistently assessed the care as very positive. But even if one uses a specific model of care, NPs still need to follow the established protocols, guidelines, and evidence-based practice results regarding the management of each patient and must remain in the NP scope of practice.

Maintaining Competency of Providers

Peer review of one's work as an APN is nothing new. In fact, defining competency has long been a challenging experience for all healthcare workers. Few tools measure NP competence. Gardner, Hase, Gardner, Dunn, and Carryer (2007) feel NPs competency standards must be met and that peer review should focus on capability, which is the ability to deal effectively with a situation as it arises.

Peer review of NPs can be conducted in several ways. Generally, the NP manager develops an annual schedule with *Review Dates, NP to Be Reviewed,* and *NP Reviewers.* The manager carefully rotates the NP Reviewers so each NP is reviewed by different members of the NP staff and not the same two NPs. Often, a random day is chosen quarterly and a random visit number is selected to identify three or four charts for the two peers to evaluate. For example, during the months of April, August, and December a random date of the 12th is chosen. Then, the chart of every fourth patient seen on April 12 of each provider under review is collected and audited. A legend checklist with specific criteria is developed by NP staff to use as a universal measure in assessing each other's charts. A template of a Peer Performance review form can be found in Section III. Reviewers assume the charts reflect care rendered and include plans for future care, management, and follow up. Table 4.1 lists seven criteria by which peers can evaluate each other.

The responses are shared among the two NPs who completed the review, and the findings (as long as the two NP peer reviewers agreed on the assessment) are written and shared with the reviewed NP. A copy of the peer review is placed in the NP's personnel file by the manager after review. Some agencies do peer review less frequently than others; quarterly is a suggestion. Others assess NP competency by having the physician collaborator follow a similar process as described. In other agencies, the manager may prepare the NP review.

The process of hospital credentialing acts as a means of peer review, since the application is extensive and includes review of competency. To obtain credentialing for hospital privileges, an NP has to apply in a way similar to a physician.

To be recertified as an APN, each NP must complete a certain number of continuing education hours; a specified number of hours must be related to pharmacology. NPs are responsible for providing employers with certificates of completed continuing education. These certificates are another way of documenting competency and are essential as evidence of competency if questions arise.

Another process related to peer evaluation of NPs is implementing a career ladder of promotion. Most institutions do not have a system that places NPs into levels, as exists with Registered Nurses (RN). Rowell, Forsythe, Avallone, and Kloos (2008) suggest a promotional ladder for NPs would be an effective model, and they provide an example of their *Professional Profile Data/Clinical Ladder Advancement Criteria/ Competencies Checklist.* This process would generate higher patient care outcomes and increased NP satisfaction.

Self-reflection is another method for evaluating competency. NPs need to look deeper and reflect on all advanced practice functions, such as leadership

4.1 Criteria for Assessment of NP Competency

- Completeness of documentation.
- Review of systems (ROS) data: This is equivalent to universal care for a specific chief complaint or follows a checklist of data identified by staff.
- A differential diagnosis is identified for each chief complaint.
- Diagnostics are appropriate and cost effective for diagnoses identified.
- Plan is appropriate for diagnoses identified.
- Health teaching is clearly documented.
- Follow-up of plan of care is documented and identified as shared with patient.

skills, management ability, and professional work. It is easy to get caught up in focusing on clinical skills and always being too busy to attend a meeting, conference, or professional event. The longer NPs go without publishing, presenting, and becoming active in professional organizations, the more difficult it becomes to reverse this process. It is similar to when one is in school; it is best to jump right into the discussion, ask questions, and not be deterred by what other people think. It is time to:

- Take a look at daily clinical practice,
- Assess strengths and weaknesses, and
- Come up with goals to work toward over the next few months.

One can use a self-portfolio program to develop a résumé or curriculum vitae. McMullan, Endacott, Gray et al. (2003) share ideas on what to include in a portfolio and how best to market oneself.

Development of a Professional Résumé and Biosketch

A curriculum vitae (CV) is a listing of one's accomplishments that is generally used when one has multiple professional and educational experiences, service presentations, consultations, projects, publications, grants, teaching, and other professional credentials. Because the customary assessment of an academician's work involves scholarly research, teaching, service (university, school, professional, and community) and sometimes, clinical work, the CV format is used. A résumé (see Figure 4.1) is a more succinct listing of employment, professional experience, education, service, and awards received. When looking for the first NP position after graduation, it is wise to list the student practica. However, once experience as an NP has been acquired, delete the practicum sites, unless you are applying for a position that requires experience in a specific clinical area related to a practica site not otherwise accrued.

A request to submit a biosketch may be made by newspapers, magazines, or community bulletins if they are writing a story about the practice or about NPs.

4.1

Example of Resume

Olivia Rusk, MSN, APRN-BC
5 Rye Road
Toret, AZ 84534
1-116-456-2343
Oliviaru@aol.com

Education

Sept., 2008	Arizona University, Graff, AZ	DNP Program
Sept., 2002	State University, Tempe, AZ	Master of Science in Nursing
May, 2005		Family Nurse Practitioner
Sept., 1980	Arizona University, Graff, AZ	Bachelor of Science in Nursing
May, 1985		Registered Nurse

Family Nurse Practitioner Experience

June, 2007   Center for Advanced Pediatrics, Newton, AZ
Current   Family Nurse Practitioner-Asthma/Allergy Specialist
Manage the care for patients in a busy pediatric office.

July, 2004   Human Service Council
June, 2007   Horace Net School Based Health Center, Newton, AZ
Family Nurse Practitioner
Serve the adolescent population rotating through the three high schools in Norwalk. Perform physical and gynecological exams; diagnose and treat common adolescent illnesses. Provide health education both individually and in group settings.

Nov., 2005   Americares Clinic, Newton, AZ
Current   Family Nurse Practitioner
Volunteer services quarterly in the women's clinic providing annual exams, reproductive health education, STI screening and treatment, family planning education, and medication.

Nov., 2002   Southeast Community Health Center, Martin, AZ
June, 2004   Homeless Department
Family Nurse Practitioner
Provided primary care to the homeless population in outreach settings, such as shelters, rescue missions, and clinics.

Teaching Experience

Jan., 2006   The Arizona University, Newton, AZ
Current   <u>Courtesy Adjunct Faculty, School of Nursing</u>
                Precept family nurse practitioner students at the school-based health centers to
                provide pediatric clinical experience for students working toward their master's
                degree in nursing.

2005–2008   Airway University Fayfir, AZ
                <u>Adjunct Professor, School of Nursing</u>
                Clinical instructor at Summit Hospital working with 4th year nursing students.
                Supervised patient care. Performed pre- and postclinical conferences; reviewed
                and corrected care plans.

Publications

Rusk, O. (in press, 2010). Celiac disease—a great masquerader: Guidelines for increasing
accurate diagnosing management *ADVANCE for Nurse Practitioner.*

Rusk, O. (2009). Management of c.difficile: Implications for nursing. *MEDSURG Nursing: the
Journal of Adult Health, 10*(9), 12–19.

Rusk, O. (2008). Peering: The Essence of Collaborative Mentoring, *Journal of Nurse Practitioner,
3*(9), 33–40.

Rusk, O. (2007). Monitoring prescription practice and microorganism resistance with patients
experiencing symptoms of urinary tract infections. *The International Journal of NPACE, 8,* 86–91.

Rusk, O. (2006). Providing self-care models for well adults can increase cost-effectiveness.
The International Journal of NPACE, 6, 2, 1–6.

Presentations

Use of Smoking Cessation Programs with Adolescents,
7/09: American College of Nurse Practitioners, Memphis, TN

Management of Celiac Disease in Young Adults,
11/08: NPACE Conference, Boston, MA

Memberships

Arizona State Nurses Association
American College of Nurse Practitioners
Sigma Theta Tau International, Mu Delta

Licenses

Advanced Practice Registered Nurse, State of Arizona
Registered Nurse, State of Arizona and New York State

A biosketch is a succinct, two-paragraph (approximately 60-word) document listing an individual's most relevant and current accomplishments. Grant Directors often request a biosketch of the writer (see Figure 4.2).

4.2

Example of a
Biosketch

Martha Burke O'Brien, MS, ANP-BC, APRN, has been the Director of the Trinity College Health Center (TCHC) at Trinity College in Hartford for 11 years. Early in her tenure, she received a commendation from the American College Health Association for her creative practice model of an all Advanced Practice Nurse staff, using physician collaboration in the "true" sense of collaboration. She received her BSN from Northeastern University and worked at the John Dempsey Hospital of the University of Connecticut Health Center after graduation. She received her MS from Boston College in Adult Primary Care. Before becoming the Director of the TCHC, she worked as a Primary Care Nurse Practitioner in the Adolescent Clinic at St. Francis Hospital and Medical Center for several years. She was involved in the Connecticut Nurse Practitioner Group, Inc., now known as Advanced Practice Registered Nurse Society, serving as President and Membership Chairperson for years. In addition, she has received multiple awards, including The Nurse Practitioner of the Year Award in 2001. As a member of the American College Health Associations' Consulting Services Program Advisory, she has also consulted with several college health clinics throughout the northeast about setting up nurse practitioner run clinics. She has done several presentations on Adolescent Health, Sexually Transmitted Diseases, and Reproductive Health, and has published in Nurse Practitioner journals.

Monitoring for Quality Improvement

The American College of Medical Quality developed *Medical Quality Management: Theory and Practice,* edited by Varkey (2009), which is a compilation of knowledge to help implement a comprehensive Quality Improvement Program. Examples of structural, process, and outcome measures, benchmarking, trends, and baseline measurements, use of fishbones (cause-and-effect diagrams), flow charts, process mapping, histograms, bar charts, and scattergrams are used to display data. They are all ways of displaying an agency's quality. Nurse practitioners also monitor quality using the Plan, Do, Study, and Act (PDSA) methodology, particularly when testing a change on a small scale and explaining how the Six Sigma philosophy generates positive outcomes. (Six Sigma is Motorola's management philosophy that high-level objectives reduce defects in products and services.) Other excellent resources to use when assessing and/or developing one's quality improvement system are *Quality by Design: A Clinical Microsystems Approach* (Nelson, Batalden, & Godfrey, 2007) and *The Healthcare Quality Book: Vision, Strategy, and Tools* (Ranson, Joshi, Nash, & Ranson, 2008).

Every agency must have methods to monitor safety and recommend higher quality outcomes of health care. The Agency for Healthcare Research and Quality (AHRQ) summarizes this focus as providing the right type of care in a timely fashion for the patient needing the care in order to maximize individual health outcomes. Taking the recommendations from two of the safety reports of the Institute of Medicine (IOM), *To Err Is Human: Building a Safer Health System* (1999) and *Crossing the Quality Chasm: A New Health System for the 21st Century* (2000), NPs must address issues that impact the quality of health care throughout the country. The following recommendations from the Institute of Medicine can be used when developing and managing quality improvement methods. *Crossing the quality chasm: A new health system for the 21st Century* (2000) recommends every healthcare agency be designed to provide care proven to be:

- Safe
- Effective
- Patient centered
- Timely
- Equitable

To Err Is Human: Building a Safer Health System (1999) makes the following suggestions for healthcare agencies:

- Develop a focus on measuring leadership, research, and outcome tools/ protocols to improve knowledge about safety,
- Evaluate experience and learn from errors using immediate and mandatory enforcements of change, and
- Develop new safety practices at the delivery level so an entire safety system is implemented throughout the organization.

The Institute for Healthcare Improvement (IHI), which also focuses on patient safety and quality, has identified *patient flow and customer service* as the two most significant parameters to track during a patient's journey through the healthcare system. IHI recommends the following qualities be attained in order to be successful:

- Efficiency, effectiveness, and good turnaround time,
- Predictability, decreased variation, and improved forecasting,
- Systems thinking, whereby people think in a less linear and more multidimensional way, as there are many interconnecting relationships and a constant sense of change (a dynamic flow exists in healthcare agencies when growth and innovation occur) (Wheatley, 2006, Peters, 2003, Senge, 2006),
- Employees demonstrating caring and individualizing care to each patient (healthcare is not just a service business—it is a personal service) (Studer, 2004). This requires creative thinking and spontaneous employee extension to our consumers (Csikszentmihalyi, 1990), and
- Innovative matching of supply with demand from consumer.

The IHI strongly supports improving patient safety through the abovementioned flow process and states that increased flow will produce higher quality care and fewer medical errors. The Joint Commission echoes this thought by requiring healthcare agencies to demonstrate they are developing ways to increase the patient flow. An example of increasing flow is (1) being able to get laboratory results back to providers and patients quickly or (2) keeping all healthcare professionals involved in and aware of the significance of improving flow and consumer satisfaction demands (Jenson, Mayer, Welch, & Haraden, 2007). The NP can function as both a leader (working with the consumer and advancing the organization's culture of being consumer friendly and receptive to change) and manager (connecting with the hierarchy and the members of the systems to maintain system functioning) in quality improvement issues (Kotter, 2002; Kenney, 2008). It certainly makes sense to follow guidelines based on methods that have been proven to improve patient outcomes. As an example of how to obtain this evidence, go to the Food and Drug Administration (FDA) Web site, which was created so that professionals and consumers could access information and evidence about how various medications have been used and how best to use them now. Professional organizations also provide resources on available evidence for assisting with patient problems. An example is the News Section of *The Journal for Nurse Practitioners,* which in February 2009 (p. 83) described several of these resources. Reycroft-Malone, Seers, Titchen, Harvey, Kitson, and McCormack (2004) offer suggestions as to what research, clinical experience, and patient experience can benefit patient outcomes.

Patient Safety and Quality: An Evidence-Based Handbook for Nurses, edited by Rhonda Hughes, PhD, MHS, RN, and published by the Agency for Healthcare Research and Quality, can be obtained at no cost in print or on CD by calling 1-800-358-9295 or downloading from www.ahrq.gov. This publication mentions specific patient safety and quality improvement issues for NPs, such as:

- Evidence-based practice and health services research
- Patient-centered care
- Family care giving and disease prevention
- Safe management of medication
- Personal safety for nurses
- Quality improvement
- Outcome management
- Prevention of hospital-acquired infections
- Computerized patient order entry
- Technology to support nurse documentation

Few reliable tools are available to measure patient satisfaction with NP care, but Bear and Bowers (1998) reported positive outcomes using the Client Satisfaction Tool, which has a reliability of 0.95. The study could be replicated in any NP setting. Safety and outcomes can be improved by developing a checklist of necessary actions for a specific patient prior to a procedure or test. Pronovost, Needham, Berenholtz, et al (2006) developed a step-by-step guide for physicians to follow in caring for specific types of patients in an ICU. This checklist was effective in Pronovost's setting where it decreased hospital-acquired infections to zero. Instituting checklists with step-by-step guidelines can be easily implemented in any healthcare setting. Table 4.2 shows checklists that save time, as well as assist in obtaining comprehensive information that otherwise might be forgotten in collecting a health history for common complaints seen in primary care. In addition, adapting the standard hard copy checklists into electronic documentation may decrease the amount of narrative needed. These forms assist

4.2 Examples of Checklists for Obtaining Health Histories

Checklist for Obtaining Health History for Abdominal Pain

☐ Yes	☐ No	1. Onset gradual/ sudden
☐ Yes	☐ No	2. Nausea/ vomiting
☐ Yes	☐ No	3. Constipation/ diarrhea/ blood in stool
☐ Yes	☐ No	4. Δ in appetite/ food intolerance
☐ Yes	☐ No	5. Recent travel
☐ Yes	☐ No	6. H/o STI/ new sexual partner
☐ Yes	☐ No	7. Vaginal odor/ itch/ discharge/ bleeding/ Δ in menses
☐ Yes	☐ No	8. Testicular pain
☐ Yes	☐ No	9. Fever/ chills
☐ Yes	☐ No	10. Urinary pain/ urgency/ frequency
☐ Yes	☐ No	11. Back/ flank pain
☐ Yes	☐ No	12. H/o injury
		13. Rate pain 1–10 _____

Checklist for Obtaining Health History for Fatigue

☐ Yes	☐ No	1. Δ in sleeping
☐ Yes	☐ No	2. Δ in appetite
☐ Yes	☐ No	3. Fever/ chills
☐ Yes	☐ No	4. Headache
☐ Yes	☐ No	5. Nausea/ vomiting
☐ Yes	☐ No	6. Constipation/ diarrhea
☐ Yes	☐ No	7. Temperature intolerance
☐ Yes	☐ No	8. Shortness of breath
☐ Yes	☐ No	9. ↑Stress/ significant losses/ crying spells
☐ Yes	☐ No	10. Sore muscles/ joints
☐ Yes	☐ No	11. Skin rash or Δ/ easy bruising
☐ Yes	☐ No	12. Recent travel
☐ Yes	☐ No	13. Δ in menses

Checklist for Obtaining Health History for Headache

(Circle)		1. Onset: gradual or sudden
(Circle)		2. Pain sharp or dull or stabbing
		3. Rate pain 1–10 scale ____
☐ Yes	☐ No	4. Precipitating factors
☐ Yes	☐ No	5. First or worst headache
☐ Yes	☐ No	6. H/O headaches/ migraines
☐ Yes	☐ No	7. S/S similar to past headaches
☐ Yes	☐ No	8. Fever/ chills
☐ Yes	☐ No	9. Visual changes
☐ Yes	☐ No	10. Sensitive to noise/ light

(continued)

☐ Yes	☐ No	11. Nausea/vomiting
☐ Yes	☐ No	12. Precipitating factors
☐ Yes	☐ No	13. Nasal cong./ cold symptoms

Checklist for Obtaining Health History for URI

☐ Yes	☐ No	1. Fever/ chills
☐ Yes	☐ No	2. Nasal congestion/ post nasal drip
☐ Yes	☐ No	3. Facial pain/ pressure
☐ Yes	☐ No	4. Ear pain
☐ Yes	☐ No	5. Sore throat/ trouble swallowing
☐ Yes	☐ No	6. Trouble breathing
☐ Yes	☐ No	7. Δ in appetite
☐ Yes	☐ No	8. Nausea/ vomiting
☐ Yes	☐ No	9. Chest/ back/ abdominal pain
☐ Yes	☐ No	10. Sore muscles or joints
☐ Yes	☐ No	11. Exposure to others with URI S/S
☐ Yes	☐ No	12. Skin rash or Δ
☐ Yes	☐ No	13. Neck pain/ trouble moving head

Checklist for Obtaining Health History for Urinary Symptoms

☐ Yes	☐ No	1. Painful urination
☐ Yes	☐ No	2. Urinary frequency
☐ Yes	☐ No	3. Urinary urgency/ hesitancy
☐ Yes	☐ No	4. Blood in urine
☐ Yes	☐ No	5. Abdominal/ back pain
☐ Yes	☐ No	6. Fever
☐ Yes	☐ No	7. Chills
☐ Yes	☐ No	8. Fatigue
☐ Yes	☐ No	9. Nausea/ vomiting
☐ Yes	☐ No	10. H/o prior Urinary Tract Infections
☐ Yes	☐ No	11. Strong urine odor
☐ Yes	☐ No	12. Vaginal odor/ itch/ dish

NPs to anticipate specific problems with certain complaints and leave space for additional documentation.

The findings of Walsgrove and Fulbrook (2005) regarding the development of NP positions in the acute care setting showed a positive correlation between having an NP and generating high-quality patient outcomes. This study can serve as a model for other practice settings. More and more NP-run practices are meeting benchmarks and receiving high-satisfaction reviews from patients. The following are examples of successful NP-started businesses:

▨ Health and Continence Institute of New England, developed by H. Carcio (2008), received start-up funding from two grants and used approximately $10,000 of her own money.

- Advanced Clinical Consultant started with $20,000 from S. Lawson-Baker, the owner. In 2008, Lawson-Baker received the NP entrepreneur of the Year award sponsored by *ADVANCE for Nurse Practitioners*.
- Angels on Call, Home Remedy, and Housecalls are businesses started by M. Lawlor (2008), with $45,000 of his own money. The business paid him back and now runs totally debt free with much success.
- The JAY Clinic, Rochester, MN, started by Jay Fotland (2009), uses a fee-for-service model and an annual membership fee for services.
- Eagan Child and Family Care, started by Gretchen Moen (2009), emphasizes care for Somali and Latin American children and families.
- Diabetes Care Management, a Telehealth technology and telephone communication service used by NPs with diabetic patients. It helps patients balance glycemic control at home (Chang, Davis, Birt, Castelluccio, Woodbridge, & Marrero, 2007).

For further information on NP-owned businesses and practices, access the NP Business Organization Web site at http://npbusiness.org/nurse-practitioner-sites, participate in NP blogs, and consult other Web sites regarding developing a NP business.

Individual Nurse Practitioner Malpractice Insurance

An increasing number of nurse practitioners are becoming involved in liability issues, sometimes even without direct involvement in the care in question. The American Association of Nurse Attorneys (2005) recommends that NPs have individual professional malpractice insurance, preferably with a carrier that has an A or excellent rating. This rating indicates financial stability. The NP with professional liability needs to be covered until the statute of limitations on a particular care episode runs out. In addition, it sometimes takes 7 to 10 years for a claim to be resolved. Therefore, it is imperative that the insurance company be capable of sustaining its business for many years. Three parts of the policy should be checked carefully:

- How much the carrier will pay regarding legal expenses even if only a settlement is needed,
- Conditions of the contract explaining the rights of the insured and the carrier, and
- Exclusionary clauses listing items not covered by the policy.

If an NP is listed in a malpractice lawsuit or if a complaint is made to the Nursing Licensing Board, the NP needs to know if the insurance carrier covers both malpractice and disciplinary issues. The average NP needs to have $1,000,000 per claim/$6,000,000 in the aggregate amount of coverage. (This amount varies by state and is delineated in the state practice act.) This means that for each incident, one million dollars would be paid, and the maximum amount covered would be six million dollars. The NP also should know to what timeframe the coverage applies. It is also prudent to determine if the insurance covers legal representation if the NP is called for a deposition and if the defendant's expenses are also covered. An NP should have a policy for malpractice, disciplinary, deposition, and defendant expense coverage (American Association of Nurse Attorneys, 2005).

In addition, an NP should know if the policy is a Claims-Made (any incident is covered as long as the policy is active) or an Occurrence (covers all claims during the period the NP was insured) policy. Because some claims require several years to resolve, an Occurrence policy seems more effective (Buppert, 2008). Some NPs, such as Family Nurse Practitioners, might need a higher amount of coverage/incident and aggregate insurance because they work with a wider population lifespan and have higher liability. All NPs may want to look into umbrella coverage, which is an add-on that increases coverage and is generally less expensive than a policy with higher coverage.

Some NPs may also choose to purchase general liability coverage, which includes compensation for medical expenses, wages lost, and general damage, such as emotional upset secondary to injury or property damage. For further questions regarding malpractice issues go to The Law Office of Carolyn Buppert, P.C. Web site at www.buppert.com.

Burroughs, Dmytrow, and Lewis (2007) describe the frequency and severity of NP professional liability claims and recommend many risk management strategies to decrease liability. They explain the NP's scope of practice is "critical with respect to any theory of liability or potential allegations that may be asserted in malpractice litigation" (p. 54). Judgments regarding negligent conduct will be based on whether the NP was working within the scope of practice.

Performing the Professional, Leader, Clinician, and Manager Roles as a Nurse Practitioner: Implications for Increasing Salary

The Bureau of Labor Statistics (BLS) predicts advanced practice nurses will be in high demand, especially in rural and underserved areas of the country (2005). One reason for this high demand is their lower cost when compared to physicians (Buerhaus, Staiger, & Auerbach, 2009). Nurse practitioner salaries differ with geographic area, gender, years of NP experience, type of education and continuing education, and the practice setting (primary or specialty care). Nurse practitioners must realize that salaries will vary across the country based on cost of living, cost of practice, local economy, and NP workforce demand and supply. The American Academy of Nurse Practitioners conducted a national survey of salaries in 2007 using a randomized sample of 7,832 responding NPs. The average salary was $81,486 for full-time NPs averaging 37 hours a week. A copy of the report is accessible to members of the AANP at http://www.aanp.org/NR/rdonlyres/AD41DD8D-FD16-4F84-968C-F7192A0E79D6/0/NPCompensation2007.pdf. Many NPs receive more compensation than just this average salary as a result of their bonuses and ownership of a share of the practice.

Knowledge of other NP salaries in the region is helpful in negotiating a beginning salary or an increase (Pulcini, Vampola, & Levine, 2005). Information from a national salary survey, such as that distributed by The American Academy of Nurse Practitioners, helps negotiate a salary that reflects an NP's responsibilities.

Multiple ways are available to augment one's salary and gain experience performing the leader, manager, and professional functions of the NP. They include the following.

Leader—Successfully applying for the senior or supervising position at a practice setting will result in a salary increase, as well as other benefits. Volunteering for projects, working with a community agency, setting up a Health Fair, developing health promotion pamphlets, working as an adjunct for a School of Nursing, or returning to school for more specialized skills or a DNP could prove financially rewarding in the future. Tutoring, developing NP Continuing Education programs, and NP certification test preparation could be lucrative, as might consulting and leading other healthcare professionals in health policy changes. An NP could run for political positions or network for an appointment, such as an NP on the State Nursing Board. An NP could also apply to be a site visitor for the Commission on Collegiate Nursing Education (CCNE). The AACN Web site provides the information to assist one in preparing this application. Although some of these leadership positions may not pay, they will serve the NP well in making connections and becoming a part of a network that may increase opportunities for paid consultant work. One could also be an Expert Witness for lawyers looking for content experts in nursing.

Manager—NPs who enjoy the managerial aspect of their work may want to explore owning a business or going into a partnership with other NPs and/or physicians. One could return to school for an MBA or, preferably, a DNP to obtain the skills and content needed to manage a business. This book is intended to help equip the NP to take advantage of the many managerial opportunities.

Professional—As an officer of a professional organization one would have good contacts with other healthcare professionals and may be asked to participate in panel discussions or other presentations, write book chapters, and participate in interdisciplinary projects. These experiences may lead to other initiatives, such as grant writing, sharing resources, consultancies, or even patient referrals. Generally, any collaboration with another agency or partner reduces expenses and possibly even generates future revenue. One could receive honorariums, consulting fees, reduced professional organization dues and conference registration fees, or author royalties. Doing volunteer or pro bono work at a clinic or School of Nursing could lead to future financial or professional rewards.

Clinical—One could also maximize a salary by doing per diem NP clinical work in an off-hours clinic or on weekends or by giving clinical instruction to NP students. Linking up with the School of Nursing could provide connections for future paid teaching as an adjunct assignment. In addition, NPs can start niche businesses, such as sports and fitness, spas, and holistic care clinics. NPs can write journal articles, chapters, and books, and then present their findings at professional organization conferences. An example of a specialized book that will assist primary care providers and specialists in offering improved care is *Primary Care for Sports and Fitness: A Lifespan Approach* (Toy & Healy, 2008).

Grant Writing

It is more important than ever that NPs acquire grant writing skills in order to obtain financial support for their special projects, research, and educational program/training. These projects may revolve around a variety of topics, including:

- Health promotion teaching,
- Health screening for specific populations in the community,
- Models of care for frequently seen problems, such as sickle cell anemia, lead poisoning, alcohol and substance abuse, or
- Development programs for NPs and staff

Health screening and health promotion initiatives are effective and serve as a positive networking bridge to communities at risk for various health problems. Today's Health Teaching and Promotion Initiatives can assist in marketing the services of the practice or to recruit people for future programs if the practice is planning to continue to offer the activities at a nominal cost.

There are six categories of grants:

- Hospital and agency-based grants,
- Federal grants,
- Corporate partnerships,
- Pre- and postdoctoral research training fellowships,
- Professional association grants, and
- Foundation grants (Holtzclaw, Kenner, & Welden, 2009).

Generally NPs are more apt to start with a professional organization or foundation grant, which provides seed funding for a project. After successfully managing a smaller project, it is more realistic to apply for a state or federal grant. The National Institutes of Health changed their philosophy of funding to one of translating new information that will directly benefit the health of people. This is termed translational research, and NPs could easily become involved in this type of work.

Grants do not fund building expansion, office equipment, or generally identified equipment in a healthcare practice. However, a special or new diagnostic tool or screening device not readily available to a population that has been shown to have excellent patient outcomes could be fundable. Generally, requests for staff positions, attending conferences, or any type of travel should be limited; these are not usually funded by a foundation grant. NPs would gain good experience if an opportunity to participate in a clinical trial is offered. Working with someone to disseminate results of one's research through publications or presentations would also be a positive learning experience.

The process of grant writing is arduous and time consuming but, in this day of cost containment, obtaining any funding helps the practice accomplish its goals, achieve high patient satisfaction, and, in some instances, sustain a practice. Every advanced practice nurse needs to cultivate grant writing skills. The steps are as follows:

■ Explain the project,
■ Identify targeted participants, and
■ Find organizations or foundations most apt to fund the project.

For example, The Commonwealth Fund, provides foundation grants regarding health and health reform. Information can be accessed using the "Grants" link at http://www.commonwealthfund.org/.

The first step is writing a letter of interest/intent, which the funding agency requests on its Web site. During this "call for letters," the criteria for the grants are specifically delineated, and the foundation's Web site has links to successful projects funded in the past. Read the funding agency's mission statement and know its goals. The reviewer who assesses your letters of intent to submit a proposal or the proposal itself will correlate your material with the agency's mission and goals. Some foundations and organizations maintain the same focus every year. Other foundations specifically spell out funding goals for each year. The grant writer should collect information from the foundation's Web site regarding the specific grant program and check with the Grant Director about any project ideas or questions not answered online. Being a member of a professional organization may allow one to submit a request for a small seed grant, generally no more than $1000.00, which would provide experience in writing the grant request, managing the work funded by the grant, and disseminating the information learned from the research funded by the grant. An example of a short letter of intent is shown in Figure 4.3.

Sometimes foundations want more detail in the letter of intent than was submitted. They may also request additional information, including biosketches and a budget. It is imperative the grant writer check the Web site of the foundation or organization to obtain appropriate directions for submitting a letter of intent. See Figure 4.4 for an example of a long letter of intent.

The second step occurs after the grant writer is selected to actually apply for the grant. The foundation or organization sends the applicant a Request for Proposal (RFP). Copies of full grants can sometimes be accessed from the funding agency. If one was to apply for a federal grant, workshops help applicants gain knowledge about grant development. It is most important to have a co-investigator, such as a faculty member who has received grants, assist with the writing of the proposal. Holtzclaw, Kenner, and Walden (2009) in their book, *Grant Writing Handbook for Nurses,* offer numerous suggestions and examples of grant proposals.

Many new opportunities for funding for healthcare projects are available as a result of the 2009 Recovery Act Funds sponsored by the National Institutes of Health. A good Web site to access for further information is http://aacn.nche.edu/Government/pdf/Stimfund (see also Table 4.3). The speaker should try to speak publicly about the project and get the public to write to local, state, and federal politicians to show support. This may lead to success with funding. Collaborating with another agency with similar goals and/or an academician will possibly improve funding outcomes.

4.3

Short Letter of Intent for Foundation/Organization Funding

Use letterhead of your agency

Date

Grant Director Name
Name of Foundation/Professional Organization
Address

Re: Call for Grants

Dear Grant Director:

This letter of intent requests your consideration of a full proposal to fund a two-year project entitled End-of-Life Care for Older Patients in Long-Term Care, which would educate staff nurses on caring for palliative care patients. It will be managed by the University School of Nursing in collaboration with two gerontology partners, Wyatt Home and Harpers Shore Home.

Studies indicate that nurses do not feel competent or confident in implementing EOL care (Ferrell, Virani, Grant, Coyne & Uman, 2000). In the late 1990s, the American Association of Collegiate Nursing (AACN) and the City of Hope National Medical Center formed the End-of-Life Nursing Education Consortium (ELNEC), with funding from the Robert Wood Johnson Foundation. This initiative is a national educational program for nurses that includes nine modules covering EOL care: introduction to palliative care, pain management, symptom management, ethics, culture diversity, communication, grief and loss, achieving quality care, and final hours of death. Since nurses spend more time with patients at the end of life than members of any other discipline (Gelband, 2001), it is the goal of this project to provide ELNEC training (program consists of a minimum of nine hours) to 75% of the nurses in the two long-term facilities.

As a certified ELNEC Trainer, our goal is to educate the nurses over a six-month period regarding the ELNEC modules. This proposed project seems to fit your mission of providing palliative care and your interest in the welfare of older adults. I am interested in submitting a proposal for the July 30 funding cycle.

Thank you for your consideration, and I look forward to hearing from you.

Sincerely,

Name
Agency

References

American Association of Colleges of Nursing. ELNEC—Graduate end-of-life nursing education consortium for graduate faculty. Retrieved June 25 2009 from http://www.aacn.nche.edu/ELNEC/graduate .htm 2007.

Ferrell, B., Virani, R., Grant, M., Coyne, P. & Uman, G. (2000). Beyond the supreme court decision: Nursing perspectives on end-of-life care. *Oncology Nursing Forum, 27*(3), 445–455.

Gelband H. (2001). Professional education in palliative and end-of-life care for physicians, nurses and social workers. In KM Foley & H Gelband (Eds). *Improving palliative Care for Cancer.* Washington, DC: National Academy Press.

Hanson, L. C., Danis, M., & Garrett, J., (1997). What is wrong with end-of-life care? Opinions of bereaved family members. *Journal of the American Geriatrics Society, 45,* 1339–1344.

Zerzan, J., Stearns, S., & Hanson, L., (2000). Access to palliative care and hospice in nursing homes. *Journal of the American Medical Association, 284,* 2489–2494.

4.4

Long Letter of Intent for Foundation/Organization Funding

Use letterhead of your agency

Date

Grant Director Name
Name of Foundation/Professional Organization
Address

Re: Call for Grants

Dear Grant Director:

This letter of intent requests your consideration of a full proposal to fund a two-year project entitled *End-of-Life Care for Older Patients in Long-Term Care.* It will be managed by the University School of Nursing in collaboration with two gerontology partners, Wyatt Home and Harpers Shore Home. The total funding required is $140,946. Please see the attached letters of support for this collaborative effort with the university. These facilities have enthusiastically agreed to participate in this initiative.

The School of Nursing mission includes a commitment to social responsibility, truth, and justice, and is an extension of the University's Jesuit ideal that underscores the need to provide care to vulnerable populations. The School of Nursing is positioned as a leader in palliative care and gerontology. Renowned nurse scientists in Palliative Care, Dr. Rod Ulzwe, and Dr. Donna Herman, as well as others in the field of gerontology, have consulted at the School and participated in the School's Annual Distinguished Lecture Series in the fall of 2006. The School has supported six faculty members to become End-of-Life Nursing Education Consortium (ELNEC) Trainers, hosted a Symptom Management Conference for training nurses throughout the state (in collaboration with CT Coalition of End-of-Life [EOL] Nurse Educators), received funding from the J Geriatric Nursing Education Project, received funding from HRSA, and obtained funding from the DP Research Foundation to conduct four research studies in EOL topics and integrate EOL into the graduate and undergraduate curricula. The receipt of grant support has provided faculty members with the opportunity to enhance knowledge development and dissemination in the nursing care of multiple populations, especially in the care of older adults at Wyatt Home and Harpers Shore Home.

The goal of the proposed project builds on the current work of the School of Nursing, Wyatt Home, and Harpers Shore Home by providing education and resources to further develop palliative care expertise for nurses. There are three distinct components of this project, which will provide the framework for the attainment of this goal:

- To educate nurses working in two long-term care facilities regarding end-of-life (EOL) care in order to provide the highest quality care for older adults at the end of life;
- To disseminate a replicable model of EOL care to nurses in other LTC facilities in the state through the Connecticut Coalition of EOL Nurse Educators, ELNEC, and other partners of the university; and
- To raise public awareness especially for low income elders in or contemplating admission to a long-term care facility dependent on Medicaid and Medicare to foster policy reforms regarding EOL reimbursement.

Studies indicate that nurses do not feel competent or confident in implementing EOL care (Ferrell, Virani, Grant, Coyne & Uman, 2000). In the late 1990s, the American Association of Collegiate Nursing (AACN) and the City of Hope National Medical Center formed the End-of-Life Nursing Education Consortium (ELNEC), with funding from the Robert Wood Johnson Foundation. This initiative is a national educational program for nurses that includes nine modules covering EOL care: introduction to palliative care, pain management, symptom management, ethics, culture diversity, communication, grief and loss, achieving quality care, and final hours of death. Since nurses spend more time with patients at the end-of-life than members of any other discipline (Gelband, 2001), it is the goal of this project to provide ELNEC training (program consists of a minimum of nine hours) to 50% of the nurses in the two long-term facilities. To sustain the EOL knowledge at each facility, an ELNEC Train-the Trainer Course (program consists of a minimum of 18 hours) will be given to four RNs from each facility. A Web site with information on obtaining ELNEC sponsorship, a full description of modules, and publications of the multiple outcomes that have been generated by ELNEC graduates is accessible at http://www .aacn.nche.edu/elnec/factsheet.

There are increasingly more deaths in long-term care facilities (Zerzan, Stearns & Hanson, 2000). Palliative care programs are either nonexistent or underutilized in nursing homes. Because of Medicare and Medicaid policies for hospice/palliative care reimbursement, many patients in nursing homes have difficulty in accessing hospice services. Hanson, Danis, & Garret (1997) found the least positive evaluations of EOL care by families and friends occurred in long-term care facilities, with 78% of families perceiving that their loved ones experienced pain at end of life. By educating more nurses in EOL care and increasing awareness of older adults and their families, increased attention to the need for quality care for all patients at end of life should occur.

The *EOL Care for Older Patients in Long-Term Care Project* will accomplish the following outcomes:

Outcome 1: To educate nurses working in two LTC facilities regarding EOL care in order to provide the highest quality of care for older adults at the end of life. Objectives include:

- Determine current knowledge base and perceived areas of need regarding EOL care.
- Contact ELNEC to obtain sponsorship of courses for ELNEC training (educate 75% of nurses in each LTC facility).
- Obtain sponsorship of one course for ELNEC Train the Trainer, so that an annual ELNEC Training Course can occur by staff in order to provide sustainability (educate 4 nurses from each facility).
- Identify personnel who will be champions of palliative care to participate in ELNEC Train the Trainer Course.
- Schedule and provide educational programs for RNs and LPNS (2 training courses and 1 Train the Trainer Course).
- Set up a resource center at each facility to house the ELNEC power points, videos, books, and other educational support.
- Evaluate the effectiveness of the program (chart reviews, pre- and posttesting of nurses, patient and family interviews).
- Facilitate the incorporation of best practices into care delivery with members from social work, pastoral care, medicine, physical therapy, occupational therapy, and recreational therapy by including representatives at the training sessions.
- Assist the new ELNEC Trainers at each agency in preparing and implementing their first ELNEC training course.

Outcome 2: To disseminate a replicable model of EOL care to nurses in other long-term care facilities in the state through the Coalition of EOL Nurse Educators, ELNEC, and other partners of the School. Objectives include:

- Communicate ongoing outcomes from this project to representatives of the Coalition of EOL Nurse Educators by email, telephone, and at periodic Coalition Meetings so that other LTC agencies can replicate this project.
- Disseminate outcomes of this project with ELNEC so that nurse ELNEC Trainers in other states can replicate this project.
- Disseminate outcomes regionally and nationally with presentations and publications at professional meetings.
- Set up a Web site to assist nurses in LTC facilities in contacting the Project Director for assistance in replicating this project at their institutions.
- Participate in state conferences, such as the Annual Aging Conference cosponsored by the School of Nursing and one of the school's partners, South Agency on Aging, to market this project for further replication.

Outcome 3: To raise public awareness, especially for low income elders in or contemplating admission to a long-term care facility dependent on Medicaid and Medicare in order to foster policy reforms regarding EOL reimbursement. Objectives include:

- Schedule experts in palliative care from area hospitals, hospice/palliative care programs, and others to speak at seminars about the National Consensus Project for Quality Palliative Care and how it impacts older adults.

- Distribute fliers (developed by nursing students in their Health Care Delivery Systems course) throughout the local community to advertise the seminar.
- Implement quarterly educational seminars for the community through the School's Health Promotion Center to promote awareness of palliative care.
- Schedule focus groups of families of older adults at the two LTC agencies before implementation of the ELNEC project and after two ELNEC courses have run to assess family awareness of palliative care.

Ms. NP will be the director of this project which will begin April 2009 and end in April 2011. Other investigator's names can be listed here. See **Attachment I** for brief biographical summaries.

The total project budget is provided in **Attachment II** and will cover staffing, travel, and materials. There are no other funds committed or anticipated for this project.

It is our hope the Foundation will look favorably on this project and a full proposal will be requested. Thank you in advance for your consideration.

Sincerely,

References

American Association of Colleges of Nursing. ELNEC—Graduate end-of-life nursing education consortium for graduate faculty. Retrieved June 5, 2009 from http://www.aacn.nche.edu/ELNEC/graduate.htm 2007.

Ferrell, B., Virani, R., Grant, M., Coyne, P. & Uman, G. (2000). Beyond the supreme court decision: Nursing perspectives on end-of-life care. *Oncology Nursing Forum, 27*(3), 445–455.

Gelband H. (2001). Professional education in palliative and end-of-life care for physicians, nurses and social workers. In KM Foley & H Gelband (Eds). *Improving palliative Care for Cancer.* Washington, DC: National Academy Press.

Hanson, L. C., Danis, M., & Garrett, J., (1997). What is wrong with end-of-life care? Opinions of bereaved family members. *Journal of the American Geriatrics Society, 45,* 1339–1344.

Zerzan, J., Stearns, S., & Hanson, L., (2000). Access to palliative care and hospice in nursing homes. *Journal of the American Medical Association, 284,* 2489–2494

4.3 Frequently Used Web Sites for Federal Funding Regarding Stimulus

- United States Department of Health & Human Services (HHS)—www.hhs.gov/recovery
- National Institutes of Health (NIH)—www.nih.gov/recovery/index.htm
- National Institute of Nursing Research (NINR)—www.ninr.nih.gov/Aboutninrdirectors page/ARRA+messag.htm
- NINR Challenge Grant—http://grants.nih.gov/grants/funding/challenge_award
- Consolidated Grant Information—www.grants.gov
- Recovery Overview—www.recovery.gov

Conclusion

This chapter's focus was to assist NPs in understanding the differences among protocols, standards of care, patient care guidelines, and disease-focused guidelines. During poor economic times, when it is difficult to obtain resources and employ enough staff, NPs need to use their creativity to accomplish goals and provide high-quality care by being efficient in business practices and raising money through grants. In fact, all NP educational programs should devote a portion of each clinical practica to the business aspect of the practice (Wing, 1998). It is a unique time to be opening one's own healthcare business and/or starting a new partnership, but opportunities are available for NPs willing to take the challenge. As more physicians retire and fewer physicians enter primary care practice, there will be more opportunities for NPs to provide care in a high-quality and holistic fashion to patients. Suggestions for determining which type of individual malpractice coverage to obtain are made. Recommendations for increasing salary by functioning in all four aspects of the NP role (Leader, Professional, Manager, and Clinician) are also discussed. Examples of a résumé and biosketch are offered for NPs to use as a model for developing their own. Grant writing is discussed, along with samples of long and short letters of intent that can be used for submitting ideas regarding a proposal for funding.

Reflective Thinking Exercises

1. Using the Federal Drug Administration (FDA) Web site for Drug Safety at www.fda.gov/cder/drugSafety.htm, develop a succinct bulletin of the information categories available at this site to share with other NPs. Specifically, cite two examples of how this site could be used by the agency where you are currently employed.
2. Develop a checklist for an NP procedure that is frequently performed at your work setting. You can download the video, *How a Simple Checklist Can Dramatically Reduce Medical Errors,* by P. Pronovost (2008), published by IHI Open School for Health Professionals at http://psnet.ahrq.gov/resource.aspx?resourceID=8743 to assist in this process. Be as succinct as possible, as this improves compliance of use by staff.
3. Develop a cause-and-effect chart (fishbone) of a potential problem you see affecting patient safety at your employment site. Share findings with a group of NPs or with your NP class on your course discussion board to develop quality improvement measures. Use the Plan/Do/Study/Act (PDSA) methodology to complete this project.
4. Use reflective practice techniques to determine if there are ways to apply your "deeper sense of self" in providing therapeutic outcomes for your patients or community populations. Describe these instances, and explain why you interpreted these encounters as therapeutic.
5. Develop a letter of intent/interest for applying for start-up funding or expansion of an existing healthcare program for a private foundation/or-

ganization. See the examples of short and long letters of intent (Figures 4.3 and 4.4).

6. Using Informed Consent, *The Clinical Advisor's* malpractice newsletter, review two cases and describe how, if the verdict was not in favor of the NP, the NP could have received a positive verdict. The Web site is http://www.clinicaladvisor.com/issue/May/01/2009/1686/. Another source that can be helpful to review legal cases involving NPs is Legal Eagle Eye Newsletter for the Nursing Professional which can be accessed at http://www.nursinglaw.com/.

References

Agency for Healthcare Research & Quality. Retrieved April 3, 2009 from www.ahcpr.gov

American Academy of Nurse Practitioners Annual Salary Survey. (2007). Retrieved June 2, 2009 from http://www.aanp.org/NR/rdonlyres/AD41DD8D-FD16-4F84-968C-F7192A0E79D6/0/NPCompensation2007.pdf.

American Academy of Nurse Practitioners Standards of Practice for Nurse Practitioners (2007). Retrieved June 2, 2009 from http://www.aanp.org.

American Association of Colleges of Nursing. ELNEC—Graduate end-of-life nursing education consortium for graduate faculty. Retrieved June 5, 2009 from http://www.aacn.nche.edu/ELNEC/graduate.htm 2007.

American Association of Nurse Attorneys. (2005). *Health law, legislation, and compliance section.* Columbus, OH: author.

Bear, M. & Bowers, C. (1998). Using a nursing framework to measure client satisfaction at a nurse-managed clinic. *Public Health Nursing, 15*(1), 50–59.

Bourbonniere, M. & Evans, L. (2002). Advanced practice nursing in the care of frail older adults. *Journal of the American Geriatrics Society, 50*(12), 2062–2076.

Buerhaus, P., Staiger, D., & Auerbach, D. (2009). *Nursing workforce in the United States: Data, trends, and implications.* Sudbury, MA: Jones and Bartlett Publishers.

Buppert, C. (2008). Nurse practitioner's business practice and legal guide. 3rd ed., Sudbury, MA: Jones and Bartlett Publishers.

Bureau of Labor Statistics. (2005). *RNs—Bureau of Labor.* Retrieved June 22, 2009 from http://allnurses.com/general-nursing-discussion/registered-nurses-bureau-102710.html

Burroughs, R., Dmytrow, B. & Lewis, H. (2007). Trends in nurse practitioner professional liability: An analysis of claims with risk management recommendations. *Journal of Nursing Law, 11*(1), 53–59.

Carcio, H. (2008). Outside the box: Restoring dignity through dryness. *ADVANCE for Nurse Practitioners, 12,* 36.

Chang, K., Davis, R., Birt, J., Castelluccio, P., Woodbridge, P.,& Marrero, D. (2007). Nurse practitioner—based diabetes care management: Impact of telehealth or telephone intervention on glycemic control. *Disease Management Health Outcomes, 15*(6), 377–385.

Cochrane Collaboration. Retrieved April 20, 2009 from http://www.cochrane.org/.

Commission on Collegiate Nursing Education. (2009). Procedures on Accreditation. Retrieved April 12, 2009 from http://www.aacn.nche.edu/Accreditation Commonwealth Foundation for Public Policy Alternatives. Retrieved April 20, 2009 from http://www.commonwealthfoundation.org/

Csikszentmihalyi, M. (1990). *Flow: the psychology of optimal experience—steps toward enhancing the quality of life.* New York, NY: Harper and Row.

Ferrell, B.,Virani, R.,Grant,M., Coyne, P. & Uman, G. (2000). Beyond the supreme court decision: Nursing perspectives on end-of-life care. *Oncology Nursing Forum, 27*(3), 445–455.

Fotland, J. (2009). Changing a broken system: Clinic design gives patients options. *ADVANCE for Nurse Practitioners, 2,* 20.

Gardner, A., Hase, S., Gardner, G., Dunn, S. & Carryer, J. (2007). From competence to capability: A study of nurse practitioners in clinical practice. *Journal of Clinical Nursing, 17,* 250–258.

Gelban, H. (2001). Professional education in palliative and end-of-life care for physicians, nurses and social workers. In KM Foley & H Gelband (Eds). *Improving palliative Care for Cancer.* Washington, DC: National Academy Press.

Hanson, L. C., Danis, M., & Garrett, J., (1997). What is wrong with end-of-life care? Opinions of bereaved family members. *Journal of the American Geriatrics Society, 45,* 1339–1344.

Hotzclaw, B., Kenner, C. & Walden, M. (2009). *Grant writing handbook for nurses.* 2nd ed. Sudbury, MA: Jones and Bartlett Publishers.

Hughes, R. Ed. (2007). *Patient Safety and Quality: An Evidence-based Handbook for Nurses* Washington, D.C.: Agency for Healthcare Research and Quality.

Institutes of Healthcare Improvement. *Transforming care at the bedside.* Retrieved April 22. 2009 from http://www.ihi.org/ihi.

Institute of Medicine. (1999). *To err is human: Building a safer health system.* Washington, DC: National Academy Press.

Institute of Medicine Committee on the quality of Health Care in America. (2000). *Crossing the quality chasm: A new health system for the 21st century.* Washington, DC: National Academy Press.

Jenson, K., Mayer, T., Welch, S., & Haraden, C. (2007). *Leadership for smooth patient flow: Improved outcomes, improved service, improved bottom line.* Chicago, IL: Health Administration Press.

Kenney, Charles, (2008). *The best practice: How the new quality movement is transforming medicine.* New York, NY: Public Affairs.

Kotter, J. (2002). *The heart of change.* Boston: Harvard Business School Press.

Lawler, M. (2008). One to watch: One business leads to another. *ADVANCE for Nurse Practitioners, 12,* 24–25.

Lawson-Baker, S. (2008). Always say "yes": Entrepreneur of the year. *ADVANCE for Nurse Practitioners, 12,* 30–33.

McMullan, M.,Endacott, R., Gray, M., Jasper, M., Miller, C., Scholes, J., & Webb, C. (2003). Portfolios and assessment of competence: A review of literature. *Journal of Advanced Nursing, 41,* 283–294.

Moen, G. (2009). Eagan child and family care. *ADVANCE for Nurse Practitioners, 2,* 18. *National Institutes of Health Roadmap.* National Institutes of Health. Retrieved June 1, 2009 from http://www.grants.nih.gov/grants/oer.htm

Nelson, E., Batalden, P., & Godfrey, M. (2007). *Quality by design: A clinical microsystems approach.* San Francisco: Jossey-Bass.

NP Business Organization. *NP business and practices.* Retrieved on June 26, 2009 from http://npbusiness.org/nurse-practitioner-sites.

Orem, D. (1980). *Nursing: Concepts of practice.* New York: McGraw-Hill.

Peters, T. (2003). *Re-imagine!* London: Dorling Kindersley

Pronovost P., Needham D., Berenholtz S., et al. (2006). An intervention to decrease catheter-related bloodstream infections in the ICU. *New England Journal of Medicine, 355,* 2725–2732.

Pulcini, J., Vampola, D., & Levine, J. (2005). Survey: Nurse practitioner practice characteristics, salary, and benefits survey, 2003. *NPACE., 9(*1), 49–58.

Ranson, E., Joshi, M., Nash, D. & Ranson, S. Eds. (2008). *The healthcare quality book: Vision, strategy, and tools.* 2nd ed. Chicago: Health Administration Press.

Rowell, R., Forsythe, P., Avallone, D. & Kloos, J. (2008). Moving up!: Implementing an effective APN promotional program. *The Nurse Practitioner, 33*(12), 39–44.

Roy, C. (1984). *Introduction to nursing: An adaptation model.* Englewood Cliffs: Prentice Hall.

Rycroft-Malone, J., Seers, K., Titchen, A., Harvey, G., Kitson, A., and McCormack, B. (2004). What counts as evidence in evidence-based practice? *Journal of Advanced Nursing, 47*(1), 81–90.

Senge, P. (2006). *The fifth discipline: The art and practice of the learning organization.* New York: Doubleday.

Six Sigma. Retrieved April 20, 2009 from http://www.isixsigma.com/.

Studer, Q. (2004). *Service excellence.* Baltimore: Firestarter Press.

Toy, B. & Healy, P. (2008). *Primary care for sports and fitness: A lifespan approach* Philadelphia F. A. Davis Company.

Uphold, C. & Graham, M. (2003). *Clinical guidelines in family practice.* 4th ed., Gainesville: Barmarrae Books, Inc.

Varkey, P. Ed., (2009). *Medical quality management: theory and practice. American College of Medical Quality.* Sudbury: Jones & Bartlett.

Walsgrove, H. & Fulbrook, P.(2005). Advancing the clinical perspective: A practice development project to develop the nurse practitioner role in an acute hospital trust. *Journal of Clinical Nursing, 14,* 444–455.

Wheatley, M. (2006). *Leadership and the new science: Discovering order in a chaotic world* (3rd ed.). San Francisco: Berrett-Koehler Publishers.

Wing, D. (1998). The business management preceptorship within the nurse practitioner program. *Journal of Professional Nursing, 14*(3), 150–156.

Zerzan, J., Stearns, S., & Hanson, L., (2000). Access to palliative care and hospice in nursing homes. *Journal of the American Medical Association, 284,* 2489–2494.

Managing a Revenue-Generating Practice

5

Learning Objectives

1. Differentiate business ownership structures used for nurse practitioner (NP) practice.

2. Consider planning process before starting a business.

3. Develop a business plan for an NP-run agency.

4. Describe the elements of the three basic financial statements.

5. Define risk management and its implications for NP practice.

6. Differentiate among various patient payer systems for healthcare delivery.

7. Describe the basic coding, billing, and reimbursement processes used in health care.

8. Describe a compliance program and its relationship to billing, coding, and reimbursement.

9. Illustrate the use of budgets as financial control mechanisms.

10. Explain cost saving mechanisms using efficiency management.

Key Words: business structures, pre-business planning, business plans, malpractice, risk management, coding, billing, reimbursement, financial management

If you wish to start an independent NP practice, a pre-business planning exercise is a prudent place to start. The Small Business Administration (SBA) has a questionnaire entitled, *Small Business Readiness Assessment Tool,* that can be found at http://web.sba.gov/sbtn/sbat/index.cfm?Tool=4. This questionnaire requires a frank analysis of personal abilities and provides resources to further prepare you for this exciting step.

Nurse practitioners interested in establishing an independent practice need to be adept at business, especially financial matters. Starting a business begins with planning, planning, and more planning. Nurse practitioners must combine their clinical skills of observation and investigation with ingenuity and creativity. This chapter will help guide the NP through the process of planning and writing a business plan. Possible business ownership structures are discussed, along with budgets, risk management, coding, billing, and compliance.

Before starting a business, realize that owning a practice or joining a practice as a co-owner entails financial risk. Therefore, the first and most important step is to consult an attorney and an accountant for guidance regarding federal and state laws that regulate healthcare businesses. Small businesses must abide by laws that can be found on state small business advocate group Web sites or that of the federal Small Business Administration (www.sba.gov). Local business groups and attorneys specializing in business start-ups can also be helpful. You will need to become familiar with many types of law, such as (www.allbusiness.com, 2004):

- Employment/Hiring Law
- Contract Law and Business Formation
- Environmental Law and Regulations
- Consumer Protection Laws
- Intellectual Property Laws
- Tax Laws

The American Association of Nurse Attorneys' guidebook, *Business and Legal Guidebook for Nurse Practitioners* (2005), can assist with understanding the legal aspects of developing an NP run practice. Reviewing *Nurse Practitioner's Business Practice and Legal Guide* (2008) by Carolyn Buppert, an NP and attorney, is also helpful.

Choosing the correct business structure can be legally challenging unless one engages an attorney and accountant to assist in determining the type of entity that best fits individual needs and situations. The attorney and accountant will provide advice about the tax advantages/disadvantages of the different structures and any legal restrictions. The Small Business Administration (https://www.sba.gov) suggests that one consider the following personal traits before consulting legal and financial counsel:

- The expected size of the practice
- The level of control the NP wants
- The expected level of profit (or loss) expected
- The NP's need to receive cash from the practice

In addition, Buppert (2008) also recommends that one consider:

- The business structure that best limits the risk of personal financial liability.

■ The requisite business and clinical knowledge to manage a practice.
■ The state law if it limits independent clinical business endeavors through NP scope of practice by requiring intervention by a physician.

Business Structures

Before choosing the business structure, the NP must decide whether the practice will be for-profit or not-for-profit (i.e., charitable entity). A not-for profit entity is "an organization formed for the purpose of serving a purpose of public or mutual benefit other than the pursuit . . . of profits. It is important to know what a not-for-profit corporation is not. It is not a way for ordinary businesses—or people—to shield assets or avoid paying income tax. It is not an alternative business form for any regular type of business" (http://www.not-for-profit.org). In a not-for-profit business, the organization keeps all profits in order to expand or improve services. Thus, there is no profit sharing. Not-for-profit organizations are generally started for civic, charitable, or religious endeavors. The tax laws for the formation of a not-for-profit are complex.

Most NPs start for-profit entities. Many business structures exist, including sole proprietorship, partnership, and corporation.

Sole Proprietorship

In a sole proprietorship, the NP is the only owner and is responsible for every aspect of the practice, including clinical care, supervision of the operations, and fiscal management. A sole proprietorship can have employees; the term "sole" just describes the ownership structure. For legal and income tax purposes, the business and the NP are the same. The business does not file an income tax return; all income and expenses are included on the NP's personal income tax return. In this type of practice, the NP is the decision maker regarding all operational and fiscal concerns. Before starting a sole proprietorship practice or "hanging a shingle," one should have previous clinical experience and be comfortable being the decision maker for a business.

If the NP is not comfortable starting a practice as a sole proprietor, an alternative might be working as an independent contractor for an established practice. This will help the NP gain clinical experience and learn about business operations. Similar to the sole proprietor, independent contractors work for themselves and report income on their personal tax returns. Independent contractors do not receive benefits from their employers and do not have income taxes withheld from their fees. Consultation with an accountant is needed to ensure tax payments are made on a timely basis to avoid penalties.

Partnership

A partnership consists of two or more owners. When entering into a partnership, the NP needs to consult an attorney to protect the interests of all owners. The partnership agreement should specify the expectations of all partners, the cash withdrawals all partners may make, how any losses will be covered, what each partner will contribute to the start up of the practice, how new partners can be admitted to the partnership, how partners can leave the partnership, how disagreements will be settled, and so on. This document is crucial if future misunderstandings or enmity are to be prevented. Technically, each partner in the practice has responsibility for oversight of the operations. Practically speaking, the partnership agreement will specify the specific duties of each partner.

As with a sole proprietorship, the business and owners are the same for legal and income tax purposes. The partnership does file its own income tax return, but all the income and expenses are allocated to the partners according to a predetermined formula included in the partnership agreement. This formula could be based on many different metrics, including hours worked, amount of new business brought in, or level of seniority. This allocation results in no profit to the partnership; the partners receive all the profit. The partners' profit must be reported on their personal income tax returns.

Several different types of partnerships can be created, and state laws differ regarding partnerships. Most partnerships are "general partnerships" and operate as described. However, if no partnership agreement exists, then all partners share equally in profits and losses regardless of participation in the practice.

In limited partnerships, most partners have limited input into the day-to-day operating decisions. These "quiet partners" receive a "dividend" on their investment if the practice is profitable. If there is a loss, the "limited" partner is not financially affected. This type of partnership is rarely used in health care.

Corporation

A corporation is a separate legal entity that receives a charter from the state in which it has headquarters. The corporation, as a legal "person," must pay income taxes, can enter into legal contracts, can be sued, and can sue others. The owners of the corporation are its shareholders. The shareholders elect a Board of Directors to serve as their representatives to supervise the management of the business. The Board of Directors hires officers of the practice. Most states require that a corporation have at least two officers: President and Secretary.

This structure has many advantages over that of the sole proprietorship and partnership structures. The most important difference is that the owners have limited legal liability. This means owners are not personally liable for the debts of the corporation. Most important is that the owners are not personally responsible for the payment of judgments resulting from the corporation being sued. This structure is quite complex and requires many documents be filed with state and federal government. Legal and accounting advisers should assist with all these filings.

Corporations usually employ many people. Hospitals, colleges, and large multiprovider healthcare companies are typically incorporated. Corporations that employ NPs pay salaries and benefits. Large, established private practices can be run by corporations, such as physician practice management companies (PPMCs), independent practice associations (IPAs), and physician-hospital management services organization (MSOs). Sometimes Preferred Provider Organizations (PPOs) offer ownership through a costly "buy-in" price to join the practice. With this arrangement, the NP can reap the benefits through a profit-sharing agreement.

Limited Liability Company

This is an interesting structure that allows the NP the protection of a corporation through the limited liability feature of LLCs. The owners of an LLC are called members. The LLC is generally taxed in a manner similar to that of a partnership.

Before meeting with legal counsel to set up an LLC, view information on such Web sites as Incorporation/Cooperation Formation Services (http://www .incorp.com) or Limited Liability Company (http://www.llc.com). These sites have information and provide details on forming an LLC in a video. LLC status protects the NP's family and personal assets from legal actions against the NP-owned business. This protection does not exist for civil litigation. LLCs are very popular with NP-run businesses since they provide liability protection and flexibility with management. They also provide protection from errors made by others acting on behalf of the business. Forms for LLCs can be downloaded from http://www.entrepreneur.com or http://www.allbusiness.com, so you can review them before meeting with an attorney.

Pre-Business Planning

Pre-business planning includes determining whether the geographic area chosen can support another healthcare practice and engaging in *financial modeling,* which identifies variables that must be accounted for in a business plan (Aboul-Encin, 2009). Most new businesses develop because the NP wants to change a current operational philosophy or create more cost-effective methods of operation. Sometimes, new businesses are created to fill a specific niche in an existing business.

Pre-Planning Phase

Examine in great detail the local business environment to ascertain whether a new business can be financially supported by the community. Many resources are available to assist in developing a successful plan (see Figure 5.1).

In addition, the SBA Web site (http://www.sba.gov/smallbusinessplanner) has free on-line training courses on the basics of starting a business, along with

5.1

Small Business
Development
Resources

- Local and state governments offer resources to encourage small business development.
- Entrepreneur.com—free forms
- Small Business Association (SBA.gov)
- Better Business Bureau (BBB.com)
- SCORE/Counselors to America's Small Business (SCORE.org)
- NurseEntrepreneurs.com
- Nurse-Entrepreneur-Network.com
- Allbusiness.com

a plethora of resources, referrals to helpful tools, and contact information to access counselors who can assist in the planning process. Some of the topics covered are:

- Small Business Primer: Guide to Starting a Business
- How to Prepare a Business Plan
- Technology 101: A Small Business Guide
- Marketing for Small Business
- How to Prepare a Loan Package

The pre-planning process is similar to reviewing the literature before writing a formal paper. The exercise serves to answer the question, "What exists in the business community already, and how will this new practice be considered in the current environment, taking into account all influential variables?"

Use these questions adapted from the Small Business Web site (www.sba .gov) and from Mackey (2005) to start the pre-planning inquiry and to begin thinking about the three major areas of the business plan: market analysis, financing the practice, and management of the practice's operations.

Market Analysis and Market Testing

This analysis surveys the local area and economy to determine if the community can support a new practice and if the local population shows interest in having one. The following questions are examples of the type of inquiry needed to complete a market analysis:

- Investigate locally to learn about existing healthcare businesses:
  - ☐ Who are the current competitors in the area?
  - ☐ Where are patients currently obtaining the service of the proposed practice?
  - ☐ Is the population large enough to maintain a new practice and realize a profit if patients don't leave their current service providers?
- Determine whether the new practice will be different from existing practices:
  - ☐ If no competition exists, why not? Do patients want/need the service of the proposed new practice? What will convince patients they want/ need the service?
  - ☐ If competition does exist, will the new practice take business away from existing practices?
  - ☐ What is different about how the new practice will operate to encourage clients to leave an existing relationship with a practice or provider?
- Assess other practices and obtain knowledge regarding how to provide services in a better way. Specifically, describe how services will be provided in a better manner.
- Identify potential or new areas from which to obtain patients:
  - ☐ Who are the patients, and what are their demographics?
  - ☐ Provide information about the patients that explains why this population needs a new healthcare practice.

Financing the Practice

Before beginning a business, calculate the anticipated costs and the projected amount of start-up funding needed. Consider expenses for these three areas: start-up and operations, sales/marketing/advertising, and revenue sources.

- *Expenses:*
  - ☐ *Start-Up:* Determine the initial costs for a market analysis, development and writing of a business plan, and consulting fees for attorneys and accountants.
  - ☐ *Operations:* Estimate the cost of opening the practice, including office space, office and medical equipment, and supplies.
    - Office space: find a location and find out the rental cost or purchase price
    - Office equipment: furniture, phones, technology needs, copiers
      - ○ Examination rooms: furniture
      - ○ Waiting room: should the furniture be new or used
      - ○ Break room furniture: provide an area for eating and meetings
      - ○ Supplies for the business office and patient exam rooms
      - ○ Medical equipment: should it be rented or purchased
    - Laboratory machines: microscope, centrifuge, refrigerator
    - Pharmacy needs for on-site dispensing to patients
    - Storage space—locked cabinets for storing valuable pharmaceuticals and prescriptions
    - Medical supplies needed
    - Recurring administrative costs and fees (annually or monthly basis)
      - ○ Licenses and other regulatory filings, physician contracts, payroll processing company, accountant, attorney, billing company, software licenses and upgrades, medical waste disposal, medical record storage, document shredding company, cleaning contractor, security
      - ○ Payroll
      - ○ Insurance: malpractice, rental, business liability, disaster, workers' compensation, health benefits
      - ○ Utilities: electricity, phones, cable, computer network
      - ○ Taxes: payroll, property, income
  - Sales/Marketing/Advertising
    - Estimate the cost of creating a logo to enhance recognition of the practice.
    - Estimate costs of promotional materials: flyers, Web site creation and maintenance, radio and television commercials, newspaper advertising newspapers
- *Revenue*
  - ☐ What fees will be charged?
    - Fee for service—collection directly from the patient with no insurance required
    - Medicaid/Medicare reimbursement—systems to submit and collect reimbursement must be initiated
    - Contractual income—patients will receive the NP's care through direct stipend payment

☐ What methods of payment will be accepted?

☐ Is direct NP reimbursement possible?

- Is a physician required for reimbursement? Determine how the physician will be compensated (hourly versus flat rate charge versus percentage of profits) and related costs.

☐ With which insurance providers will the NP be associated?

☐ How will the billing process be completed? If the business is small, consider outsourcing to a billing company rather than using an employee.

- Funding options

☐ Are grants available?

☐ Small Business Administration Web site (www.sba.gov) provides leads on funding and grants for start-up businesses.

☐ Donations from benefactors who share a similar vision.

☐ Small business loans from local banks or credit unions (personal loans): local lenders know the community better than national banks and may be more willing to provide loan approval

☐ Investors or partners who might want to share in the financial benefits of the business' success

Management of the Practice's Operations

- *Daily Operations*

☐ Explain the operational philosophy guiding the practice.

☐ How will the practice be organized, so that it will run efficiently and effectively?

☐ How will the practice operate differently from the competition to fill the needs previously identified?

- How will the operational difference benefit the practice in terms of cost savings, efficiency, patient satisfaction, healthier patients, and other considerations?

- *Networking*

☐ What relationships need to be forged with local businesses, schools, parent-teacher associations, local government, social service agencies, religious and community leaders, and politicians?

☐ Talk with local business owners who may become associated with the practice (e.g., local pharmacy, medical supply or durable medical equipment (DME) supplier).

- *Marketing/Advertising*

☐ What strategies will be employed to advertise the new practice?

☐ Estimate the cost of periodic advertising

☐ Estimate the cost of Web site maintenance

☐ Estimate costs of co-sponsoring events or teams for publicity (e.g., a breast cancer walk or softball team).

(Mackey, 2005; Cardamone, Shaver, and Werthman, 2004; www.SBA.gov, 2009)

For example, suppose you are considering opening a cosmetic dermatological practice. The first question is whether sufficient business is available. Determine if your practice can survive even though the same geographic area already has two physician dermatology practices and a spa business. In a large metropolitan area, the market could possibly support another cosmetic dermatology practice. In a smaller suburb, however, it probably could not, unless the population has a particular demographic component to explain a higher than normal demand for this type of service (e.g., a subset of the population that may be particularly interested in looking youthful). Use this pre-planning exercise to determine the demographic composition of the local population. The question promotes investigation and fact finding to support or negate the viability of introducing a new and competing practice to the market area.

Be mindful of determining the size of the market available for a new practice and what revenue is needed to sustain profitable operations. This pre-planning phase can take a while to complete, especially if the NP is currently employed. Alternatively, take into account how long it will take to obtain the cash needed to have someone else do the analysis. Anticipated population and economic changes can influence this analysis. The closing of factories, changes in public financing of transportation, or other changes in the local environment will influence the analysis and success of the new practice.

The NP may consider hiring a business consultant to conduct the pre-planning tests and analyses, but it will be costly. The answers found during the pre-planning phase are used directly in the official business plan. An official business plan is necessary as it is circulated to prospective funding sources as well as to potential partners and employees.

Developing a Business Plan

The goal of a business plan is to articulate the vision and mission of the business to others to secure support or financial assistance. Those reviewing the plan look for clear and succinct descriptions of the proposed venture. Be prepared to share detailed information (see Figure 5.2).

5.2

Business Plan Elements

Summary	**Financial Information**
Cover Page	Projected Income Statements (5 years)
Executive Summary	Projected Statements of Cash Flows (5 years)
Table of Contents	Projected Balance Sheets (5 years)
	Loan Applications
Business Outline	Alternative Funding Sources
Mission Statement	
Business Description	**Supporting Documents Section**
Market Research and Market Analysis Results	Personal Financial Information
(competition outlined)	Licenses
Management Plan	Insurance Documents and Certificates of
Marketing Plan	Insurance
Timeline	Legal Documents
Identified Risks and Problems	

A business plan is generally divided into four elements: Summary, Business Outline, Financial Information, and Supporting Documents.

Summary

The summary includes a cover page with the name and demographic information of the practice and the owner. A logo can be created and included on the cover page to help create a business identity. This logo should be used on all stationery items, business cards, and letterhead for easy identification of the practice.

The Executive Summary follows and is an overview (up to two pages) of the business proposal, including the purpose of the practice and background information about the healthcare provider(s). The Executive Summary is the "first impression" of the practice. Everyone knows you only have one chance to make a first impression. It MUST highlight the distinguishing points about the practice, excite readers about the practice and its opportunity for success, convey the expertise of the provider(s), and accurately and succinctly convince the readers this is an opportunity NOT TO BE MISSED. The Executive Summary section culls important points from throughout the business plan and succinctly briefs the reader on those important points.

The Executive Summary is followed by the Table of Contents, which allows the reviewer to go directly to the section of interest. Financial groups will look to the financial section to consider the bottom line and the level of risk involved in a potential investment. Consulting physicians may look to the management section to see how their role may evolve in the business overtime.

Business Outline

The Business Outline, the second section of the plan details information about the practice and includes the seven parts explained below.

Mission Statement: A mission statement answers the question "What is the purpose of the practice?" It articulates the overarching operational goals of the practice and may describe some operational principles. Because the mission statement is the foundation of the practice and its operation, time should be spent investigating, documenting, and clearly explaining the reasons for the practice. This statement can also be used to answer questions from start up to expansion and growth. For example, if your mission is to provide cost-effective accessible health care to an underserved population, a buyout offer from a large health system conglomerate would most likely be refused. Why? Because the mission statements differ diametrically: accessible cost-effective care versus profit-making health care. When crafting a mission statement, consider all of the initial motivations that led to wanting to open this new practice. A template of a mission statement is provided in Section III.

Business Description: A description of the practice comes next. Explain specifically why the new practice is a valid idea. Include:

- What services are to be offered, to whom, and why.
- Why the specific location was chosen.

The operational process is described next. Articulate points such as:

- The hours of operation.
- The healthcare service provided.
- The types of staff needed.
- The specific services or procedures setting the practice apart from others.
- The structures to be put into place to assure quality and to monitor patient satisfaction and employee commitment.

This information is used to produce and define policy regarding the eligibility for and available services through the business.

Market Research and Market Analysis Results: Results from the analysis of local practices and marketing procedures are summarized next. Include:

- An overview of how the practice differs from its competitors.
- Demographic information about the area.
- Findings from the market analysis indicating a receptive business environment.
  - ☐ Evidence (statistics) of the need for a new practice in this geographical location.
  - ☐ An assessment depicting the need for additional or different health care services.
- Challenges the practice can overcome with the new operational model.
- Market strength(s) of the new practice.
- Estimates of provider utilization based on population and currently available services.
- Evidence the market will produce enough revenue to offset expenses of the practice.

Management Plan: The next step is to articulate the details of the practice's business structure and management of daily operations. The following should be included:

- The business structure: sole proprietorship, partnership, or corporation.
- Identification of all owners, practitioners, and staff positions with names (if known).
- How daily operations of the practice will be managed (office manager, business manager, etc.).
- If the practice is organized as a corporation, list the members of the Board of Directors.
- The person ultimately responsible for business decisions.
- An Organizational Structure Chart showing the flow of authority in the practice.

This information can be diagrammed as shown in Figure 5.3.

If the practice is structured as a corporation, a Board of Directors may be able to assist with governance issues and to guide the practice in fulfilling its mission. The Board should be composed of community representatives with var-

5.3

Organizational Structure Chart

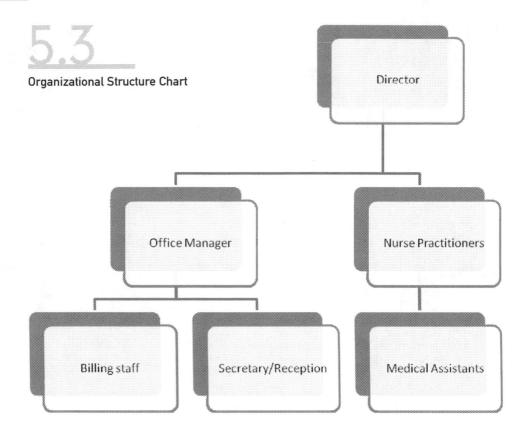

ied expertise in health care, education, and business. Lockee (2008) identified the three functions most important functions of a Board of Directors as:

- Responsibility for the interests of the patients and the community.
- Duty to follow the rules and policies of the practice.
- Responsibility for representing the practice's best interests.

Members of the Board should be knowledgeable about their duties and expectations regarding attendance at meetings and participation in decision making.

Marketing Plan: The marketing plan is the next component. Again, use your pre-planning work and summarize the advertising methods that will provide the best "bang for your buck." If new to the area, you need to establish credibility not only with potential patients but also with local business owners and the local medical community. In addition, good relationships with the department of education, daycare providers, police and fire departments, ambulance services, pharmacies, groceries, banks, and other public entities can reap untold rewards. Inform local emergency rooms and subspecialists that your practice is open to referrals. Sending thank you cards and referrals helps to cement working relationships with other local healthcare providers. If the community lacks primary care providers and/or established practices no longer accept new patients, the NP should forge relationships to announce a new source of care that is accepting primary care referrals (Shute, 2008).

Nurse practitioners and new practices need to be visible in the community too. Ways to accomplish this include:

- Volunteering in community organizations.
- Establishing a booth at the annual healthcare fair.
- Having a Web site marketed in community papers, church bulletins, etc.
- Hosting grocery store and restaurant events and other creative avenues to increase visibility.

Include all your marketing ideas and methods in the business plan.

Timelines: Timelines are next. Describe when the pre-planning process began, when funding will be obtained, and when the new practice will open. Target dates are listed to supply goals and help readers measure progress toward opening. Goals and dates can later be used for outcome evaluations.

Risk assessment: In this section, report any potential barriers to achieving goals included in the plan. Report short-term problems, such as road closures as a result of construction, that will hinder access to the practice. This sharing demonstrates excellent communication and shows realism in the planning process.

Financial Information

The last element of the business plan is finances. Many inexpensive software programs are available to help with this stage, but simple spreadsheets can be easily prepared. All business owners benefit from knowing how to use spreadsheets. Computer literacy is necessary to keep track of the practice's financial condition.

The financial section should show the three basic financial statements: income statement, statement of cash flows, and balance sheet. Because this is a new practice, all statements will be projections. These projections will estimate practice earnings over the next five years and are based on assumptions made based from the information in the previous sections. Be sure to explicitly state all assumptions. The projection for the first year should present monthly information; for all other years, quarterly or yearly information is acceptable.

Remember that for accounting purposes, the practice is separate from the NP. Starting a bank (checking) account for practice transactions is a must; it must be kept separate from personal accounts.

Income Statement

The annual income statement provides information about the practice's operations, specifically whether or not the operations have been profitable. The financial information collected previously will be used to project income and expenses. The major components of the income statement are revenues and expenses. Revenues are practice earnings for completing work. Revenue in healthcare businesses comes mainly from the reimbursement of patient visits, as well as dividends from business investments. This means every patient seen is a revenue source for the practice. Expenses are all the costs of running the practice, including salaries, supplies, medicines, equipment rental, and so on. Figure 5.4 is an example of how to report income and expenses.

Projected Income Statement

	Year 1				December	12 Months	Year 2	Year 3	Year 4	Year 5
	January	February	March	April						
Revenue:										
Services Provided	70,000	70,000	70,000	70,000	75,000	875,000	950,000	950,000	950,000	950,000
Expenses:										
Accounting	5,000	1,000	1,000	2,000	1,500	18,500	10,000	10,000	10,000	10,000
Legal Fees	8,000	5,000	1,000	1,000	5,000	27,000	2,000	2,000	2,000	2,000
Advertising	200	200	200	200	200	2,700	2,500	2,500	2,500	2,500
Salaries	35,000	35,000	35,000	35,000	35,000	420,000	420,000	450,000	450,000	450,000
Benefits	8,000	8,000	8,000	8,000	8,000	96,000	96,000	96,000	96,000	110,000
Conferences	0	0	1,000	1,000	0	8,000	8,000	8,000	8,000	8,000
Credit Card Fees	250	250	250	250	300	3,350	3,500	3,500	3,500	3,500
Depreciation	1,500	1,500	1,500	1,500	2,100	19,900	24,000	40,750	57,500	59,000
Insurances	1,500	1,500	1,500	1,500	1,500	18,000	20,000	20,000	20,000	20,000
Internet Access	200	200	200	200	200	2,400	2,500	2,500	2,500	2,500
Lab Fees	1,000	1,000	1,000	1,000	1,200	13,000	15,000	15,000	15,000	15,000
Licenses	200	200	200	200	200	2,400	2,500	2,500	2,500	2,500
Medical Supplies	1,500	1,500	1,500	1,500	1,500	18,000	18,000	18,000	18,000	20,000
Office Supplies	400	400	400	400	500	5,200	5,200	5,200	5,500	5,500
Rent	2,500	2,500	2,500	2,500	2,500	30,000	30,000	30,000	35,000	35,000
Repairs/Maintenance	250	250	250	250	250	3,000	3,000	3,000	3,000	3,000
Subscriptions	250	0	0	0	0	250	300	300	300	300
Taxes	700	700	700	700	700	8,400	9,000	9,000	9,000	9,000
Telephone/Answering Service	800	800	800	800	800	9,600	10,000	10,000	10,000	10,000
Travel	0	0	250	250	0	2,000	2,000	2,500	2,500	3,000
Utilities	500	500	500	400	500	5,600	5,600	6,000	6,000	6,000
Total Operating Expenses	67,750	60,500	57,750	58,650	61,950	713,300	689,100	736,750	758,800	776,800
Operating Profit	2,250	9,500	12,250	11,350	13,050	161,700	260,900	213,250	191,200	173,200
Interest Expense	1,375	1,410	1,345	1,335	850	13,915	9,000	6,700	4,200	1,535
Income before Taxes	875	8,090	10,905	10,015	12,200	147,785	251,900	206,550	187,000	171,665
Income Tax Expense	263	2,427	3,272	3,005	3,660	44,336	75,570	61,965	56,100	51,500
Net Income	613	5,663	7,634	7,011	8,540	103,450	176,330	144,585	130,900	120,166

Statement of Cash Flows

The annual statement of cash flows indicates sources of income and how the money was spent. This sounds simple, and it is. The statement of cash flows is basically a reorganized check register that provides valuable information to potential investors and the practice owner(s). The three sections of the statement correspond to the three main business functions: operating activities, investing activities, and financing activities. Operating activities show the cash flows for the main operations of the practice: income received for patient care and moneys paid to run the practice. Investing activities represent investments in the practice, such as purchasing a new X-ray machine. These investments are meant to improve the practice by expanding the services offered. Financing activities explain how the practice is financed: owner investments in the practice and debt financing. See Figure 5.5 for a sample statement.

Balance Sheet

This financial statement is a picture of the practice as of a specific date. The balance sheet provides information about the practice's resources (assets) and debts (liabilities). The difference between the assets and the liabilities of the practice is your residual equity in the practice. An example of a Projected Balance Sheet is shown in Figure 5.6.

Documents Section

The Documents Section includes all supporting legal papers and documents accumulated in the pre-planning process. Be sure to keep original documents safe and have copies notarized for authenticity if necessary. Copies of the following documents should be included:

- Rental or purchase agreement for building space, along with pictures of the space.
- Curriculum vitae for all owners and service providers.
- Licenses: RN, APRN, operational license, DEA, CLIA.
- Partnership agreement or documents of incorporation.
- Business agreements with vendors.
- Insurance Certificates: Malpractice, business, disaster, business umbrella, liability, and renters/owners.
- Advertising materials.

If the practice is a sole proprietorship, the following additional items should be included: owner income tax forms, personal financial records, and banking information

The length of the business plan varies greatly depending on the detail and how involved the operations of the business are. All four sections are needed to provide a complete overview of the business. Clearly, the pre-planning work assists in the compilation of the business plan. Reviewing sample business plans can be done at the following Web sites:

Projected Statement of Cash Flows

	Year 1						Year 2	Year 3	Year 4	Year 5
	January	February	March	April	December	12 Months				
Operating Activities										
Cash received from patients	7,000	7,000	7,000	7,000	7,500	87,500	95,000	95,000	95,000	95,000
Cash received from insurance companies	12,600	50,400	63,000	63,000	67,500	720,000	846,500	855,000	855,000	855,000
Payments to employees	−35,000	−35,000	−35,000	−35,000	−35,000	−420,000	−420,000	−450,000	−450,000	−450,000
Payments to vendors	−26,563	−25,088	−21,663	−22,015	−24,175	−269,673	−212,059	−245,896	−250,515	−265,314
Income tax payments				−11,084		−19,336	−67,761	−65,366	−57,566	−52,650
Interest payments	−1,375	−1,410	−1,345	−1,335	−850	−13,915	−8,970	−6,690	−4,210	−1,535
Total cash provided by operating activities	−43,338	−4,098	11,993	566	14,975	84,576	232,710	182,048	187,709	180,501
Investing Activities										
Purchase new medical equipment	−110,000				0	−150,000	−10,000	−25,000	−25,000	−40,000
Purchase office equipment	−5,000					−10,000	−5,000	−5,000	−5,000	−5,000
Purchase office furniture	−30,000					−30,000			−10,000	
Total cash used by investing activities	−145,000	0	0	0	0	−190,000	−15,000	−30,000	−40,000	−45,000
Financing Activities										
Cash received from bank	150,000					150,000				
Draw down on line of credit	45,000	5,000				50,000				
Repay line of credit			−5,000		−5,000	−63,915				
Principal repayment for note payable	−2,040	−2,060	−2,070	−2,080	−2,200	−25,420	−27,525	−29,810	−32,285	−34,960
Total cash provided by financing activities	192,960	2,940	−7,070	−2,080	−7,200	110,665	−27,525	−29,810	−32,285	−34,960
Change in cash	4,623	−1,158	4,923	−1,514	7,775	5,241	190,185	122,238	115,424	100,541
Cash balance at beginning of period	0	4,623	3,465	8,388	−2,534	0	5,241	195,426	317,664	433,088
Cash balance at end of period	4,623	3,465	8,388	6,874	5,241	5,241	195,426	317,664	433,088	533,629

5.6

Projected Balance Sheet

	Year 1					Year 2	Year 3	Year 4	Year 5
	January	February	March	April	December				
ASSETS									
Cash	4,623	3,465	8,388	6,874	5,241	195,426	317,664	433,088	533,629
Accounts Receivable	50,400	63,000	63,000	63,000	67,500	76,000	76,000	76,000	76,000
Office Equipment	5,000	5,000	5,000	5,000	10,000	15,000	20,000	25,000	30,000
Office Furniture	30,000	30,000	30,000	30,000	30,000	30,000	30,000	40,000	40,000
Medical Equipment	110,000	110,000	110,000	110,000	150,000	160,000	185,000	210,000	250,000
Accumulated Depreciation	-1,500	-3,000	-4,500	-6,000	-19,900	-43,900	-84,650	-142,150	-201,150
Total Assets	198,523	208,465	211,888	208,874	242,841	432,526	544,014	641,938	728,479
LIABILITIES									
Accounts Payable	4,689	3,597	3,183	3,321	3,724	36,796	36,910	37,684	40,174
Line of Credit	45,000	50,000	45,000	45,000	0	0	0	0	0
Income Tax Payable	263	2,690	5,961	-2,118	11,084	18,893	15,491	14,025	12,875
Note Payable to Bank	147,959	145,903	143,835	141,752	124,584	97,058	67,248	34,964	0
Total Liabilities	197,910	202,190	197,979	187,954	139,391	152,747	119,649	86,673	53,049
OWNER'S EQUITY									
Owner's Capital	613	6,276	13,909	20,920	103,450	279,780	424,365	555,265	675,430
Total Liabilities and Equity	198,523	208,465	211,888	208,874	242,841	432,526	544,014	641,938	728,479

- www.bplans.com/sample_business_plans.cfm
- www.myownbusiness.org/
- www.score.org/template_gallery.html

Despite all of the detailed planning and hard work, businesses can fail. Motivation, determination, and self-reliance can only get one so far. Most businesses fail because of insufficient financial planning. The most difficult part of starting a new practice is estimating the financial need for outside funding, the amount of credit required, and the costs of running the practice. It is impossible to consider all possible financial pitfalls. Unexpected items do occur, such as the closing of local businesses, patients losing their insurance coverage, or interest rates rising without notice. The NP needs to be a consummate professional and an astute manager. To succeed, the NP needs to combine solid clinical and leadership skills with constant monitoring of the practice's finances.

Risk Management for the Practice

Risk management involves an examination of current processes for potential liability and modifying processes to avoid errors. Preventive in nature, it serves to protect patients and practitioners from the impact of errors. Retaining an attorney, as well as an insurance expert, to assist in managing potential risk is a wise business practice. Two areas of risk that should concern the NP are clinical and operational errors, as well as malpractice and business liability concerns (Crowe & Carlyle, 2003). Insurance is necessary to protect both the clinical practice and the personal assets of the provider(s) (Barry, 2006).

Malpractice coverage is essential when delivering any kind of health care. Malpractice is a complaint against NP actions that violate the Scope of Practice or Nurse Practice Act and result in patient injury. An example of malpractice or liability at the business level would be failing to obtain patient consent before releasing medical records, thereby revealing personal health information without the patient's consent. Another example is fraudulent billing. When owning and operating a business, the owner has responsibility for all areas of the practice and must therefore be knowledgeable about all operations.

General liability insurance coverage is also necessary. This protects the practice from lawsuits resulting from injury, such as might be obtained if a chair in the waiting room collapses. An insurance professional can best guide the owner on the level and types of protection necessary for the practice. See Figure 5.7 for a brief listing and description of types of insurance.

Risk management also includes consistent documentation of healthcare. Using the following tools can help ensure this goal:

- Clinical guidelines
- Standard documentation forms
- Detailed job descriptions clearly articulating expectations
- Thorough policy and procedure manuals
- Documentation of preventive actions taken

All these are examples of sound risk management techniques, and implementation is encouraged.

5.7

Types of Business Insurance

General Liability—covers claims of negligence for bodily injury.

Business Umbrella Coverage—has a larger financial cap to cover claims against businesses.

Product Liability—covers injury if business provides a service or product and warnings or instructions were not properly explained.

Home-Based Business Insurance—covers home office if homeowner's policy excludes business related liabilities such as theft, injury, property loss, or disability.

Internet Business Insurance—covers damage incurred by viruses, malware, or hackers.

Criminal Insurance—covers against losses incurred by employees (theft, criminal activities, etc).

Business Interruption Insurance—covers expenses if unable to operate due to natural hazards.

Directors Coverage—covers management personnel in the event decisions resulted in harm.

Errors & Omissions Insurance—covers liability if something is missed or incorrectly implemented causing expense to someone.

Renters Insurance—covers property and belongings if business is located in rental space.

From www.sba.gov

Many practices now maintain medical records electronically. For practices using manual records, the use of a standard documentation form by all providers for all visits will help to ensure thorough and consistent documentation. The following statement in a medical record, "the physical exam was within normal limits," is legally inadequate because it does not document what body parts were evaluated or what is considered "normal." Rather, consider using a checklist documentation form that can save time and provide thorough documentation of care. Refer to the template in Section III as a guide or Figure 5.8. Because these forms are comprehensive, they assist in the coding and billing process as well.

Using a system of checks and balances for daily operations is also a good risk management approach. In the event of an emergency, all of the equipment in the emergency box needs to be current and in good working order. Expired or missing medications from the box will impede successful outcomes. Using a sim-

Sample Documentation Form

Name:_____ **Date/Time:** _____

S:
  C/C:
  HPI:

ROS: line through negatives & circle if positive and explain

Constitutional:	fever weight loss:
Eyes:	discharge itch redness vision change
ENT/mouth:	hearing loss ear pain congestion runny nose epistaxis sore throat dysphagia lymph nodes sores
Cardiovascular:	CP palpitations decreased circ
Respiratory:	SOB CP cough phlegm wheezing hemoptysis dyspnea
Gastrointestinal(GI):	N V Diah Abd pain GERD loss appetite p.o. fluids
Genito-Urinary(GU):	dysuria hematuria polyuria hesitancy nocturia discharge:
Musculoskeletal:	numbness tingling pain weakness swelling joint pain
Skin:	itch rash hives ulcers pain
Neurological:	headache dizziness LOC numbness tingling pain weakness
Psychiatric:	depression anxiety panic loss of sleep excessive sleep attending class
Endocrine:	weight loss weight gain moodiness hunger thirst inability to concentrate

Meds & OTCs:
Allergies :
Pt Med Hx:// Fam Med Hx :
Smoker: (No) // #_____/day___:yrs *ETOH*: (No)// #/wk: _____ *Drug use*:(No) (Yes)_____
Encouraged cessation/moderation   Encouraged cessation/moderation   Encouraged cessation/moderation

O:
HT: _____ WT: _____ T: _____ Pulse: _____ Resp: _____ BP:_____ LMP:

	circle each if normal	**describe abnl**
Appearance:	WDWN Alert cooperative in NAD	
SKIN:	Warm dry intact no lesions no erythema	
HEENT:	PERRLA EOM x 6 cornea clear no papilledema	
Eyes:	Sclera and conjunctiva clear anicteric without d/c	
Ears:	canals clear TMs: no bulging nl reflex nl landmarks	
Nose:	membranes wnl no exudates sinus not tender	
Oro/Post:pharynx	membranes wnl no erythema no exudate no lesions tonsils not enlarged	
Neck:	FROM supple no adenopathy no thyromegaly	
HEART:	RRR S1/S2 no murmur pulses equal: groin/DP/PT ____+	
LUNGS:	clear gd aeration no crackles no wheeze no rhonchi	
ABDOMEN:	audible BS soft nontender no masses no HSM no CVA tenderness	
MUSC/SKEL:	FROM all extrem no bruising no pain gd CSM strength = bilat joints: no pain no swelling no erythema	
NEURO:	A&O x 3 CN II-X grossly intact nl gait Romberg WNL	

	circle each if normal		describe abnl
RECTAL:	Skin clear no lesions no masses no hemorrhoid		
GU: Male: Penis:	__circumcised no lesions no d/c		
	Scrotum: no masses no hernias testicles ↓↓ bilat		
GYN: Female			
Breasts:	no axillary nodes no skin retractions no abnl mass		
	no lesions no expressible d/c		
Ext. genitalia:	nl hair distribution no lesions		
BUS/Vulva:	no tenderness no redness no d/c no lesions		
Vagina:	pink rugated no lesion no d/c		
Cervix:	pink no CMT no d/c nonfriable		
Uterus:	firm no masses nontender		
Adnexa:	no masses nontender		

IN OFFICE testing	Urine Dip:		Wet Prep
Urine HCG:	color:	blood:	pH:
Rapid Mono:	leuks:	Sp Grvty:	whiff:
Rapid Strep:	nitrites:	ketone:	Clue cells:
Rapid Flu:	Urobili:	bili:	WBC's:
Rapid HIV:	protein:	glucose:	RBC's:
	pH:		trich:
			yeast hyphae:

A/P:

Education/follow up instructions/ Handout(s) given and discussed:_____

(Y) (N) Patient has given me permission to leave a voicemail/email message about this visit.

Examiner's Signature: _____Date:_____ Contact Phone: _____

Interim/Phone Notes:

ple checklist monthly, as demonstrated in Section III, provides easy oversight and makes the task easy to delegate to others for completion. These checklists can be used for all routine tasks.

Patient Payer Systems

Currently, the healthcare system uses three major types of payer systems. The first, the Fee-for-Service system, has gained and lost popularity over the years. It is still a viable option for NP practices because there are fewer barriers to obtaining reimbursement. The Third-Party Payer system is the second and most frequently used system in the United States. The final system, the Contractual system, entails a written agreement to render care for a designated population for an agreed-upon stipend or payment (Tashakkori & Aghajanian, 2000).

Fee-for-Service systems are easily understood, as the patient makes payment directly to the care provider. No insurance forms are filed, so no reimbursement issues exist. Limitations to care are determined by the patient's perception of its necessity and ability to pay. Since an insurance company is not involved in the decision process, multiple conversations with the insurance company are avoided, which results in lower overhead costs.

A Third-Party Payer system means that a business or entity pays a healthcare provider for services on behalf of the patient. These payers include the government, Medicaid and Medicare, and private insurance, such as indemnity plans and Health Maintenance Organizations (HMOs).

As far back as 1988, NPs, serving as primary care providers, have understood the importance of gaining access to third-party reimbursement. Caraher (1988) pointed out the public's use of NP providers would climb if direct reimbursement were available to NPs as primary care providers. Currently, NPs are only a bit closer to achieving the goal of recognition as independent primary care providers. Most large insurance companies and state Medicaid programs follow the lead of the federal Medicare system in terms of the reimbursement process. Since 1977, federal legislation has been enacted allowing direct reimbursement to NPs, but there are always accompanying caveats in the legislation (see, for example, the 1977 Rural Health Clinics Service Act [PL95-210] and the Omnibus Reconciliation Act of 1980 [PL-96-499] of 1988 and 1990). Interpretation and implementation of laws allowing direct reimbursement to NPs have varied because opposing entities fear overbilling or loss of control if reimbursement directly to NPs is achieved (Caraher, 1988).

Direct stipend for Contracted Care delivered by NPs is the last reimbursement method. The NP is paid directly by the party entering into the contract with the NP, so no claims are filed for payment. The system exists primarily when a subpopulation, such as the sheltered homeless, desires healthcare coverage. The subpopulation may not have insurance or may not be able to access network coverage because of circumstances such as incarceration. For example, an NP business negotiates to provide primary care services to incarcerated youth or to students at a college health clinic for an agreed-upon fee. In these cases, the contract price covers all care rendered. Contract care does not require billing or empaneling of insurance. At the end of the year, a report is prepared for the contracting agency showing the services provided.

Billing, Coding, and Reimbursement

The Center for Medicare and Medicaid Services (CMS) is part of the U.S. Department of the Health and Human Services (HHS). The Center is responsible for creating and interpreting Medicare laws. Part A and Part B define Medicare reimbursement. Part A covers reimbursement for hospitalization, hospice, skilled nursing facilities, and some aspects of home health care. Part B covers physician services, outpatient services, laboratory, medical equipment, and other aspects of home health care. Parts A and B are governed by different reimbursement rules. Medicaid programs are federally funded but controlled through state-administered contractual programs different from those run by the federal government for Medicare. Nurse practitioners with individual National Provider Identifier numbers (NPIs) who meet certain qualifications may submit bills using the *Current Procedural Terminology (CPT) codes,* 4th edition (American Medical Association, 2004) and the *International Classification of Disease, 9th Revision, Clinical Modification (ICD-9) codes* (Hart and Hopkins, 2004) to describe care provided during a visit. By regulation payment is made ONLY for services that are:

- Defined as physician (level) services
- Medically necessary
- Actually provided
- Documented accurately
- Submitted correctly (Frakes & Evans, 2006)

The ICD–10 is scheduled for publication in 2010. Most private insurance companies base payment on similar parameters using these same codes. Medicaid contracts in some individual states are more NP friendly and will reimburse directly to NPs if the Practice Act allows. But, this acceptance of NP practice is not universal.

The process begins when an NP completes and documents a clinical visit in the medical record. The NP then completes an internal billing or encounter form that the office staff uses to charge the patient's insurance according to the care provided as documented by the NP. The patient is responsible for the required copayment. To obtain the maximum allowable reimbursement, the documentation needs to include the chief complaint, pertinent history gathered for both the patient and the family, physical exam, diagnosis, and plan of treatment. The submitted information includes the diagnosis assigned (ICD-9 code), as well as the level of acuity encountered and documented in the medical record using a CPT code. Typically, office staff or the billing company, if outsourced, transcribe the codes onto a Center for Medicare and Medicaid Services (CMS) 1500 form and submits it for reimbursement electronically. A comprehensive review, including guidance for this process can be found by reading Evaluation and Management Services Guide (2009) found at http://www.cms.hhs.gov/MLNProducts/downloads/eval_mgmt_serv_guide.pdf.

The key to responsible billing is twofold. First, the NP must thoroughly document the medical record to justify the level of acuity noted in the Evaluation and Management (E&M code) that is used to decide the CPT value. Coding techniques use acuity or relative work values to determine the level of medical decision necessary to work up the chief complaint, the level of clinical investigation necessary to diagnose the patient, and the time spent with the patient (Allen, Reinke, Pohl, Martyn, & McIntosh, 2003). As an illustration, if the presenting complaint is a sore throat and the history of present illness (HPI) documents only throat pain for two days, a low acuity or brief "problem-focused" level history will be completed. Conversely, if the HPI documents a chronological description of the development of the patient's pain, including characteristics like location, quality, severity, duration, timing, context, and associated signs and symptoms, an "extended" HPI (having four descriptors) is captured. If the complexity of the decision making surrounding the diagnosis is intricate because of an underlying illness requiring a complex physical exam that results in spending more time with the patient, a higher level of acuity can be billed. This must all be documented in the medical record. Reimbursement takes into account the complexity of the care rendered using the CPT code and the E&M code as noted on the CMS1500. Another factor taken into account in determining the CPT code is how well the patient is known to the practice. If the visit is the first encounter, the "new patient code" is used. If the patient had been seen at any time in the last three years, the visit is considered a returning patient (Frakes & Evans, 2006). A chart illustrating the complexity level needed to increase billing is found in Figure 5.9.

In the past, V code billings, which denote preventive or routine care, were not reimbursed, but V code charges are now reimbursable to an extent (www.CMS.gov). This illustrates the necessity of keeping current about changes in clinical practice and business management. Both evolve as information changes.

5.9

Complexity Chart for Evaluation and Management Services

E & M Category (new pt/returning pt)	Chief Complaint (C/C)	History Elements: Past Medical/ Family/Social	Review of System Elements	Physical Exam Elements
Problem Focused 99201/99212	1	None	1	1 to 5
Expanded Problem Focused 99202/99213	1	1 to 2 areas	2 to 9	6 to 11
Detailed 99203/99214	1 to 3 C/Cs	2 to 3 areas	12 to 14	12
Comprehensive 99204/99215	1 to 3 C/Cs	2 to 3 areas	12 to 14	14

In addition, a modifier can be added as a suffix to a CPT code. A modifier indicates a second complaint different from the identified chief presenting complaint. Modifiers, which indicate additional complexity or more time spent with a patient, can change the level of reimbursement. The addition of a modifier also may indicate which provider saw the patient. Using appropriate subterms or suffix identifiers adds information to the claim and can increase reimbursement rates by increasing the complexity of a visit (Alexander, 2009). Whoever completes the forms for reimbursement must be familiar with all the nuances to maximize reimbursement on the first attempt.

The second key to responsible billing requires that the NP must not knowingly allow inaccurate billing, which constitutes fraud. Fraudulent billing includes:

- Allowing staff to overstate the acuity on billing.
- Underbilling for services on the CMS 1500.
- Using "incident-to" billing with the physician's NPI to increase revenue when "incident-to" parameters are not met.
- Unbundling services to charge for each service individually.
- Upcharging, which is filing for care more difficult than the medical record indicates was necessary (Abood & Keepnews, 2000).

Federal rules state that **receipt** of the CMS 1500 form for reimbursement implies the **clinician knows and attests to accurate billing.** More information can be found at www.CMS.gov, in the Federal Register Guidelines, or in the 1997 Documentation Guidelines for Evaluation and Management Services that lists the parameters of coding and billing (http://www.cms.hhs.gov/MLNProducts/Downloads/MASTER1.pdf).

CMS administrators conduct audits and are always watching for fraudulent billing. If fraud is found, large fines can be levied against the practice. One recent case of fraud resulted in a fine of $50,000, with an additional fee of $1 million in restitution. This case involved an attempt to increase reimbursement by ordering a higher level of care than was needed for the patient (www.oig.hhs.gov).

"Incident-to" billing can legally occur *only* when the physician is physically in the office and the NP, who is employed by the physician or an independent contractor (not a practice partner), performs a visit under the supervision of the physician on an established patient of the practice. In addition, the physician must intend to see the patient in a follow-up visit. "Incident-to" cannot be billed if the physician is not present, if the patient is new to the practice, or if the patient will stay on the NP panel and not see the physician in the future. "Incident-to" billing is favored by practices because it garners a higher reimbursement rate (income) for the practice. Currently, the fee schedule (reimbursement level) is set by Medicare. The reimbursement rate is 80 percent of the fee schedule, with the patient responsible for paying the remaining 20 percent. Billing done using the physician's NPI number receives the full reimbursement. Bills submitted under the NPI number of the NP receive only 85 percent of the physician reimbursement or 68 percent (85% * 80%) of the fee schedule (Frakes & Evans, 2006; Counts & Mayolo, 2007).

Just as practicing nursing is both an art and a science, accurately coding and billing to achieve the maximum allowable reimbursement is both an art and a science. All healthcare professionals must learn coding. Coding has many rules and nuances that make it quite complicated. Formal training programs last 18 to 24 months.

Compliance Programs for Reimbursement

A billing compliance program is a "checks-and-balances" system for documentation and billing to prevent fraud. Compliance guidelines can be found at http://oig.hhs.gov/authorities/docs/physicians.pdf and are printed in the Federal Register (64 FR 48846). A compliance program is a voluntary program implemented to provide oversight of billing and reimbursement activity to ensure accurate and legal conduct. Implementation of such a program is recommended by the American Association of Nurse Attorneys (2005) for all healthcare practices, and it is especially advised if an outside vendor is used to perform billing functions on behalf of the practice. Even though billing may be done by a vendor, the healthcare practice and the provider listed for reimbursement on the CMS 1500 are held accountable for any erroneous activity. Billing is legal only when requesting payment for actual care rendered that is appropriately documented.

Creating a compliance program begins with appointing a "Compliance Officer;" in a small practice, this is usually the director. A compliance program consists of an internal audit, during which random checks ensure the practice is submitting honest claims for payment. Internal audits accomplish three tasks. First, they look for consistency and accuracy of billing by comparing coding and billing forms to documentation in the medical records. Secondly, they assess services provided to ensure they are "reasonable and customary" and necessary for care (i.e., no unnecessary care/visits are ordered). Finally internal audits allow directors to review policies, standards, and procedures for claims submissions to ensure they are current and acceptable (www.cms.gov).

The compliance officer reports items of concern to the appropriate party in the practice and helps to develop corrective actions. The federal Office of the Inspector General (OIG) oversees billing and shares models of compliance plans for healthcare practices (www.oig.hhs.gov). The OIG also audits private offices and practices for fraudulent billing practices. The fines for noncompliance can be hundreds of thousands of dollars. OIG looks for consistency between the billed coding and the documentation in the medical record. The OIG also offers an Annual Work Plan that gives suggestions and ideas to implement a compliance plan (American Association of Nurse Attorneys, 2005).

OIG has shown particular interest in the policy and actions taken once the practice finds a problem in a self-audit. In other words, OIG is interested in how a billing error is corrected and, more importantly, what safeguards are enacted to avoid recurrence. For example, if an outside firm does billing and "incident-to" was charged, but the physician was on vacation during that time, billing "incident-to" is inappropriate. How did the practice fix the error? What safeguards were enacted to prevent a repetition of this error? The appropriate response is to re-bill all patient encounters during the physician's vacation using the NP's NPI. In addition, a new policy should require that all CMS 1500 forms completed when the physicians are out of the office be bundled and sent to the billing company with a cover sheet stating that the physician was not in the office and to emphasize that the NP's NPI should be used.

Common errors that have been uncovered through internal audits include:

- Billing for services not rendered
- Double billing
- Billing for noncovered services
- Knowingly misusing provider identification numbers
- Unbundling: separating charges that are grouped together as one charge
- Failing to use modifiers to accurately identify providers

Medicare regulations suggest an effective compliance program include an annual review of five records per provider per payer (Medicare, 2005).

Another fraudulent activity to avoid is giving kickbacks. Kickbacks are a business arrangement among providers in which payment or compensation is paid for pre-arranging referrals to particular practitioners or laboratories. This type of arrangement is illegal because it interferes with objective medical decision making for the patient's best interest. It can also result in objections from other vendors claiming the "favored" vendors have unfair access to the practitioners and thus the resulting charges.

Cost-Savings Management

Cost-savings opportunities in running a business are attainable only if the "that's how it's always been done" theme is not part of the practice's mantra. Innovations in technology, changes in patient expectations, and fluctuating economies all make evaluation and improvement necessary to maintain a thriving practice.

Simply stated, efficiency is the foundation of running a practice at its highest potential. Although potential isn't always synonymous with profit maximization, it is related to how smoothly daily tasks are accomplished. If tasks are done on time by the right person, efficient production will allow the practice to achieve its financial potential.

Cost review and bargain shopping for office supplies and medical supplies is an area for possible savings. Many vendors offer each product, and cost comparisons among them should be done at least annually. Purchasing supplies wisely can lead to savings. In many cases, vendors will offer contract deals and "across-the-board" savings for purchases made in volume.

Reviews of services offered and associated profitability should be periodically evaluated. For example if a patient is seen for a verruca (wart) removal and the visit takes longer than a standard visit without increased complexity, the reimbursement may not match the time spent or the cost of necessary equipment. The service review should highlight those services that generate a profit and are synchronous and vital to the stated mission of the practice. Not every practice can do everything for everyone. Practice only what you excel at, and don't hesitate to refer to a specialist colleague.

The practice director/owner needs to be aware of the practice's finances. This means revenues and expenses, as well as cash flow must be monitored. The use of a monthly budget can help the owner evaluate individual staff performance and the overall practice. A budget can also serve inform all practitioners as to what level of work is expected. Compelling budget projections use reliable data to provide confident estimates rather than "guestimates," and they forecast levels needed to achieve the fiscal goals for the next year (DeSilets & Pinkerton, 2004).

Henderson (2005) listed the importance of budgeting by highlighting the skills needed to complete the process:

- Planning: the ability to forecast future business activity.
- Communication: the ability to brief superiors and staff on funding needs and how available funding will impact the practice's ability to complete daily activities or forego them.
- Coordination: allocation of funds between staffing and equipment needs.
- Motivational: the skill to inspire staff to embrace standards to complete the task even when resources are decreased.
- Management: controlling the flow of resources in an attempt to collaborate without making staff vulnerable.
- Evaluation: determining whether staff utilization patterns are appropriate and whether managers meet annual goals.

Contino (2001) explains the process of budgeting succinctly: it "entails reviewing revenues and expenses, projecting patient volumes, and estimating the revenues needed to cover necessary staffing, supply, and capital equipment costs" (p. 16). The budget must clearly represent the needs of the practice. Many types of budgets can be prepared. The most valuable lists all projected services (revenues) and costs (expenses). The actual results should be compared to the budget at least monthly. Any deviation from the budget should be investigated to explain any issues that need to be resolved. This exercise will help the owner understand the financial aspect of the practice. Figure 5.10 illustrates a simple budget that will help achieve financial goals.

The Capital Budget details the equipment needs of the practice. It imposes restraint on the practice when deciding what equipment to purchase or rent and when to make that commitment. Because most equipment is very expensive, the practice needs to identify those cost-effective screening devices and equipment that are absolutely essential for everyday use in a specific practice. As the practice matures, additional equipment can be purchased.

Provider and patient flow also need to be considered. The floor plan and use of space should be evaluated. If possible, have separate examination rooms and offices, rather than a joint office/examination room. The reason is that when a practitioner is not present, the office/examination room may remain unused. No one feels comfortable using another practitioner's office. The office of the NP who has the most weekly sessions should be closest to the examination rooms. Less time will be lost walking to see patients and then walking back to the office to chart. Each examination room should be set up identically for efficient use by any staff member. Assigning a specific exam room to an NP will result in time savings as a result of familiarity with the quirks of the room. Set up a communication system/intercom allowing for communication, so staff members won't need to search for each other. Understandable signs will facilitate traffic flow and allow patients to find bathrooms, examination rooms, or laboratory/testing areas without direction from the staff (Malkin, 2002).

5.10

Sample Budget

	Budget January	Actual January	Difference	Explanation
Revenue:				
Services Provided	70,000	68,000	−2,000	Fewer pt than expected
Expenses:				
Accounting	5,000	6,000	1,000	extra training for office staff
Legal Fees	8,000	8,500	500	
Advertising	200	500	300	
Salaries	35,000	25,000	−10,000	one nurse position open
Benefits	8,000	7,000	−1,000	one nurse position open
Conferences	0	0	0	
Credit Card Fees	250	150	−100	fewer pt using charge card
Depreciation	1,500	1,500	0	
Insurances	1,500	1,000	−500	one bill not received yet
Internet Access	200	175	−25	
Lab Fees	1,000	2,000	1,000	more tests needed
Licenses	200	300	100	down one nurse
Medical Supplies	1,500	1,500	0	
Office Supplies	400	350	−50	
Rent	2,500	2,500	0	
Repairs/Maintenance	250	150	−100	
Subscriptions	250	100	−150	
Taxes	700	500	−200	
Telephone/Answering Service	800	700	−100	started business in second week
Travel	0	0	0	
Utilities	500	500	0	
Total Operating Expenses	67,750	58,425	−9,325	
Operating Profit	2,250	9,575	7,325	
Interest Expense	1,375	1,375	1,375	
Income Before Taxes	875	8,200	5,950	

Business principles highlight the importance of having the right people work together using their knowledge efficiently (Collins, 2001). This means the appropriate person should complete each task. This is sometimes difficult because of personal preference or lack of skill, but having an NP file charts or an office manager empty trash is not an efficient use of personal skills.

Technology has increased efficiency tremendously. Ready access to the Internet to inquire about drug interactions is more efficient than paging through the *Physician's Desk Reference.* Systems of registration and patient education have become electronic as well. Making a copy of an insurance card on a copy machine for the patient chart is an obsolete practice. Insurance card scanners smaller than pens are now used; the card is scanned and stored as a portable document format (PDF). This can be used over and over for laboratory work, inquiries for referrals, and reimbursement.

Electronic Medical Records (EMRs) are reputed to be the center of efficiency for healthcare practices. The start-up costs can be as high as $40,000 per provider, which is a large investment for a small practice. Another obstacle to their use in small practices is an on-site computer specialist is needed to choose, implement, and quickly solve technical problems. Even if the charting software is not operating, patient visits must still be documented. A reliable back up is necessary. Approximately 24 percent of physician offices across the country use EMRs, but in practices of fewer than three providers, only approximately 12 percent use them (Kane, 2009).

The federal government is funding studies to see how electronic records can improve the efficiency of practices to realize cost savings and better health care. Specifically, how EMRs can improve communications between providers and practices, decrease duplicative care, and provide improved management of complicated cases. CMS incentives are available if a practice can show "meaningful use," with implementation defined as:

- E-prescribing
- Exchange of health information with other providers
- Quality of care improvement
- Capacity improving clinical decision making

The government has identified the above points as meaningful indicators. Most believe smaller practices won't be able to implement these indicators and, therefore, they will not be eligible for the CMS incentives (Kane, 2009).

If a practice is not maintaining records electronically, then dictation programs or dictation companies can help increase efficiency. Personal computer-based dictation programs are affordable and save time. They have a medical dictionary installed, so they comprehend the subject matter and vocabulary and are easily installed on any office computer to assist in efficient charting of medical records. If paper charts are used, a standard documentation form can increase efficiency.

Ergonomics is another area to consider. Having an ergonomically correct desk and computer station can help decrease injuries from overuse syndromes and may actually increase productivity and efficiency (www.OSHA.gov). Setting up each station with items in the same place on each station can decrease time wasted in the hunt for the stapler or paper clips.

Choice of personnel is another area where savings can be realized. Hiring "occasional" or per-diem staff can save salary and benefits. Often, individuals who work per-diem need flexible schedules and cannot or do not want regular work schedules. In turn, per-diem workers also give the practice flexibility; they can be engaged during high demand times without overstaffing during lower demand times. Per-diem staff do not receive benefits, so they do receive a slightly higher hourly rate. Per-diem staff can cancel or be let go at any time. These workers are, in essence, independent contractors. Another staffing option is the use of nursing employment agencies. One difference is that per-diem staff have a relationship directly with the practice, whereas nursing employment agency staff have contractual agreements with the agency. The hourly rate for an agency nurse is generally greater than that of a per-diem staff person because agency nurses receive benefits from the agency.

As discussed, revenue can be increased by coding maximally and eliminating denials through submission of valid and accurate data. Instruction manuals found on the CMS Web site may assist in accurate submissions and timely reimbursement (http://www.cms.hhs.gov/Manuals/IOM/itemdetail.asp?filterType =none&filterByDID=-99&sortByDID=1&sortOrder=ascending&item ID=CMS018912&intNumPerPage=10). The American Medical Association offers a free monthly newsletter, called the *CPT Assistant,* that helps keep NPs updated with coding tips (Hildebrand, 2005). The monthly journal *Family Practice Management* always has helpful tips and suggestions for practice savings and efficiency.

Conclusion

The NP has many options and opportunities for employment or ownership of a healthcare practice. Business literacy, especially financial literacy, is a necessary foundation for an NP practice. If interested in starting a business, pre-planning analyses and writing a business plan are crucial. Nurse practitioners can use all their clinical talent and creative problem-solving skills to inspire a business venture to achieve professional goals and freedom. Experts in law, accounting, and insurance will help protect the NP and the proposed practice. More and more NPs are venturing into practice ownership, either alone or in conjunction with another professional. Understanding a business plan and the information it contains will assist the NP in starting a practice, joining a privately owned practice, or becoming a partner of an existing business. Elements and documents of a business plan reviewed here are essential. Receiving payment for NP services has also been discussed through the payer systems, empaneling, coding, billing, and reimbursement. Comprehensive and compliant coding was stressed to ensure legal and speedy reimbursement. Finally cost savings opportunities and the importance of a budget to the financial health of the practice and its owner were pointed out.

Reflective Thinking Exercises

1. Imagine contact from an attorney for a long-lost relative about an inheritance. The bequest included paid start-up expenses for any business, but the attorney had to be informed how much would be needed. The one caveat on the bequest is that the business must make a profit or the start-up funds need to be repaid. What type of business should be pursued? How would you begin researching the business possibilities?

2. Research the local healthcare scene and list examples of each of the major patient payer systems used in the area.
3. Review a recent personal healthcare encounter:
   a. Consider elements of the visit needing improvement if offered in a new business?
   b. Was the environment for the visit efficient? Was there a long wait to be seen?
   c. Document the visit long hand on lined paper, on the documentation form included in this chapter, and read it into a tape recorder. Which documentation process is more efficient?
   d. Using the documentation form, perform coding and billing. Find an ICD-9 code and CPT code for the visit.

References

(2004, October) Important laws for small businesses retrieved from http://www.allbusiness.com/legal/laws-government-regulations-business/385-1.html

http://www.cms.hhs.gov/MLNEdWebGuide/25_EMDOC.asp http://www.cms.hhs.gov/National ProvIdentStand/

The House Agriculture Committee approved amendments to the Federal Crop Insurance Act. (H.R. Rep. No. 300, 1991).

Abood, S. & Keepnews, D. (2000) *Understanding payment for advanced practice nursing services: Volume one: Medicare reimbursement.* Washington, DC: American Nurses Association.

Aboul-Enein, N. F. (2009). *A mobile clinic's financial model on ADVANCE for Nurse Practitioners.* Retrieved June 25, 2009, from ADVANCE for Nurse Practitioners: http://nurse-practitioners.advanceweb.com/editorial/content/editoria l.aspx?cc=7305.

Alexander, N (2009). Personal interview June 18, 2009 (M. O'Brien, Interviewer).

Allen, K., Reinke, C., Pohl, J., Martyn, K., McIntosh, E. (2003, May). Nurse practitioner coding practices in primary care: a retrospective chart review. *Journal of the American Academy of Nurse Practitioners, 15(5),* 231–236.

American Association of Nurse Attorneys, (2005). *Business and Legal Guidebook for Nurse Practitioners.* Lenexa: author. Retrieved from (www.taana.org)

American Medical Association (2004). CPT 2004: *Current Procedural Terminology: Professional Edition.* Washington, DC: Author.

Balanced Budget Act of 1997. (1997). 42 USC 4511, 4512.

Barry, P., (2006, August). Perspectives on private practice. Professional malpractice insurance and practicing within professional guidelines. *Perspectives in Psychiatric Care, 42(3),* 201–203. Retrieved July 3, 2009, from CINAHL with Full text database.

Buppert, C. (2008). *Nurse Practitioner's Business Practice and Legal Guide.* Sudbury: Jones and Bartlett Publishers.

Buppert, C. (2002). "Billing for nurse practitioner services: what benefits does an NP bring to a medical practice?" *Medscape Nurses from WebMD.* Retrieved June 17, 2009 from http://www.medscape.com/viewarticle/422935_2.

Caraher, M. (1988, April). The importance of third-party reimbursement for NPs. *The Nurse Practitioner, 13(4),* 50, 52, 54.

Cardamone, M. Shaver, M., Werthman, R. (2004, April). Business planning reasons definitions, and elements. *Healthcare financial management,* 40–46.

Chen, C., McNeese-Smith, D., Cowna, M., Upenieks, V., & Afifi, A. (2009, May–June). Evaluation of a nurse practitioner-led management model in reducing drug utilization and cost. *Nursing Economics, 27(3).* p.160 (9). Expanded Academic ASAP. Gale. Trinity College. 3 July 2009.

Collins, J. (2001). *Good to Great: Why Some Companies Make the Leap . . . and Others Don't.* New York: HarperCollins Publishing.

Contino, D. (2001, August). Financial management. Budget training: it's overdue. *Nursing Management, 32*(8), 16–17. Retrieved August 16, 2009, from CINAHL with Full Text database.

Crowe, M., & Carlyle, D. (2003, July). Deconstructing risk assessment and management in mental health nursing. *Journal of Advanced Nursing, 43*(1), 19–27. Retrieved August 20, 2009, from CINAHL with Full Text database.

Crumbie, A. (2006, May). Nurse partnership for a nurse practitioner. *Primary Health Care, 16(4),* 14–16. Retrieved July 5, 2009 from CINAHL with Full text database.

Counts, M. and Mayolo, R. (2007, June). Growing revenue with APNs. *Nursing Management,* 49–50.

DeSilets, L., & Pinkerton, S. (2004, March). Administrative angles. budget$!! budget$!! budget$!! *Journal of Continuing Education in Nursing, 35*(2), 52–53. Retrieved August 16, 2009, from CINAHL with Full Text database.

Frakes, M., and Evans, T. (2006, March-April). An overview of medicare reimbursement regulations for advanced practice nurses. *Nursing Economics, 24(2).* 59–66.

Goolsby, M. (2005, September). 2004 AANP national nurse practitioner sample survey, part I: an overview. *Journal of the American Academy of Nurse Practitioners, 17(9),* 337–341. Retrieved July 5, 2009 from CINAHL with Full text database.

Hart, A and Hopkins, C. (2004). *2004 ICD-9-CM: Professional for physicians: International Classification of Diseases, 9th revision, Clinical Modification.* Los Angeles: Practice Management Information Corporation.

Henderson, E. (2005, February). Balancing the books: budgeting within residential care. *Nursing & Residential Care 7(2),*

Hildebrand, P. (2005, May). Learn the business skills of advanced nursing practice. *The Nurse Practitioner, 30(5),* 55–56.

Horrocks, S., Anderson, E., and Salisbury, C. (2002). Systematic review of whether nurse practitioners working in primary care can provide equivalent care to doctors. *British Medical Journal, 324,* 819–823.

Kane, L. (2009). Best EMRs for small practices. *Medscape Business of Medicine.* Retrieved August 10, 2009 from http://www.mcdscape.com/viewarticle/702950.

Kaplan, L. and Brown, M. (2009, February). State and local APN salary data: the best evidence for negotiations. *The Journal for Nurse Practitioners, 5(2),* 91–97.

Kleinpell, R., and Perez, D. (2006, May). Negotiation strategies for ACNP practice. *The Nurse Practitioner, 31(5),* 6–11.

Mackey, T. (2005, December). Planning your nursing business. *Journal of the American Academy of Nurse Practitioners, 17(12),* 501–505.

Mackey, T., McNeil, N., Klingensmith, K. (2004, January-February). Outsourcing issues for nurse practitioner practices. *Nursing Economics, 22(1),* 21–32.

Malkin, J., (2002). *Medical and dental space planning: a comprehensive guide to design, equipment, and clinical procedures.* New York: John Wiley.

Miller, M., Snyder, M., Lindeke, L. (2005, September). Forces of change. nurse practitioners: current status and future challenges. *Clinical Excellence for Nurse Practitioners, 9(3),* 162–169. Retrieved June 14, 2009, from CINAHL with Full text database.

Mundinger, M., Kane, R., Lenz, E., Totten, A., Tsai, W., Cleary P., (2000). Primary care outcomes in patients treated by nurse practitioners or physicians: A randomized trial. *JAMA: The Journal of American Medical Association, 283(1),* 59–68.

Newland, J. (2006, May). 2006 Nurse practitioner salary & practice survey. *Nurse Practitioner, 31(5),* 39. Retrieved July 5, 2009 from CINAHL with Full text database.

Rollet, J. and Lebo, S. (2007, October). 2007 Salary Survey Results: A Decade of Growth. *Advance for Nurse Practitioners.* Retrieved June 29, 2009 from http://nurse-practitioners.advanceweb.com/editorial/content/editoria l.aspx?cc=105177

Rural Health Clinics Service Act (1977) Public Law No. 95-210.

Sharp, K. (2006, March). Salary survey results from the northeast Tennessee nurse practitioner association. *The Tennessee Nurse, 69 (1),* 1. Retrieved July 5, 2009 from CINAHL with Full text database.

Shute, N. (2008, March) Can't find a doctor? you are not alone. US News and World Report, USNews.com. Retrieved August 8, 2009 from http://health.usnews.com/articles/health/living-well-usn/2008/03/19/cant-find-a-doctor-youre-not-alone.html.

Tashakkori, Z., Aghajanian, A. (2000, April) Reimbursement issues in advanced practice nursing: an overview. *MedSurg Nursing*. FindArticles.com. 03 Aug, 2009. http://findarticles.com/p/articles/mi_m0FSS/is_2_9/ai_n18609885/

The Omnibus Reconciliation Act of 1980. (1980). Public Law No. 96-499.

U.S. Small Business Administration. (2009). *Small Business Assessment Tool*. Retrieved July 24, 2009, from http://www.sba.gov/smallbusinessplanner/plan/getready/index.html

U.S. Small Business Administration. (2009). *Get Insurance*. Retrieved August 3, 2009, from http://sba.gov/smallbusinessplanner/manage/getinsurance /SERV_INSURANCE.html)

Role of the Nurse Practitioner Director/Owner: Implications for Strategic Planning and Management

6

Learning Objectives

1. Describe the components of the strategic planning process.

2. Describe how the director actively employs a mission statement, vision, and goals in an organization.

3. Discuss the process and develop an organizational design for a small business.

4. Articulate key points of the director/owner's job description as a professional, clinician, leader, and manager.

5. Examine federal agencies and regulations regarding compliance in healthcare businesses.

6. Define standards in terms of obtaining practice agency accreditation.

7. Develop a policy and procedures manual to guide operations using templates.

8. Identify components of a disaster/emergency plan of an agency and integrate the surrounding community's plan.

Key Words: organizational structure, job description, mission statement, strategic plan, risk management, regulatory compliance, practice accreditation, disaster and emergency plan

In many practice areas, nurse practitioners (NPs) have capitalized on opportunities to employ their leadership, professional, and management skills as directors of health services. Examples of NP-run practices include college health centers, retail clinics, and primary care practices. These can serve as frameworks

137

to demonstrate the responsibilities of an agency director. In this chapter, the word "director" denotes the role of owner in a privately owned practice or of a leader in a clinical practice or agency.

Directors need to understand the practice's organizational design and structure. Therefore, identifying and illustrating governance structures and communication mechanisms for the practice are important skills. As described in Chapter 5, planning is necessary for a practice to succeed. Strategic planning is an exercise that enables the practice to reach its short- and long-term business goals. The duties and responsibilities of the NP director/owner should be delineated through a job description. The chapter describes the documents that guide both clinical and regulatory oversight. Examples of relevant policy and procedures are given, along with a discussion of their importance to the smooth operation of a practice. Section III provides relevant templates. Finally, the regulatory compliance process at a practice level is presented. This chapter demonstrates how NPs can be autonomous providers using professional, clinical, leadership, and management skills.

Organizational Design

More than 50 percent of healthcare businesses operate in out-patient settings, and projections indicate that in 10 years, more than 70 percent of healthcare services will be provided outside the hospital setting (Dunham-Taylor & Pinczuk, 2010). In fact, advances in technology already enable more interaction between providers and patients through telephone and computer functions. Innovation and implementation of technology is rising steadily, as electronic documentation becomes increasingly available and easier to use (Porter-O'Grady & Malloch, 2007). Thus, the NP director needs to determine how to operate the practice in a patient-friendly and cost-effective manner. Virtual interactions and resources can be used for follow up, specific screenings, and other healthcare needs. Studer's book, *Hardwiring Excellence: Purpose, Worthwhile Work, and Making a Difference* (2003), shares ideas about "jumpstarting" an organization in realigning its mission, philosophy, and strategic plan.

Strategic Planning

Strategic management is crucial because it provides guidance and direction for the practice. It applies to all business activities of a practice and flows from the strategic planning process. Mosely (2009) describes strategic planning as crucial to be a successful business as it guides growth and operations.

He explains that *strategy* has many dimensions, including:

- Steering the direction of operations for a specific period of time, usually three to five years.
- Building a reputation for the business.
- Integrating the business vision throughout the entire organization.
- Balancing the organization's mission to adapt to the external environment.
- Ensuring decisions are based on true long-term commitments.

- Having and being comfortable with a sense of risk and uncertainty.
- Seeking change and growth for the business.
- Refusing to accept the status quo.

If the practice has a Board of Directors, its members will participate with the director in the strategic planning process. The strategic planning process involves integrating the information obtained in the business plan into a useful strategic plan. The strategic plan articulates a vision for the practice's future and describes how that vision will be achieved. Many models exist for the strategic planning process (http://managementhelp.org; http://score.org; http://netmba.com; https://sba.org); all result in a relevant practice that responds to the needs of its patients. The first step in the strategic planning process is defining the practice's core values, mission, and vision.

Core Values

Core values are the foundation of the practice. They do not describe the practice nor do they change with circumstances; rather, they are the principles guiding everyday conduct of the business. Dunham-Taylor and Pinczuk (2010) describe core values as the overarching beliefs that constitute the "backbone" of policy of an organization. The following need to be considered when articulating core values:

- What makes the practice special?
- Is there a special niche that the practice wants to enter?
- What reputation does the practice want to acquire?

For example, in a college health center, the core values revolve around teaching decision making based on health and healthy values. The clinician must acknowledge the patient is in a developmental stage and is experimenting with self-imposed boundaries instead of those dictated by an authority figure. In addition, providers of college health must be mindful that students frequently make poor health decisions because of peer influence. The NP must invoke a nonjudgmental acceptance of patients despite "risky behaviors" that result in the need for medical care. Education is crucial not only for self-care, but also for healthy lifestyle choices that may not have been modeled at home.

For a primary care practice, the core values may be similar: respectful and nonjudgmental primary care. However, the emphasis is to provide efficient, evidence-based, profit-producing care. Providers must accept a patient's self-determination and independence and provide education as needed.

Mission Statement

The mission statement communicates the practice's fundamental purpose. It is different from a vision statement in that a mission statement focuses on the practice's operation as presented to the public, while a vision statement is for internal planning and focuses on the practice's future. The mission statement is a succinct statement describing what the practice does, its specific competencies, and why it exists. A summary of the practice's values should also be included.

The mission statement can be referred to as a steadfast resource for decision making and should guide the conduct of all operations.

A college health clinic's mission may be to deliver primary health care to newly autonomous patients, thereby encouraging development of these individuals with special emphasis on teaching health self-advocacy and self-care. This is accomplished one on one by incorporating self-care education in each visit and, in a larger context, by incorporating campus wide health education on self-care for common illness.

For a primary care practice, the mission statement may consider providing accessible, cost-effective, nonjudgmental, evidence-based, patient-centered healthcare methods that include the patient in all healthcare planning and decision making. Section III includes a template of a mission statement.

Vision Statement

The vision statement flows from the core values. It describes the practice's future and how it will differ from the way it currently runs. It should "also reflect [the] kind [of] organization we intend to become in order to have [the] hoped for impact" (http://www.createthefuture.com). The strategic planning participants should consider the following attributes of the practice: its future size, reputation, scope of activities, and types of programs. More specific considerations are budget issues and resources, the targeted population, and staff size and composition.

Goals/Objectives and Strategies

The practice plan helps accomplish the stated mission and vision. Goals and objectives are statements describing the results the practice wants to achieve during the planning period. They derive from the mission and vision statements and can include topics such as growth, profitability, cost-effective operations, resources needed to reach goals, staff utilization and performance, and relationships with the community. Goals and objectives are typically stated in terms that can be measured quantitatively. Strategies explain the approach the practice will take to reach the stated goals and objectives. The strategies will specify who is responsible for achieving a specific goal, when the goal must be achieved, and how progress toward attaining the goals and objectives will be measured.

In this phase, choices must be made, because the practice can't do everything. A decision must be made about which of the possible goals and objectives the practice will pursue. Other goals need not be discarded, but they will have to be pursued at a later time.

Monitoring

This phase is as important as planning because progress toward goals and objectives must be monitored regularly. Monitoring allows the practice to review progress to date and to focus on obstacles and issues encountered. Changes in the external and internal environment of the practice may have changed, and resolution of issues encountered may require adjustments to the goals/objectives and strategies. The strategic planning process does not guarantee survival or growth of the practice. The plan must be dynamic and should be updated as necessary to accommodate innovative ideas and keep the focus on the agency's vision and mission.

Organizational Structures

One must consider the business foundation and current operations to identify and articulate the organizational structure. The organization chart is a graphic representation of who reports to whom; it is required documentation for some licensure and accreditation processes. The strategic plan assists in creating the appropriate structure of an agency. Organization charts provide graphic guides of the governing hierarchy and a clear illustration of each position's relationship to the organization as a whole. It shows reporting lines and depicts where decision making authority lies within a practice. Nurse practitioner-run businesses often appear horizontal because each NP usually has the authority to make decisions at the point of care. An organizational chart must be updated as the practice changes (Randolph, 2008). Chapter 5 had an example of an Organizational Structure Chart. Such charts diagram authority and communication within a practice.

In a sole proprietorship, the structure is uncomplicated, as one person receives all daily operation reports and is ultimately responsible for final decisions. In partnerships and corporations, the structure can become complex. For example, a college health practice may have up to three reporting lines for decision making or governance overseeing its operations. Each line deals with a different aspect of daily operations. Reporting consists of:

- *Medical care* reporting to a collaborating physician, or an NP director.
- *Operational information* reporting to the appropriate authority or the position in the organizational chart responsible for oversight of day-to-day operations.
- *Business affairs* reporting to the owner(s): In the case of a corporation, the Board of Trustees or Board of Directors represent the owners. They are not interested in reviewing medical case reports or daily operational information. They are interested in reviewing financial information and reports regarding operational concerns.

Director's Job Description

The Director frequently feels like a jack-of-all-trades. Whatever responsibilities are not assigned to someone else belong to the director. In a large practice, the director tends to be more involved in achieving the broad goals of the agency. In a smaller practice, the director is responsible for monitoring progress toward broad goals, as well as day-to-day operations. One of the director's primary foci is awareness of environment influences and competitors. The director must also embrace and encourage change. In addition, a director must maintain clinical competence. The NP's reputation as a clinician may be what attracts people to the practice. Success is often both exhausting and yet exhilarating. Duties are as diverse as setting standards through actions and policy, as complex as hiring and staffing appropriately, and as challenging as preparing for regulatory inspections. The following is a nonexhaustive list of tasks for the director within the four aspects of the ANP role: Professional, Clinician, Leader, and Manager.

Professional

1) *Role Model*—The director of the practice sets the tone for all others. As "the boss," the director is a role model for every staff member, so the director's energy and approach to treating patients will be judged acceptable and emulated by others. Therefore, the director needs to have high energy and act efficiently, confidently, and competently. The director should have a professional look and demeanor. Wearing a well-fitting lab coat and clean professional clothing is important. Budney, Rogers, Mandracchia, and Lascher (2006) found lab coats and professional attire encourage patient confidence. Coats can be embroidered so patients can see a name and title, but it is important to introduce yourself at every visit and to explain the NP role each time to highlight and clarify the credential of a nonphysician provider. Further, all clinical staff should also wear lab coats or scrubs. Front desk staff should dress as if they are scheduled to have a lunch with *the* most influential person in the community, as they are the first impression patients receive of the practice. If you need to establish a dress code policy to achieve this objective, use the blank policy form at the front of Section III for guidance. Greeting each patient at the front desk in a respectful manner does wonders for patient satisfaction and creates a positive reputation and excellent word-of-mouth advertising for the practice.

2) *Leader*—The director leads the entire organization by overseeing the mission, vision, and tone of the business. The NP director should focus energy and time in implementing the vision in a creative manner. Using Senge's (2006) ideas about building learning-oriented cultures rather than staying in one's comfort zone, the NP director can maximize resource use, expand the business, and successfully fulfill the vision.

    Over time, the NP director learns to trust and follow intuition by doing things in ways others may not always think is "best," particularly if it conflicts with preserving or enhancing the bottom line. But, many steps forward have begun with one small financial step backward. This thinking is similar to the classic statement by Bennis and Nanus (1985), in which they differentiated between managers and leaders: "managers are people who do things right and leaders are people who do the right things" (p. 21). The NP director should also be aware of the importance of the concept of emotional intelligence, which states that emotions impact one's life more than one's intelligence. Goleman (1998) suggests ways to assist in increasing one's emotional intelligence to maximize leadership abilities to make connections and partnerships with others. This requires connecting with the emotions of others. This skill also augments the leader's ability to motivate people to actively participate in change and embrace new modalities leading to improved outcomes.

3) *Mentor*—Once the practice is open and running smoothly, consider becoming a preceptor for an NP student for a semester or a mentor for a newly employed

NP. Finger (2005) suggests that mentors are very useful in helping others transition from RN to ANP roles. Mentors do not have the weekly commitment that academic preceptors do. Instead, they serve as long-term guides who share knowledge and experience with new NPs in expressions of a role, in advancing clinically in a specialty field, or in starting as an entrepreneur (Hayes and Kalmakis, 2007). In defining mentoring in nursing, Grossman (2007) points out the importance of more NPs taking on the role: "mentoring in nursing encompasses a guided experience, formally or informally assigned, over a mutually agreed-on period, that empowers the mentor and mentee to develop personally and professionally within the auspices of a caring, collaborative, culturally competent, and respectful environment" (p. 28). Remember that the mentor also develops, changes, and grows. So mentoring includes collegial relationships through which the mentor helps the mentee and the mentee helps the mentor. This type of organizational culture is ideal and something both the director and the other employees can strive to create.

Clinician

1) *Expert*—During the hectic period of starting or managing a business, the director must maintain clinical expertise through active practice and continuing education. The director should embrace and provide an example of the highest standards of patient care, evidence-based practice, and consciousness of outcomes and areas for potential improvement. An effective technique for achieving these goals is reflective-based practice. Take fifteen minutes a day to reflect on care delivered, interactions with others, and patient experiences. Through this reflection, one assesses the practice. The assessment can use skills learned in the nursing process, whereby one: [A]ssesses business action and offerings, [D]iagnoses whether they were effective/positive or in need of improvement, [P]lans an intervention to improve or change operations, [I]mplements the planned change, and [E]valuates or reflects again on the status of the business for ongoing improvement (American Nurses Association, 2009).

2) *Quality Administrator*—Decisions for setting guidelines or acceptable clinical interventions reside with the director. Be sure chosen clinical guidelines are current and, if available, use evidence-based practice in care regimens. Become a role model and inspire peers, students, and educators to also use them (Adams & McCarthy, 2007). An administrator who understands the priorities of the practice will stay in tune with its operations and earn the respect of the staff. Clinical guidelines, as well as strategic plans, should be reviewed regularly. Conway-Morana (2009) suggests that this be done quarterly.

3) *Collaborator*—All NPs must collaborate with clinical peers within and outside the agency. Directors lead by example and collaborate with staff members in front desk operations or on referrals off-site. In some states, collaboration is required by law. In any event, collaboration should always occur if the NP deems it necessary. Collegiality, which is noted as an APN Standards of Practice by the ANA (Standard 10), means that APRNs are always participants on a larger multidisciplinary healthcare team for consumers. This infers constant collaboration with peers in all sites (ANA, 2004).

Leader

1) *Consultant*—Staff will request regular consults regarding operational, clinical, legal, and employee issues. Being open and available is of utmost importance, as staff members need to know the director is available for support and to answer questions.

2) *Scribe*—Attendance, information shared, and suggestions received at governance and staff meetings must be documented. The meeting's agenda is set by the director, and communications regarding the meeting must be kept in a safe place. These meetings should be long enough to communicate with employees and discuss changes in the operation. Templates for documenting policy about topics to be covered can be found in Section III.

3) *Change Agent*—As director, this aspect of leadership means seeking to improve systems and efficiency at all available opportunities. Covey (1989) explains that leadership is not management. Each role encapsulates different qualities, but leadership must come first. Leaders manage well. Another point Covey stresses is that success happens twice: once in the mind's eye as a creative vision and once in reality. This is consistent with reflective practice theory.

4) *Facilitator*—As a director and leader listening intently and communicating with staff members are essential. Encouraging suggestions empowers staff and helps facilitate individual growth by increasing staff commitment. Helping staff members find educational opportunities to broaden their skill sets or gain confidence is another tool that can help facilitate growth.

5) *Supporter*—Staff members respond positively to encouragement and supporting their independent and creative solutions pays dividends. Staff satisfaction depends on trusting and feeling confident about the leader (Laschinger, Finegan, Shamian, & Casier, 2000). Even very short, but immediate, feedback can produce valuable results and raise staff morale (Blanchard and Johnson, 1982).

Manager

Management of the organization is probably the most time consuming part of the director's role. Operational management means overseeing the daily operations of the facility and all its intricate operations. Figure 6.1 presents a sample job description divided into pieces that highlight the relevant policy for each section of the job description. In the list below, every policy marked with an (*) has a template in Section III that can be edited and easily incorporated into any practice. Items marked with an (∧) are explained in greater depth elsewhere in the chapter; those *italicized* have sample forms available in Section III.

The director can be a successful manager by using fairness, common sense, positive attitude, and organizational skills. The following documents are necessary in every practice:

1. *Policy and Procedures Manual*—The policy and procedure (P&P) manual is an essential office tool. Most dread the need to review this long document annually, but a comprehensive manual is a helpful communication tool. P&P manuals prepared in a uniform manner and properly organized and cata-

logued served many purposes. P&P manuals communicate all operations of the practice in a policy fashion.

The manual needs to be written by the director because it forms the basis of all operations by conveying the practice's values, mission, and vision through policy (Randolph, 2006). The P&P manual can be divided into administrative, clinical, and important documents, and it should contain all the necessary paperwork to operate smoothly. Consider burning CDs for staff members so they have ready access if a question arises. Writing, updating, ensuring distribution, and acknowledgment of annual review by each staff member is the responsibility of the director. Suggestions for policy include:

Administrative Policies and Forms

- Mission Statement*∧
- Governance Policy*∧—describes specifics of reporting and operational structure of the business and *Governance Meeting Documentation form*
- Staff Meeting Policy*—describes specifics of how staff will receive communications and *Staff Meeting Documentation form*
- *Organizational Chart*∧
- Official Documents Policy*—informs everyone where operational documents are located
- Policy and Procedure Policy*—proclaims the authority of the P&P manual
- Eligibility to Receive Services Policy*—describes who can seek care from the practice. This is a helpful document if a complaint of discrimination or negligence arises.
- Notice of Available Services Policy*—describes the services available from the practice. This is a helpful document if a complaint of favoritism or neglect arises. It also delineates how the services will be publicized.
- *Patient Bill of Rights*—informs patients what to expect from the practice
- *Patient's Responsibilities*—informs patients of the practice actions expected of them.
- Patient Complaint and Grievance Policy*—informs patients how to file a complaint about any aspect of the practice and informs staff how to manage the complaint.
- Medical Records Policy*—ensures consistent compilation and storage of medical records.
- Chart Order Policy*—ensures consistency among charts.
- Release of Information Authorization Policy*—ensures lawful release of protected health information from a private medical record and *Release of Information form*
- *Referral Form*—provides a standard communication process between the primary care office and the specialist.
- *Problem Oriented Medical Record form*
- *New patient health questionnaire*
- Disposal of Medical Records Policy*—ensures the consistent disposal of protected health information.
- Appointment to Medical Staff Policy*∧

Director's Job Description

Job Description

Title   Director of Health Services
Department   Health Center
Reports to
Supervises   XXXXXXXX
                Advanced Practice Registered Nurses
                Registered Nurses
                Coordinator of Health Services
                Coordinator of Insurance Services and Referrals
                Secretary
                Billing Personnel

Date
Complete/Revised
Statement of Purpose

The Director is responsible for all operations of the business to serve the needs of the practice populations. The Director serves as the focal point for promoting a creative, collaborative health services model. The Director will promote the integration of services provided by the business and community educational, health, and counseling resources. Serving as the chief administrator of the business the director, will also be expected to provide clinical care. The Director reports to the Board of Directors.

Minimum Qualifications

Must have:

1. Current Advanced Practice Registered Nurse licensure in XXXXX
2. National certification as a nurse practitioner,
3. Prescriptive authority in _____ and State and Federal DEA licenses.
4. Master's degree in nursing required, Doctorate or advanced degree in Administration preferred.

Duties and Responsibilities

1. Coordinate, update, and supervise application of policy and procedures.
2. Coordinate the assigning of clinical guidelines.
3. Hire clinical staff and verify licensure and credentials.
4. Supervise and regularly evaluate on-site health care providers.
5. Maintain adequate staffing on a daily basis and prepare schedules.
6. Arrange for continuing education for all staff.

7. Function as a clinician.
8. Function as a consultant to staff members regarding clinical, legal, and employee issues.
9. Serve as liaison with insurers regarding service utilization and risk management issues.
10. Evaluate and recommend changes as needed in community consultation arrangements.
11. Chair clinical staff meetings.
12. Orient new staff members.
13. Facilitate training of employees regarding emergency interventions and OSHA.
14. Oversee budgets, supplies, equipment, and operation of the physical facility.
15. Create all necessary documents for medical records of students.
16. Maintain the Webpage.
17. Maintain statistics on utilization of health care services; keep client logs, medical reports, and incident reports; and prepare reports as directed and as needed.
18. Provide methods for evaluating the quality of the services and client satisfaction.
19. Oversee the coding and billing of insurance program.
20. Arrange and participate in the compliance of billing practices.
21. Integrate Emergency Planning of the business with the community.
22. Delegate responsibilities as appropriate to other staff members.

Physical Demands

The above statements are intended to describe the general nature and level of work being performed by people assigned to this classification. They are not to be construed as an exhaustive list of all responsibilities, duties, and skills required of personnel so classified. All personnel may be required to perform duties outside of their normal responsibilities from time to time, as needed.

Additional Information

- Orientation Policy*∧
- Credentialing upon Hire Policy*∧
- Annual Credential Policy*∧ and *Personnel file checklist form**
- Staff Performance Review Policy*∧ and *Staff Performance review form**
- Peer Performance Review Policy*∧ and *Peer Performance review form**
- Collaboration Agreement*∧
- Hours of Operation/Staffing Policy*
- Contact Phone List Policy* and *Contact Phone List form**
- On-Call Policy*

Clinical Practice Policies

- Clinical Guideline Policy*—names a reference for everyone to use as a clinical guide.
- Infection Control Policy*∧
- Cleaning and Decontaminating Spills Policy*—describes the location of personal protective equipment (PPE) and ensures safety for all who clean contaminated fluids.
- Handwashing Policy*—advises behavior expectations.
- Medical Waste Policy*—explains identification and disposal procedures for medical waste.
- Clinic Cleaning Policy*—advises expectations of worksite cleanliness.
- Mandatory Reporting Policy*—clarifies actions to be taken in legally required reporting instances.
- Emergency Equipment Policy*—states the requirement of checking all emergency equipment to ensure proper functioning.
- Emergency Equipment/Medication Box Policy* and *Emergency Equipment/Medication Box checklist form**
- Eyewash Policy*—ensures proper eyewash use, care, and maintenance.
- Oxygen Tank Policy*—ensures proper oxygen tank use, care, and maintenance.
- Fire Drills Policy*—describes procedures for mandatory fire drills and *Fire Drill Documentation form**
- Fire Policy*—states expected behaviors in the event of a fire.
- Fire Extinguisher Policy*—ensures proper extinguisher use, care, and maintenance.
- Discarding of Expired Pharmacological Agents Policy*—ensures safe and proper disposal of unused medications.
- Stocking of Exam Rooms—ensures consistency in placement of medical exam supplies in exam rooms.
- Prescription Pad Policy*—ensures lawful and safe keeping of this valuable clinical tool.
- Referral to Subspecialist Office*—ensures consistency with the procedure of referral and allows for a system of checks and balances for follow up of recommended clinical care.
- *Fax Cover Sheet Form*

Important Documents—This section includes the storage of any business licensure, business association agreements (HIPAA) with vendors, contracts for services with vendors, business insurance certificates, copy of license, and Fire Marshall Inspection Certificate.

2. *Staff Oversight*
   a. *Staff*—Hiring clinical and support staff is an important decision made by directors. Although several retail clinic companies established in pharmacy locations have streamlined services to allow just one NP to work alone, this is not traditional. Hiring the right candidate for any and every position is crucial for the smooth operation of a practice. All clinical and support employees need to possess similar philosophies to promote a trouble-free work environment.

Interviewing can be as anxiety provoking for the director as it is for the job candidate. Strasser (2005) encourages behavioral-based questioning in order to become acquainted more thoroughly with the candidates. This technique allows for evaluation of responses through open-ended questions and helps to elicit candidate competencies through the questioning process. Strasser also emphasizes the need to be mindful of questions that cannot be asked and refers interviewers to Human Resource departments for guidance. If no Human Resource department exists to help with setting limits, avoid asking about personal demographics, such as age, citizenship, religion, personal family arrangements, and disabilities, except when the disability may affect the requirements of the position. Asking about these areas in interviews may lead to a complaint of discrimination if the candidate is not chosen. To avoid liability, Strasser recommends keeping the interview content and style as similar as possible among candidates and taking notes on whether or not a position is offered. It helps the conversation if a job description for the position is readily available. The candidate should present a résumé or curriculum vitae and a list of references at the start of an interview. After the interview, take the time to call references and listen to how the inquiries are answered: is it a "politically correct response" or an opinion stated with ease based in truth?

   b. *Credentialing upon Hire**—The first day of work for new employees is busy with paperwork. The director is responsible for (or, the delegation of) the credentialing of each clinical staff member before allowing direct patient care to ensure patient safety. Credentialing is completed either before making a job offer or upon starting, with the understanding that the position is contingent on an uneventful credential review. Credentialing involves verifying all of the applicant's professional historical information, including licensure, educational achievements, and malpractice history. See the Credentialing upon Hire form* for a full list of items to be checked during this process.
   c. *Appointment to Medical/Clinical Staff**—Send appointment letters confirming assignment to Medical Staff annually. Some hospitals require copies if an NP wishes to acquire staff privileges.
   d. Orientation*—At the start of service, the director or designee conducts an orientation that includes physical space, policies and procedures, and expectations for each employee. Benner has documented the steps from Novice to Expert. Starting in a new position, regardless of previous expe-

rience, resets the clock to zero. An orientation is a necessary introduction to new circumstances an employee may encounter.

e. *Performance Reviews*

   i. Staff Performance Review/Evaluation*—The director completes annual performance reviews for each staff member. The leadership style of the director dictates whether it is a formal or an informal process. An annual evaluation provides feedback so that the employee understands how his or her performance measures up to expected standards. It is also a good communication opportunity. It also presents a chance for directors to increase staff responsibilities or compliment and praise effort and performance.

   ii. Peer Review/Chart Audits*—Peer review allows feedback from staff other than the director. The director facilitates the process, but the audit or review is done with clinical peers. The exception is if the review is done as part of the compliance program for billing. Compliance review is done by the compliance officer, who is usually the director.

g. *Collaboration Agreements*—If required by statute in the Nurse Practice Act, a Collaboration Agreement must be signed by each clinical staff member. The director ensures the presence of an executed agreement for all clinical personnel. The particular components of an agreement are discussed in Chapter 7.

h. *Scheduling Staff*

   i. Weekend coverage—should be distributed evenly among all eligible staff members. Weekend and evening hours are beneficial to the practice because they increase patient satisfaction and provide increased access for working patients.

   ii. Time-off requests—should be submitted in writing preferably by email, so there is a date/time stamp of the correspondence. If adequate staffing allows, requests are granted in the order they are received.

   iii. On-call scheduling—should be distributed evenly among staff members or outsourced to an established call company. Often, existing local practices will take on-call duties for other practices for a financial consideration. If staff covers call, consider one night per week rather than a full week at a time because calls can be disruptive to daytime functioning. Sharing weekdays (i.e., each Monday night for 7 weeks) can also help keep staff healthy.

   iv. On-call correspondence—Each call received while on-call is considered care rendered/advice given and needs to be documented in the medical record.

i. *Chair Staff Meetings*—These meetings ensure communication about operations and changes in operations. As stated previously, staff meetings are one of the most important functions of the director. Meetings set and improve the standards of operations by keeping staff up to date about healthcare trends. Any and all changes to operations, regardless of size, must be communicated to staff members in meetings. Take notes of the meeting, highlighting the positive and negative issues reported by the staff. Meeting minutes should then be distributed to all staff members regardless of whether they attended the meeting. After distribution, check with staff members who were present to ensure that they understand any changes. Keep a binder or electronic file of minutes for easy access.

    j. *Annual Credentialing**—Before the annual performance evaluations, the director should review all personnel files. Each staff member's should receive a list of all credentials that need updating.

3. *Finance*

    a. *Budget*—Oversight of the day-to-day operations makes the process of monitoring budget and fiscal operations the director's responsibility. Directing an office or running a practice requires an understanding of financial planning, budgeting, coding, reimbursement, and financial analysis. Outsourcing accounting tasks is frequently done in small practices, but knowledge about day-to-day operations and budgeting is crucial to the success of the practice.

       The budgeting process can be overwhelming at first (see Chapter 5 for greater detail), but the budget serves as an excellent control document. It shows the expected results for each month, each person, and/or each department depending on the level of detail needed for the practice. These expected results are then compared to the actual results. The director's monthly budget review helps monitor utilization and see trends in the practice's operations. Needed adjustments to processes and actions to increase productivity can be made more quickly when fiscal operations are monitored monthly. The Director should also jot down trends (both favorable and unfavorable) to assist in the next planning cycle (Cohen, 2006).

       Planning is the best preparation for success in budgeting. The Strategic Plan should be used as a guide when planning for new programs, staff, or the addition of services. The plan can also be used to validate requested increases to meet expectations for the upcoming year.

4. *Operations*

    a. *Ordering Supplies and Equipment*—Clearly, healthcare facilities must have the diagnostic tools necessary to provide the services within their scope of practice. Primary care clinics need supplies and equipment, such as exam tables, stools, clocks, otoscopes, opthalmoscopes, blood pressure measuring equipment, scales, Snellen eye chart with a 20-foot distance marked for easy use, fluorescein dye for determining eye injuries, pulse oximetry, cerumen removers, sterile scalpels and scissors, blood glucose testing apparatus, pap smear containers and instruments for gynecological examinations; speculums, lubricant jelly, slides, KOH and normal saline, urine dipsticks, rapid strep and influenza tools, mononucleosis tests, guaiac testing for blood in stools, and pregnancy tests. Machines such as an ECG, nebulizers for asthmatic treatments, spirometers, and forced expiratory Volume Measurers are also needed. Laboratory equipment, such as an autoclave or other sterilization equipment, a refrigerator for specimens, biohazard waste disposal containers, locked cabinets to house chemical reagents, testing supplies, timers, microscope, Wood's or slit lamp, laboratory requisitions for local laboratories used by the patients' insurance, release forms for patients to sign to request laboratory findings from previous providers and to share current results, tubes and needles for veni-puncture, culture tubes for urine transport, and all types of blood and body tissue specimens, centrifuge for spinning blood specimens, sharps box, gloves, and adequate lighting must be available in the laboratory area.

b. *Order Disposable Supplies*—the director or designee is responsible for ordering all disposable supplies needed to operate the clinic. This includes gloves, gauze, bandages, table paper, disposable single use testing or equipment.

c. *Oversee Physical Plant*
   i. Cleaning and Decontaminating Spills of Blood or Body Fluids Policy*
   ii. Bloodborne Pathogens Exposure Control Plan (OSHA)∧
   iii. Infection Control Information*∧
   iv. Infection Control Policy*
   v. Handwashing Policy*
   vi. Clinic Cleaning*

d. *Oversee Regulatory Compliance* ∧
   i. Health Insurance Portability and Accountability Privacy Act (HIPAA) Statement∧
   ii. Occupational Safety and Health Administration (OSHA)—Medical Waste Policy∧
   iii. Discarding of pharmacological therapeutics Policy*
   iv. Clinical Laboratory Improvement Amendments (CLIA)∧
   v. Inspection/Licensure∧

e. *Maintain Equipment*
   i. Electrical Safety and Accuracy Checks—Electrical safety checks are conducted annually on all electrical equipment used for patient care. This ensures that no harm can come to the patient and no fire hazard is present because of faulty wiring or lack of grounding. Examples of equipment that needs to be checked include Wood's lamps, exam lights, exam tables, etc. Diagnostic equipment must be checked annually for accuracy and diagnostic validity, as well. Automatic external defibrillator (AED), scale, blood pressure cuff, and pulse oximeter for example all need annual calibration to ensure diagnostic validity.
   ii. Emergency Equipment*—is checked quarterly for appropriate use, care, and maintenance. Check functioning and ensure expiration dates are valid.
   iii. Eyewash*—is checked weekly for use, care, and maintenance. Flush the station for 10 minutes weekly to remove sediment that may have settled in plumbing from nonuse.
   iv. Oxygen*—is checked monthly for use, care, and maintenance. Check for remaining levels and expiration. Oxygen canisters have an expiration date that signifies when the internal tank compression can no longer be guaranteed.

f. *Maintain Statistics*—the director is responsible for maintaining statistics on utilization of healthcare services by keeping client logs, medical reports, and incident reports, and preparing reports as directed and as needed.

g. *Quality Control and Improvement*—the director is responsible for providing methods to evaluate the quality of services provided by the business. See Chapter 4 for a discussion of quality control and improvement.

h. *Patient Satisfaction*—the director is responsible for providing methods to evaluate patient satisfaction either through formal or informal surveys (see Chapter 4).

5. *Maintain Emergency Planning for the Business*
   a. Emergency Management Plan
   b. Material Safety Data Sheets∧*
   c. Disaster Plan∧
   d. Emergency Equipment/Medication Box Check List*—Most small health-care delivery businesses have emergency equipment on hand, including an AED, electrocardiograph (ECG) machine, oxygen and oxygen dispensing equipment, fire extinguishers, eye wash stations, and a quick grab emergency box. (The contents of this box can be found on the checklist in Section III.) If these items are on site, they require a routine check to ensure they are operational and that medications have not expired. Difficult liability issues can result from having these items on premises, but not in working order or not being used properly. OSHA regulations dictate requirements regarding the required frequency of operational checks; a checklist makes recordkeeping easy.
   e. Fire Drills with Documentation*—As an employer, remember that staff safety is a top priority. OSHA recommends regularly scheduled mock fire drills to keep staff trained in the event of a fire. Here, repetition is the key to success. Fire Drill Policy, Fire Policy, Fire Extinguisher policy, and Fire Drill documentation can all assist in meeting this recommendation.
   f. *Accident Reporting*—may be required by the general liability insurance carrier. Check with the individual carrier. Other mandated reporting based on the delivery of health care, such as suspected child and/or elder abuse and infectious disease reporting, are also mandated by state law.
   g. Contact Phone Policy*—having access to staff contact information is helpful during weather or other emergency situations.
   h. *Marketing*
      i. Web site—create and maintain a Web site. Domains are relatively inexpensive (i.e., yahoo small business). Advertising online will increase business revenue.
      ii. Maintain Advertising and Brochure—create a logo for stationery and advertisements used in newspapers and flyers. The director should oversee marketing projects and monitor results.

Regulatory Compliance of the Practice

Licensure

The state's Public Health Code enumerates regulations concerning licensure and inspection requirements from the state Department of Public Health (DPH). The Health Code will define the level of license required based on the types of services offered by the practice. Often, private practices are not required to have a license. In Connecticut, for example, privately owned physician practices do not require licensure or inspection. If the practice conducts any type of surgical-related care, an Outpatient Surgical Clinic license is required. If the practice is run by an institution of higher education and offers gynecological services, an Outpatient Clinic license is required. If a license is required by the DPH, an inspection to prove compliance with the Public Health Code occurs on a regular basis. The Code will dictate the parameters that need to be met to pass inspection. Review the Public Health Code in the state of interest to learn its requirements for practice oversight.

OSHA Workplace Safety and Infection Control Requirements

The OSHA Web site is the best place to become familiar with regulations (http://www.osha.gov/dcsp/smallbusiness/index.html). A handbook with detailed instructions about compliance and checklists to assist in the process are available. OSHA exists to promote workplace safety by setting requirements and standards for employers. OSHA's focus is to require employers to provide tools, equipment, and training so that employees remain safe on the job. OSHA also requires employers to report accidents to employees and provide historical information about infractions.

OSHA regulations cover many areas of employment, including fire safety requirements, electrical safety, building safety, ergonomics, medical waste, bloodborne pathogens and personal protective equipment, chemical handling and information, and sexual harassment and violence in the workplace. These areas require training, reporting, and oversight.

OSHA regulation 1910.1200(b)(3)(ii) states that employers who receive or work with chemicals shall maintain material safety data sheets (MSDS) readily available for employees. MSDSs accompany almost every chemical, including routine soap and liquid eraser used by office staff. The MSDS sheets include information on the molecular composition of the product and instructions for care if unexpected exposure occurs. MSDS information can be found at www.ehso.com/msds.php.

OSHA also sets forth regulations on medical waste for the safety of employees and the public. Regulations governing health care facilities can be found at http://www.osha.gov/pls/oshaweb/owasrch.search_form?p_doc_type=STANDARDS&p_toc_level=1&p_keyvalue=1910. The regulation, 1910 Standard, is explained and illustrated in detail.

Developing a Blood Borne Pathogens Exposure Control Plan and a Waste Removal Plan are required for every healthcare business. Most hazardous waste removal companies sell plans to personalize for your practice site. Important considerations for the plan include:

- A list of all job classifications in which employees have occupational exposure to blood or body fluids and are classified in an "at-risk-for-exposure" position.
- An explanation of how you will monitor the requirements of compliance to include:
  - ☐ Use of universal precautions.
  - ☐ Availability and required use of personal protective equipment (PPE) by employees.

- ☐ Distribution methods of PPE for those in the "at-risk-for-exposure" roles.
- ☐ Availability of hand washing facilities and required use of them.
- ☐ Handling of blood specimens or other potentially infectious materials.
- ☐ Housekeeping standards for spills and routine cleaning to decrease chance of contamination/exposure to Blood Borne Pathogens (BBP).
- ▦ Blood Borne Pathogen training and protection includes:
  - ☐ Plan for annual BBP training.
  - ☐ Medical evaluation for protection for BBP, vaccine availability within 10 days of employment and after training.
  - ☐ Postexposure medical evaluation.
  - ☐ Confidential medical recordkeeping for inoculations.
  - ☐ Communicating hazards to employees and others who occupy the office space.
  - ☐ Easily interpreted consistent warning labels.
- ▦ Recordkeeping for Annual Training
  - ☐ Annual documentation that each employee has access to a copy of the regulatory text of the standards, Federal Register, Vol. 58., No. 235, Dec. 6, 1991, and an explanation of its contents.

Clinical Laboratory Improvement Amendments and Laboratory Resources

In 1988, the Clinical Laboratory Improvement Amendments was passed by the U.S. Congress. These regulations are the universal standards regarding accurate collection and testing of patient laboratory results. Each facility completing diagnostic testing on-site must have a CLIA certificate. The Center for Medicare and Medicaid Services (CMS) is the federal regulatory body that empowers CLIA to certify laboratories and/or lab areas. Certification levels are based on the type and quantity of laboratory testing done on-site. Certification may include an inspection of the laboratory by CMS or by a private agency, such as The Joint Commission or the College of American Pathologists.

Bennett, Cervantes, and Pacheco (2000) explain the potential point-of-care testing errors occurring in laboratories. Dumas (2009) shares the three most frequent reasons for citations during from the 2008 CLIA inspections. He reinforces the importance of having solutions for common problems stated clearly in the policy for CLIA management of the laboratory. Howerton, Anderson, Bosse, Granade, and Westbrook (2005) explain the importance of monitoring testing practices in CLIA-waived practices. They recommend personnel involved in the testing be trained and receive all updates regarding safety, physical and environmental requirements, staffing, and documentation. The three phases of testing are:

- ▦ Test ordering and specimen collection.
- ▦ Control testing, performance of test, and interpretation and recording of results.
- ▦ Reporting of results, documentation, and biohazard waste disposal.

These three phases can be used to create a policy regarding management of laboratory testing for CLIA-waived settings. By accessing the CLIA Certificate of Waiver Fact sheet at http://www.cdc.gov/hiv/topics/testing/resources/factsheets/roltCLIA.htm, one can determine which level of CLIA Waiver certification the practice needs to acquire. Many states have additional regulations that apply to laboratory testing, and some states require separate applications to the state agency along with the CLIA federal certificate. For those healthcare facilities needing CLIA certification, Lessig and Ehrmeyer (2005) discuss quality improvement as equivalent to quality control and provide recommendations regarding the significant role of the director in insuring quality control.

The Health Insurance Portability and Accountability Privacy Act (HIPAA)

Enacted in 2004 by the federal government, HIPAA regulations are pertinent to healthcare delivery in the United States. The agency protects the patient by requiring that all medical record information be available on a need-to-know basis. It requires patient consent to disclose any personal health information (PHI), except that information necessary for ongoing treatment or payment for services. HIPAA regulates several areas of patient care, such as protection of PHI in medical records, submitting financial electronic interactions, and security and maintenance of Internet access and computer-based storage on businesses considered "covered entities." Practices are considered "covered entities" if any type of electronic billing is done by the office or on the office's behalf. Entities are bound to dispense *Notice of Privacy Rights* to each patient of the practice. This *Notice* includes information stating the patient's specific rights in regard to their medical record oversight. The practice is also legally bound to obtain written acknowledgement that the patient received such notification. Lusis (2008) guides practices by suggesting that help can be found in crafting the notice at http://www.hrsa.gov/servicedelivery/language.htm. The standards can be found at http://www.hhs.gov/ocr/privacy/hipaa/understanding/coveredentities/index.html.

Frank-Stromborg and Ganschow (2002) list the groups of business or "entities" that require practice agreements. This agreement, called a business associate agreement, clearly states the efforts made and what vulnerabilities have been assessed in the intent of protecting patients' PHI. These entities are:

- Health plans, which provide or pay for the cost of medical care in the private or public sector.
- Healthcare clearinghouses, which process health information, such as billing services.
- Healthcare providers that conduct certain financial transactions electronically.

The essence of HIPAA is to make all healthcare industry personnel aware that the use and exchange of information as it relates to a real person must be handled with care and respect. HIPAA compels all individuals working with the PHI of a patient to do so confidentially.

Templates of a Release of Information Form and Referrals Form are provided in Section III. Disposal of Medical Records under HIPAA must be done with great care, again to ensure the confidentiality of the information. If shredding is not done on-site, a business associate agreement is requested from all vendors who handle items of identifiable patient PHI. This agreement ensures that the vendor intends to be compliant with HIPAA as well. The agreement binds the vendor in securing records against loss, access, or reproduction until destruction is accomplished. Sample Business Associate Agreements are available at http://www.sba.gov.

Preparing for Disaster and Emergency Coverage

Nurse practitioners must be prepared to manage a variety of disaster-related contingencies (Tichy, Bond, Beckstrand, & Heise, 2009; Cole, 2005). From a possible local release of biological agents to a train or plane disaster, communities and businesses need to have a Disaster or Casualty Incident Plan available. Nurse practitioners can play a role in all four phases of a disaster because of their advanced clinical diagnostic reasoning ability and skills. The four phases of Disaster/Emergency coverage (Tichy, Bond, Beckstrand, & Heise, 2009) are:

- *Prevention, Planning, Preparedness*—information skills, communication, and training assistance for emergency preparedness.
- *Response, Mitigation*—all of the activities performed during and immediately after the disaster that provided care to the victims, as well as prevent further injuries.
- *Recovery*—care provided to victims and providers to prevent physical/psychological trauma from occurring—planned over a long-term span.
- *Evaluation*—a thorough review of the plan identifying what went well and how outcomes could be improved regarding the disaster/emergency plan.

Drills must be conducted on a regular basis to ensure that staff is familiar with the plan. The chain of command is very important in a disaster. Drills should cover the duties of all positions in case someone is not available when a disaster occurs. The assigned essential staff must be aware of and prepared to perform their responsibilities. The disaster response system must include the practice staff, along with local first responders, government agencies, and outside healthcare agencies. There is a national organization (sponsored by the California Nurses Association) of volunteer registered nurses called the Registered Nurse Response Network (RNRN). It is comprised of approximately 4,000 RNs who will assist in a national disaster if needed. The Web site for the organization is http://www.calnurses.org/rnrn/.

The NP Competencies (NONPF, 2002) and the Master's Essentials Education Core Competencies (1996) indicate that all graduates of master's programs in nursing must be competent in emergency situations. Still, Tichy, Bond, Beckstrand, et al (2009) found that most master's programs do not teach specific competency skills to manage disasters. Nurse practitioners must follow the guidelines of the National Incident Management System (NIMS) regarding preparation and response to emergencies (Federal Emergency Management Agency, 2006). When NPs need to develop emergency-related policies, multiple resources are available to help, starting with the Centers for Disease Control at http://www.cdc.gov/. This site guides private health offices, school-based healthcare programs, and hospitals and community-level services in emergency preparedness. It includes a module on employer readiness and on readying employees to handle a disaster. Local and state health departments are also excellent resources for free literature and guidance. Every practice or business needs to familiar with local emergency room facilities. Meeting the directors of the emergency room, the director of emergency medical services, and medical, nursing, and administrative staff will provide an opportunity to discuss how the referral process will be handled in an emergency.

Common Areas of Concern

Several areas common to every practice present issues that can impede the smooth running of a practice. They include the physical condition of the site, proper documentation, and billing. Attention to them may be delegated to others to ensure a seamless operating practice.

It is easy to focus on the operations of the practice and lose sight of the facility's condition. Dirty carpeting, old magazines in the waiting room, and scuffed paint on the walls occur regularly and create a poor impression. Keeping the facility clean and fresh positively affects patients and employees.

Comprehensive documentation often takes more time than is available; it can become the albatross of clinical practice. Lack of comprehensive and consistent systems for charting can lead to legal vulnerability and, more important, to poor patient care. If documentation is illegible or incomplete, providers will not be able to provide the best possible care. Instituting standard forms or electronic charting is highly recommended to prevent incomplete documentation.

Incomplete or incorrect billing will definitely have a negative impact on your practice. Coding correctly can ensure maximum reimbursement. Billing correctly and thoroughly on the first attempt is not only efficient, but it can maximize profits. The compliance officer should hold staff meetings regularly to instruct NPs on accurate and complete billing. Small businesses should consider outsourcing this crucial function to experts.

Conclusion

This chapter discussed how the director oversees the day-to-day operations of the business, with a detailed job description as a guide. With so many responsibilities, the director needs an arsenal of tools to complete all the tasks successfully. Starting with the strategic plan of the practice, goals are set to improve the practice. These goals are consistent with the practice's mission and vision statements. Successful oversight involves awareness of budget allocations for daily supplies and operations, capital expenditures, and personnel need to maximize the profit goals. Day-to-day operations are enumerated in a Policy and Procedure Manual for distribution to all staff members. The Policy and Procedure manual is the "how-to" guide for expectations of activities, such as documentation, handwashing, and holding staff meetings. Templates in Section III are provided for use. Effective communication along with the Policy and Procedure manual help provide a high-quality and efficient operation. The organizational chart provides information about the practice's structure. Appropriate reports ranging from budgets to clinical care to overseeing emergency operations in the practice and community are discussed.

Federal and state agencies set regulations for compliance in the healthcare industry. The OSHA, HIPAA and CLIA regulations are discussed and must be monitored and enforced by the director. The director is responsible for determining practice standards are met in order to gain compliance with health and safety standards.

Reflective Thinking Exercises

1. As the director you become "underwhelmed" with the care and communication from the local Emergency Room concerning patients in your practice. How do you address this problem? Cite rationale to do so using the roles of the director reviewed in this chapter.
2. Consider a clinical situation in a current or past position that frustrated you because of a lack of resources or ineffective implementation. Create and write a "change of policy/procedure" to address the deficits with the goal of improved patient care.
3. Quality of care provided by each staff member is the responsibility of the director. Imagine a staff member who does not complete an assessment for abdominal pain or a front desk staff member who does not assist the patient in the waiting room who is in obvious pain. Devise a plan (what to say, what resources to use, how to hold the conversation) to address the issue with the staff member. State expectations and review the newly presented expectations in a month's time.
4. Evaluate the pros and cons of having the director demonstrate and complete the entire orientation process of a new clinician versus having a staff member lead/mentor new staff.

References

Adams, S., & McCarthy, A. (2007, June). Evidence-based practice guidelines and school nursing. *Journal of School Nursing (Allen Press), 23*(3), 128–136. Retrieved August 16, 2009, from CINAHL with Full Text database.

Adelman, D. & Legg, T. (2009). *Disaster nursing: A handbook for practice.* Sudbury: Jones & Bartlett Publishers.

American Association of Colleges of Nursing (1996). Essentials of master's education for advanced practice nursing. Washington, DC: Author.

American Nurses Association (2004). *Nursing: scope and standards of practice.* Silver Springs: Author.

American Nurses Association (2009). The Nursing Process: A Common Thread Amongst All Nurses from: Nursing World, Caring For Those Who Care http://www.nursingworld.org /EspeciallyForYou/StudentNur ses/Thenursingprocess.aspx retrieved August 22, 2009

Bennett, J. Cervantes, C., & Pacheco, S. (2000). Point-of-care testing: inspection preparedness. *Perfusion, 15*(2), 137–142.

Bennis, W. & Nanus, B. (1985). *Leaders: The strategies for taking charge.* New York: Harper & Row.

Blanchard, K. and Johnson, S. (1982). *The One Minute Manager.* New York: William Morrow and Company.

Budney, A., Rogers, L., Mandracchia, V., & Lascher, S. (2006, March). The physician's attire and its influence on patient confidence. *Journal of the American Podiatric Medical Association, 96*(2), 132–138. Retrieved August 1, 2009, from CINAHL with Full Text database.

Cohen, S. (2006, April). Best of the basics. Take the fear out of the figures. *Nursing Management, 37*(4), 12–12. Retrieved August 16, 2009, from CINAHL with Full Text database.

Cole, F. (2005). The role of the nurse practitioner in disaster planning and response. Nursing Clinics of North America. 40, 511–521.

Conway-Morana, P. (2009, March). Nursing strategy: what's your plan? *Nursing Management, 40*(3), 25–29.

Covey, S. (1989). *The seven habits of highly effective people.* New York, NY: Simon & Schuster

Dumas, T. (2009). Plan for 2009: learn from 2008. *Medical Laboratory Observer, 41*(1), 35.

Federal Emergency Management Agency (2006). NIMS implementation activities for hospitals and healthcare systems. Retrieved June 30, 2009, from http://www.fema.gov/pdf/emergency/ nims/imp_hos.pdf.

Federal Register/Vol. 65, No. 194/ Thursday, October 5, 2000/notices 59434. Department of Health and Human Services Office of Inspector General OIG Compliance Program for Individual and Small Group Physician Practices. Agency: Office of Inspector General (OIG), HHS. Action: Notice. Retrieved 7/3/09.

Finger, L. (2005, June). Nurse shares what she would have done differently. *AACN News, 22*(6), 5–6. Retrieved August 1, 2009, from CINAHL with Full Text database.

Frank-Stromborg, M., & Ganschow, J. (2002, September). How HIPAA will change your practice.. Health Insurance Portability and Accountability Act of 1996. *Nursing, 32*(9), 54–57. Retrieved August 16, 2009, from CINAHL with Full Text database.

Friedman, L., Engelking, C., Wickham, R., Harvey, C., Read, M., & Whitlock, K. (2009, April). The EDUCATE Study: a continuing education exemplar for clinical practice guideline implementation. *Clinical Journal of Oncology Nursing, 13*(2), 219–230. Retrieved August 2, 2009, from CINAHL with Full Text database

Goleman, D. (1998). *Working with emotional intelligence.* New York, NY: Bantum Books.

Grossman, S. (2007). *Mentoring in nursing: A dynamic and collaborative process.* New York: Springer Publishers.

Hawkins-Walsh, E., and Stone, C. (2004, Jan–Feb). "A national survey of PNP curricula: preparing pediatric nurse practitioners to meet the challenge in behavioral mental health." *Pediatric Nursing, 30*(1), 72 (7). Expanded Academic SAP. Gale. Trinity College. 14 June 2009 <http://find.galegroup.com/itx/start.do?prodId=EAI M>. Gale Document Number: A114698455

Hayes, E., & Kalmakis, K. (2007, November). From the sidelines: coaching as a nurse practitioner strategy for improving health outcomes. *Journal of the American Academy of Nurse Practitioners, 19*(11), 555–562. Retrieved August 1, 2009, from CINAHL with Full Text database.

Howerton D., Anderson N., Bosse D., Granade S., & Westbrook G. (2005). Good laboratory practices for waived testing sites: survey findings from testing sites holding a certificate of waiver under the Clinical Laboratory Improvement Amendments of 1988 and recommendations for promoting quality testing. *Morbidity & Mortality Weekly Report, 54,* (RR-13), 1–25.

Joint Commission (2008) *Emergency Management in Healthcare.* Retrieved June 30, 2009 from http://www.jcrinc.com/Books-and-E-books/EMERGENCY-MANAGEMENT-IN-HEALTH-CARE-AN-ALL-HAZARDS-APPROACH/1424/.

Landro, L. (2008, April 2). The Informed Patient: Making Room For 'Dr. Nurse'. Wall Street Journal (Eastern Edition), p. D.1. Retrieved June 14, 2009, from ABI/INFORM Global database. (Document ID: 1455412271).

Laschinger, H., Finegan, J., Shamian, J., Casier, S. (2000, September). Organizational trust and empowerment in restructured healthcare settings: effects on staff nurse commitment. *JONA: The Journal of Nursing Administration, 30* (9). 413–425.

Lessig, R. & Ehrmeyer, S. (2005). Lab management: CLIA 2003's new concept: equivalent quality control. *Medical Laboratory Observer, 37*(1), 32–34.

Lusis, I. (2008, September 2). Private practice and HIPAA. *ASHA Leader, 13*(12): 3. Retrieved August 16, 2009, from CINAHL with Full Text database.

Moseley, G. (2009). *Managing health care business strategy.* Sudbury: Jones & Bartlett Publishers

National Organization of Nurse Practitioner Faculties & American Association of Colleges of Nursing (2002). *Nurse practitioner primary care competencies in specialty areas: Adult, family, gerontological, pediatric, and women's health.* Rockville, MD: U.S. DHHS, HRSA, DON

Pediatric Nursing Certification Board (PNCB) (formerly the National Certification Board of Pediatric Nurse Practitioners and Nurses). (2001). *New PNP test blueprint and outline for 2002.* Gathersburg: Author.

Randolph, S. (2006). Developing policies and procedures. *American Association of Occupational Health Nurses Journal, 54*(11), 501–504.

Roberts, R., Roberts, C., Attkisson, C., & Rosenblatt, A (1998). Prevalence of psychopathology among children and adolescents. *American Journal of Psychiatry, 155*(6), 715–25.

Senge, P. (2006). *The fifth discipline: The art and practice of the learning organization.* (2nd. Ed.). New York: Currency Doubleday.

Schafer, D., Lopopolo, R., & Luedtke-Hoffmann, K. (2007, March). Administration and management skills needed by physical therapist graduates in 2010: a national survey. *Physical Therapy, 87*(3), 261–281. Retrieved August 15, 2009, from CINAHL with Full Text database.

Strasser, P. (2005, April). Management file. Improving applicant interviewing: using a behavioral-based questioning approach. *AAOHN Journal, 53*(4), 149–151.

Tichy, M., Bond, A., Beckstrand, R. & Heise, B. (2009). NP's perceptions of disaster preparedness education: Quantitative survey research. *The American Journal for Nurse Practitioners. 13*(1), 10–22.

United States Department of Labor website accessed August 2, 2009 at www.dol.gov. Regulations (Standards—29 CFR) Standard 1910.9 of the Occupational Safety & Health Administration website accessed August 2, 2009 at http://www.osha.gov/pls/oshaweb/owadisp.show_document?p _table=STANDARDS&p_id=14019 and www.osha.gov.

Roles of Nurse Practitioner Providers, Interdisciplinary Providers, and Physician Collaborators

7

Learning Objectives

1. Describe available practice settings for possible employment.

2. Articulate employment considerations when beginning the interview process.

3. Discuss negotiating points when considering an employment contract and salary.

4. Describe positive and negative outcomes from obtaining provider status (empanelling) on insurance roles.

5. Describe the usefulness of comprehensive job descriptions and employee evaluations.

6. Discuss components of a Collaboration Agreement.

Key Words: business practice sites, contract and salary negotiations, job descriptions, employee evaluations, collaborative agreements

Nurse Practitioners (NPs) need to consider many factors when deciding on a suitable position, including type of business, type of setting, contract, and salary. This chapter explains how to evaluate practice settings (e.g., not-for-profit, government), types of fiscal relationships (e.g., employee, contract staff, or business partner), and the process of negotiation to achieve a desired fiscal relationship.

New nurse practitioners should first reflect on personal goals and work values, as well as seeking opinions from experienced NPs on what type of work environment might be the "best fit." An NP who is considering establishing an independent private practice should carefully review his or her personal finances because new businesses often experience cash flow problems. When that occurs, a business personal salary is only drawn after all other expenses are paid.

However, new NPs usually do not begin a solo private practice right after graduation. The first few years of practice are better spent under the guidance of an experienced NP, where the new NP can master the skills learned in advanced education programs and then cement those skills through repetition. As a result, the NP will gain confidence in making clinical decisions. Note, for example, that the state of Maine allows independent practice under the Nurse Practice Act, but a two-year residency under the tutelage of an experienced NP is required (Pearson, 2009). During this period, the new NP should engage in exercises to assess and evaluate:

- What is done,
- How it's done, and
- If what is done can be improved, or completed more efficiently.

This chapter also presents examples of job descriptions and employee evaluations used in healthcare settings directed by NPs with collaborative physician relationships. Recommendations for maximizing employee teamwork and increasing staff morale are shared, as is a model of a collaborative practice agreement.

Employment Consideration

Every NP needs a workplace that meets his or her professional goal, which is usually employment in a desired practice type that offers a productive employment relationship and serves as a business model. Sometimes, the provisions of the state's Nurse Practice Act may limit options in finding the desired position. Therefore, begin by determining what type of practice is desired: private, community based, not for profit, hospital based, government or military based; the spectrum is endless. Seek a practice with values that match your own. If your personal values are at odds with the practice's values (e.g., weekend work hours are required or the practice does not provide needed care because of reimbursement limitations), conflicts arise that directly affect job satisfaction (Hansen, 2009). If values are shared, the setting may provide a smoother transition for the NP to become an effective clinician. Although compromise is always necessary, the NP who sacrifices personal beliefs to secure a position will meet with discord and dissatisfaction.

Employment Relationships

As a first position, the new NP may join a private practice with other clinicians. NPs gain fruitful experience in this environment, where they enjoy working with other NPs. Three classic employment relationship and compensation arrangements are available:

- Becoming a full partner of the practice.
- Becoming a salaried partner of the practice with a bonus.
- Becoming an employee of the practice.

Practice Partner

Whether equal or fixed, a partnership is generally two or more individuals—either NPs or physicians—who own and run the business together. They share liability, income, and expenses, and have input into and authority over day-to-day operations. They are expected to invest financially in the business and contribute to its viability by seeing patients and participating in the management of the business. Partners receive base salaries throughout the year and then split profits, if any, at the end of the fiscal year.

Salaried Partner

An NP can also join a practice as a salaried partner or as an employee, rather than as a partner with full ownership interest. A salaried partner is different from a salaried employee. If joining as a "salaried partner," the NP earns a "base pay." When the business balance sheet is prepared at the end of a fiscal cycle, the NP receives a bonus calculated by a formula that is usually based on productivity. The formula can vary, as many creative reimbursement packages are available. One formula calculates the NP bonus by computing the gross income received from an NP's reimbursements, subtracting all overhead, salary, benefits, and employee costs, and then dividing the net profit by the number of partners plus one. The more the practice earns through reimbursement, the higher the bonus the salaried practice partner receives. The NP is motivated to bring in income for the business while providing patient-focused health care. The owners of the practice also receive an equal portion of the NP's profit. Salaried partners are under pressure to maintain practice styles and income levels similar to their peers, as income information from each member of the practice is compared and shared among all partners.

Employee of Practice

If an NP chooses to be an employee of the practice, the NP receives a salary and benefits package without the financial risk or gain that comes with ownership. The pay is based on an annual salary or an hourly rate. An NP can start out as an employee of a practice while becoming acquainted with the functioning of the practice. As confidence and comfort increase, the practice owners may be willing to entertain a shift to a partnership arrangement. This possibility can be written into the original contract or, if the change is possible without mention in the original contract, a new contract should be negotiated.

Employment Contracts

Historically, NPs were hired in the same fashion as RNs. However, because the NP Scope of Practice allows autonomy, different terms should be negotiated. A written contract enumerating all expectations and compensation will protect all parties. Each item that is important to the NP or the employer should be spelled out in writing. Because each practice is established and maintained differently, each employee of a practice may have a contract with different stipulations. Input from a lawyer and/or financial expert will protect the NP from employment contract errors.

An NP's experience is obtained clinically and by learning the business of healthcare delivery. As a result, the NP should reflect carefully on what type of practice offers the "best fit." The NP's original plans may need to be refined. This is the essence of professional growth and development.

After the NP determines the right practice type and employment relationship, the NP needs to determine the best business model to suit his or her needs. Is it to open a new business or to join a business as co-owner or some other option? Pulcini, Vampola, and Levine (2005) cite the four most common practice configurations reported by NPs as:

- An NP/MD joint ownership practice,
- Private MD practice hired as an employee,
- Outpatient hospital practice, and
- Community health clinic practice.

In their survey completed in 2003, the authors also note that NP private practice or NP-owned business was the tenth most frequent practice setting employing NPs. In 2009, these practices are continuing to grow. In the national AANP survey, Goolsby (2005) found more than four percent of respondents nationwide were in private NP practice and nearly 33% were in physician-owned practices. The numbers of NPs in NP-owned practices are increasing, as more NPs become business literate and strive to fulfill the autonomous NP role.

Contract Negotiations

Contract negotiations are difficult for most NPs. Before nursing became an organized profession, nurses just hoped to be hired at a large hospital. This goes back to the days of wearing caps and standing to give a physician the chair. As the nursing shortage deepens and as NP practice becomes more accepted by the public and more requested by patients who have a positive "NP visit experience," NPs need to approach employment and negotiations with greater confidence. Nurse practitioners need to become savvy negotiators and work from a position of authority. They have skills that are in demand, provide quality care that is unmatched, and generate positive patient outcomes. It is time for NPs to bargain from a position of strength, since they are a valuable asset to any organization and a precious commodity in the healthcare arena (Chen et al., 2009; Horrocks, Anderson, & Salisbury, 2002; Mundinger et al., 2000).

The NP should gather the following information to use during the employment negotiation process:

- Business information on the company,
- Historical perspectives of employment trends in the agency,

■ Numbers of employed NPs,
■ Number of patients on a typical provider panel,
■ Normative numbers of visits per day per provider,
■ Process by which "no shows" are handled and billed,
■ Hours the business is open for the NP to see patients,
■ Support staff available for NPs, and
■ Expected on-call responsibilities and compensation.

These provide the basis for interview questions that will assist the NP in becoming familiar with the business and serve as "talking points" during contract negotiations.

Salary Negotiations

Salary negotiations are an essential component of the decision to accept a position in advanced nursing practice, whether you work for someone or are an owner in a shared practice. Salary surveys are conducted periodically by national nursing organizations and by nonnursing entities, such as Salary.com. Results of surveys can be found on the Web sites listed in Figure 7.1.

Advance for Nurse Practitioners completes a survey every other year and offers not only a salary range, but also lists common benefits reported by respondents. This list can be used to compile a "complete benefit package." Note that salaries vary widely by geographical, specialty, and practice site parameters. Nurse Practitioner Associates for Continuing Education (NPACE) conducted biannual salary surveys at its national conferences from 1997 through 2003. The American Academy of Nurse Practitioners (AANP) also began collecting data to provide NPs with comparison studies and statistics regarding compensation. The salary survey results from 2007 are available to members on the AANP Web site.

Interestingly, Kaplan and Brown (2009) found NPs reluctant to report salary data, even on an anonymous research-driven assessment tool. The authors couldn't explain this reluctance, but state salary reports from surveys generally use voluntary, self-report instruments, which may affect the validity of the data.

Salaries are improving as more NPs open their own practices. In a Fall 2005 survey of Tennessee and Virginia (between Knoxville and the Roanoke area), Sharp (2006) found NPs at NP-owned practices earned almost 23% more than those employed at physician-owned practices and 14% more than those working in a hospital-owned practice. Sharp (2006) and Newland (2006) found that gender difference still plays a role in the pay scale. Males earned nearly seven percent more than their female counterparts in non-NP-owned practices. These

7.1

**Salary Survey
Web sites**

■ www.salary.com
■ www.nurse.net
■ www.eriri.com
■ www.nurse-practitioners.advanceweb.com, and
■ www.aanpnet.org

points should be considered when investigating the best setting for employment. Kaplan and Brown (2009) suggest finding the right mix of occupational challenge and compensation—a mix that closely matches individual expectations. This is the best road to job satisfaction.

When working as an NP employee of a practice or business, compensation can come in different packages and can be compiled individually for each employee according to their needs. Different items go into a "package," and each item can be a point of negotiation. Items frequently listed as part of a benefits package include those in Figure 7.2.

Before opening negotiations, an NP should list the items being offered, rank them according to importance, and determine which can be sacrificed. For example, some NPs may not require full medical coverage because a spouse or partner can provide that coverage. Perhaps this expensive benefit could be used as a bargaining chip to secure a higher salary or to acquire more paid educational days. Once the benefits are rank in terms of significance to the NP, negotiations can begin. Salaries and bonuses are the most difficult to negotiate, so NPs should be prepared with up-to-date information on salary trends and bonus negotiations. Ask state nursing organizations to provide up-to-date information about your specialty in your geographic region. Once you have an idea

7.2

Benefits Menu

- Salary
- Bonus or incentive salary
- Profit sharing
- Health insurance
- Dental insurance
- Vision plan
- Long-term disability insurance
- Short-term disability insurance
- Life insurance
- Malpractice insurance
- Retirement benefits (401k and 503b)
- Educational benefits, including continuing education and subscription allowance
- Sabbatical time/professional leave (research time set aside in a practice day)
- License payment (including state practice licenses and DEA licenses)
- Certification renewal payment
- Technology tools (cell phone, PDAs, laptops, or computers)
- Vacation time
- Personal time
- Sick time
- Travel allowance for conferences
- Professional dues

of salary, add on benefits or exchange items for salary according to personal preference. All agreed upon negotiations need to be written and signed by all practice partners/owners (Kleinpell & Perez, 2006).

Noncompete Clauses

Increasingly, when practicing as a shareholder or practice partner, an employment contract includes a noncompete clause. If signed, these clauses essentially ban the NP from beginning a new (and potentially competitive) practice in the same geographic area for a specific period of time, say within 5 miles for 3 years. This clause deters NPs from leaving a practice and taking patients or panels with them. Because a practice is a business, it wants protection against the migration of patients (read as potential income) to follow an NP. This restriction makes such migration difficult. This clause is negotiable, but only in terms of parameters, mileage, or time (Alexander, 2009).

Obtaining Provider Status

Empanelling is the process of credentialing by insurance companies. Credentialing means verification of all documents and authority pertaining to clinical practice, including diplomas for all completed education, licensure from all states at all clinical levels, licensure from all federal and state agencies, certifications, previous employment sites, previous empanelling, and all privileges granted by a hospital or clinic. Each insurance company and payer agency mandates credentialing before accepting a professional relationship with an NP. Once credentialing is completed, NPs can begin to submit bills for reimbursement. Empanelling also generally allows the practice and/or NP to appear in a Provider Directory or to be considered "in-network," so patients can choose to receive care from the practice. Reimbursement is based on a negotiated contract with the individual companies. Contracting is done with "groups or practices" based on an agreed-upon reimbursement rate in accordance with Current Procedural Terminology (CPT) codes. The reimbursement rate for NP providers is commonly 80 to 85% of the approved physician fee schedule, but this varies by insurance company.

Contracting also provides insurance companies with the opportunity to invoke and impose many governing rules on providers and practices. These rules can range from mandating copayment collection to how billing must be submitted to verification of patient coverage systems to mandated quality indicator reporting. Because the practice or provider wants access to patients covered by the company and reimbursement for care rendered, these contracts are often seen as cost intensive, but compliance is assumed. The insurance companies are in the position of power in these contract negotiations.

Federal law allows NPs to be empanelled as independent providers, but a matching piece of legislation regarding reimbursement was never enacted, so NPs are sometimes not identified as the provider of care on reimbursement rosters. This invisibility is hurting the NP profession, because numbers of visits, quality of care, patient outcomes, and patient satisfaction are not attributed directly to NP care. The Nurse Practitioner Data Bank (APRNDB) was created to begin capturing this information to support NP practice, but it can only be effective if billing and reimbursement are completed using the NP's National Provider Identifier Number (NPI). The NPI is a federal system whereby each provider regardless of role has a unique number issued through the Centers for Medicaid and Medicare Services (CMS) for tracking practice habits and outcomes. These numbers are used in all electronic reimbursement transactions with CMS. This new system may result in lower reimbursement rates in the short term, but in the long run can support the NPs struggle for recognition for care provided. Some insurance companies are adding a modifier to the CPT, so NP delivered care can be identified in the office billing of physician reimbursement. This is a step in the right direction.

Job Descriptions

Job descriptions and evaluations are necessary tools that should complement each other in defining the functions and evaluating the performances of employees. Job descriptions articulate expectations related to all aspects of a position. Evaluations evaluate how successfully the employee executes those functions when compared to expectations. Job descriptions should be as thorough as possible, with comments on each aspect of the position. Copies of job descriptions and evaluations should be given to each employee at the time of hire, with the message that the tools are used to guide and evaluate job completion in the annual evaluation process. Employee evaluations or annual reviews should address each point in the job description in terms of level of success or level of improvement needed (Shaneberger, 2008). An easily understood scale of assessment can be used to "rate" performance in each portion of the job. See Figure 7.3 for an example of a grading scale.

Essentially an evaluation is a report card that shows how well an employee has met the expectations listed in the job description. Evaluations should always be reviewed with employees. Asking for an employee for a self-evaluation can help set the tone for this review. It can be a scary or defensive time for the employee. Use **examples of behavior** on the back of the form and ask the employee to do the same in order to provide a basis for the conversation. Conduct at the review can provide positive reinforcement for work well done and can encourage behavior change where performance needs to be improved. Figures 7.5 through 7.8 illustrate examples of job descriptions.

Shaneberger (2008) also agrees that annual evaluation criteria should derive directly from the job description. See Figures 7.9 and 7.10 for examples leading directly from the previous job description.

Collaborative Practice Agreements

Some states allow NPs to work without clinical supervision or oversight. Others have written protocols that mandate limitations on NP practice. Most states, however, mandate some sort of collaboration agreement. These practice agreements are legal documents that establish a working relationship between an NP and a physician. The agreement stipulates how the physician will monitor the performance and competency of the NP's practice.

7.3

Assessment Scale for Evaluations

> *Rating 1:* Receiving a rating of 1 indicates the job function being evaluated was *consistently completed entirely independently and accurately* throughout the review period, and the function was *improved upon by initiative shown by the employee.*
>
> *Rating 2:* Receiving a rating of 2 indicates the job function being evaluated was *consistently completed entirely independently and accurately* throughout the review period by the employee.
>
> *Rating 3:* Receiving a rating of 3 indicates the job function being evaluated was *completed accurately with intermittent supervision* throughout the review period by the employee.
>
> *Rating 4:* Receiving a rating of 4 indicates the job function being evaluated was *completed accurately only with supervision* throughout the review period by the employee.
>
> *Rating 5:* Receiving a rating of 5 indicates the job function being evaluated was *not able to be completed* by the employee.

NPs use a collaborative agreement to structure oversight requirements with a physician. Without such an agreement, the NP cannot practice. In these agreements, the physician places limitations on the NP's scope of practice. In addition, the agreement covers such issues as malpractice insurance and medical records review. The physician's fee is written into either a "contract for services" or it can be mentioned in the collaborative agreement. Each agreement should be based on the competencies of the NP and the confidence of the MD in those competencies. Figure 7.4 is an example of the language and items covered by an agreement. These areas can be redefined (added to or limited) by the two professionals signing the agreement.

Conclusions

A Nurse Practitioner should search internally and externally for an appropriate position. Internal searching means determining the best type of setting to meet the personal needs of the NP. External searching means finding that setting and then negotiating a sound fiscal relationship. This process can be difficult, but this preliminary work will help the NP transition easily into the new role. This is especially true if the NP and the practice share common values and the NP is comfortable with the type of site.

7.4

MD/APRN Collaborative Practice Agreement

Collaboration is an agreement concerning the working clinical relationship between an Advanced Practice Registered Nurse (APRN) and a Physician who is credentialed with relevant experience related to the work of the APRN.

I, _____ MD, and I _____ , APRN agree to enter into a collaborative agreement in the provision of health care at _____ Practice.

The APRN will provide services consistent with the Scope of Practice for the preventive care, diagnosis, and treatment of acute episodic, short-term and/or chronic illnesses, health maintenance, and patient education. This includes but is not limited to diagnosing, managing, and treating [ordering, performing, and interpreting laboratory tests, diagnostic procedures or medical therapeutics necessary] consistent with the APRN's training. Care beyond the scope of the APRN will be referred, such as life threatening conditions of airway obstruction or cardiac arrest, immediately via ambulance.

The APRN will prescribe pharmacotherapeutics, including controlled substances, schedule II through V medications in the provision of care as related to current practice standards of care. This includes but is not limited to categories of medications such as bronchodilators, antibiotics, antifungals, hormones, and analgesics. The APRN must have an independent DEA (state and federal) and an NPI number.

Consultation and referral shall be warranted by patient condition, level of expertise, and clinical judgment of the APRN. Circumstances requiring consultation with the MD or a specialist are agreed upon and listed on the bottom of this agreement. Physician oversight will be by observation during APRN consultation and by structured review of patient care via ten (10) clinical charts which will be randomly chosen, reviewed, and discussed each _____ . Clinical care will be evaluated by patient outcomes, by clinical response in laboratory data, and by chart review.

Coverage for patients during non-office hours and vacations will be arranged and mutually agreed upon and written in contractual arrangements known to all parties.

Disclosure of Physician-APRN collaboration will be by written declaration in the waiting room.

Each Party of this agreement will provide own malpractice insurance coverage to be not less than (fill in to state mandate) per aggregate.

Date:

Signed, _____   _____

Physician/Medical Director Job Description

Statement of Purpose

The Physician/Medical Director provides oversight and direction in the provision of comprehensive primary health care for acute and chronic alterations in health and preventive screenings. The physician documents clinical practice and is available to collaborate/consult with healthcare professionals in the practice as needed. The position includes 24/7 on-call responsibility while the business is open for patient care.

Minimum Qualifications

The Medical Director shall be:

- Graduated from an accredited school of medicine in the United States.
- Qualified in experience to work in this specific type of healthcare business.
- Certified by a board of medical authority to practice primary care or a compatible field for this type of healthcare business.
- Licensed as a physician in the state of (fill in) without any action against the license in this or any other state.
- Licensed by the state of (fill in) and by the federal government to prescribe medications of all types.
- In possession of an NPI number/UPIN number.
- Able to be covered by a policy of malpractice insurance.

Duties and Responsibilities of the Medical Director Shall Include:

- Oversight of medical care rendered in (fill in) as detailed in the collaborative agreements with staff.
- Consultation by telephone/pager twenty-four hours per day while business is open.
- Designation of another licensed physician to act in his/her place during his/her absence (sick, vacation, or otherwise).
- Receiving reports from the COO or office manager of significant clinical developments in patient care or business operations and assist in resolution of problems.
- Development and review of policy and procedures annually.
- Direct patient care.
- Reviewing hospital care, medical referrals, and other clinical services through chart reviews on a regular basis.
- Advising the governing board on all matters of health pertaining to the function of (fill in).
- Working collaboratively with the clinical staff of (fill in) including NPs, RNs, and ancillary administrative staff.
- Delivering comprehensive primary care using quality, evidence-based, and safe-care practices.

(continued)

- ▨ Obtaining complete medical history and immunization record.
- ▨ Performing comprehensive physical assessments (examinations).
  - ☐ Use in-office diagnostic procedures (e.g., Wood's lamp, "rapid" diagnostic tests).
  - ☐ Document results.
- ▨ Diagnosing alteration in health status/medical condition by compiling and documenting thorough differential diagnosis list.
- ▨ Planning an appropriate, cost-effective, evidence-based treatment regimen.
  - ☐ Maintain up-to-date practice standards through continuing education.
  - ☐ Explain in detail the limitations and utilization of insurance to cover cost of treatment plan.
- ▨ Implementing treatment regimen.
  - ☐ Prescribe pharmacotherapeutics (e.g., a antibiotics, narcotics, durable medical equipment).
  - ☐ Order diagnostic testing (e.g., blood work, X-rays, CT scan).
  - ☐ Educate patient regarding health/diagnosis (i.e., medication, side effects, self-care).
  - ☐ Refer to outside providers/vendors as appropriate.
  - ☐ Advocate for patient in obtaining needed services.
- ▨ Evaluating effectiveness of treatment regimen and/or alter plan to ensure desired outcome.
  - ☐ Complete appropriate follow-up of patient conditions.
  - ☐ Monitor and comply with recommendations from any referral site.
  - ☐ Provide continuity of care for chronic conditions.
  - ☐ Complete appropriate follow-up of any abnormal findings/results.
- ▨ Documenting the entire process detailed above.
  - ☐ Write legibly.
  - ☐ Document desired outcomes of care.
  - ☐ Document desired patient follow-up and patient agreement and acceptance of the plan.
  - ☐ Document abnormal diagnostic results and plan of care on how to proceed.
  - ☐ Thoroughly complete requisitions.
  - ☐ Document patient education and use of handouts/pamphlets.
- ▨ Maintaining up-to-date care standards of each step of the process above by attending continuing education offerings.
- ▨ Accepting referrals for care.
- ▨ Maintaining strict confidentiality of patient care.

Statement of Purpose

The Nurse Practitioner (NP) provides comprehensive primary health care for acute and chronic alterations in health and preventive screenings. The NP documents clinical practice that independently assesses, diagnoses, treats, and/or refers to collaborating/consulting healthcare professionals. The NP educates the patient population on preventive care and healthy lifestyle choices. The NP coordinates all care rendered in a case management framework. Work hours include weekend shifts and on-call responsibility.

Minimum Qualifications

- Graduation from an accredited school of nursing with a Bachelors and Master's degree in Nursing.
- Current certification from a national certifying body.
- Current state licensure for both Registered Nurse and Advanced Practice Registered Nurse.
- Federal DEA licensure.
- State DEA licensure.
- NPI number.
- Malpractice coverage.
- Three years experience in the delivery of primary health care in a similar population.
- Ability to practice independently.
- CPR certification.
- Gynecological experience.
- Experience and comfort with use of computer and computer programs (Office Suite, email, scheduling), office machines, building and grounds equipment.

Duties and Responsibilities of the NP Include:

- Delivery of comprehensive primary care using quality, evidence-based, and safe-care practices.
- Obtaining complete medical history and immunization record.
- Performing comprehensive physical assessments (examinations).
  - ☐ Use in-office diagnostic procedures (e.g., Wood's lamp, "rapid" diagnostic tests).
  - ☐ Document results.
- Diagnosing alteration in health status/medical condition by compiling and documenting thorough differential diagnosis list.
- Planning appropriate, cost-effective, evidence-based treatment regimen.
  - ☐ Collaborate with peers as needed.
  - ☐ Maintain up-to-date practice standards through continuing education.
  - ☐ Explain in detail the limitations and utilization of insurance to cover cost of treatment plan.
- Implementing treatment regimen.
  - ☐ Use office therapeutic procedures (e.g., asthma nebulizers, histofreezer).
  - ☐ Prescribe pharmacotherapeutics (i.e., antibiotics, narcotics, durable medical equipment).

(continued)

- ☐ Order diagnostic testing (i.e. blood work, X-rays, CT scan).
- ☐ Institute therapeutic regimens (e.g., dressing changes, soaks).
- ☐ Educate patient regarding health/diagnosis (i.e. medication, side effects, self-care).
- ☐ Refer to collaborating physician/outside providers/vendors as appropriate.
- ☐ Advocate for patient in obtaining needed services.
- ▓ Evaluating effectiveness of treatment regimen and/or alter plan to ensure desired outcome.
  - ☐ Complete appropriate follow-up of patient conditions.
  - ☐ Monitor and comply with recommendations from any referral site.
  - ☐ Provide continuity of care for chronic conditions.
  - ☐ Complete appropriate follow-up of any abnormal findings/results.
- ▓ Documenting the entire care process detailed above.
  - ☐ Write legibly.
  - ☐ Document desired outcomes of care.
  - ☐ Document desired patient follow-up and patient agreement and acceptance of the plan.
  - ☐ Document abnormal diagnostic results and plan of care on how to proceed.
  - ☐ Thoroughly complete requisitions.
  - ☐ Document patient education and use of hand-outs/pamphlets.
- ▓ Maintaining up-to-date care standards of each step of the process above by attending continuing education offerings.
- ▓ Accept referrals for care from outisde providers as well as self-referrals.
- ▓ Maintain strict confidentiality of patient care.

Provide Preventive Screenings and Health Education
- ▓ Perform routine physical exams; for travel, college entrance.
- ▓ Perform routine gynecological exams.
  - ☐ Utilize all equipment necessary to complete an exam (i.e. speculum, microscope).
- ▓ Perform sexually transmitted infection testing (both male and female).
  - ☐ Utilize all equipment necessary to complete an exam (e.g., speculum, microscope).
- ▓ Conduct assessments and provide educational information on contraceptive options.
- ▓ Distribute health education materials to patients.
- ▓ Conduct discussions with patients (prevention, healthy life style choices, immunizations for travel).
- ▓ Conduct oral communication with patient concerning general medical information.

Coordinate/Manage All Care Rendered in a Case Management Framework
- ▓ Obtain, prepare, and ship biohazardous samples (e.g., venipuncture, paps, cultures, shave biopsy).
- ▓ Assure the complete documentation of all diagnostic testing and referrals in the medical record.
- ▓ Contact patient with results and need for follow-up.
- ▓ Contact insurance and next of kin as permitted by the patient.
- ▓ Comunicate with superior of collaborative physician on complex/ill patients.
- ▓ Communicate with on-call staff if patient may contact them overnight.
- ▓ Communicate with health professionals from other offices when indicated/appropriate as permitted by patient.
- ▓ Coordinate (Contact, schedule, and confirm documentation).
  - ☐ Referrals to peers in practice as needed.
  - ☐ Referrals to outside providers (e.g., consulting/collaborating physicians, subspecialists).

- Referrals to outside vendors (e.g., X-ray, Hospital ER, agencies).
- Contact insurance companies when questions arise for coverage of patient care.
- Communicate to patients limitations of insurance coverage and cost anticipated to come from patient.
- *Provide on call services;* 24 hours a day 7 days a week when business is closed.
- *Complete administrative and clerical functions* as assigned.
- Administrative
  - ☐ Understand and incorporate the limitations and utilization of health insurance to provide clinical care.
  - ☐ Clean exam rooms between patients and at the end of the day.
  - ☐ Complete annual training in bloodborne pathogens.
  - ☐ Monitor temperature controls of vaccination refrigerator.
  - ☐ Monitor expiration dates/oxygen levels/emergency equipment as needed.
- Clerical
  - ☐ Stock exam rooms with daily supplies.
  - ☐ Monitor inventory for adequate amounts and communicate needs.
  - ☐ Sterilize equipment with autoclave **as** needed.
  - ☐ Answer phones as needed.
  - ☐ Schedule daily appointments as needed.
  - ☐ Reschedule missed appointments.
  - ☐ Operate office equipment—faxes, copiers.

Professional Functions

- Confidentiality maintained throughout care delivery.
- Evidence of continuing education.
- Comply with federal, state, OSHA, and office policy, regulation and standards.
- Complete annual OSHA and medical proficiency trainings.
- Maintain documentation standards.
- Conduct Quality Assurance/Quality Improvement reviews and assessments as assigned.
- Review peer's documentation.
- Monitor and suggest improvements in current policy and procedures.
- Develop and update policy and procedures as assigned.
- Maintain neat professional appearance.

Physical Demands

- Physical activities will include sitting/extensive standing/walking/squatting and rare heavy lifting.
- Using a computer keyboard to type.
- Reaching overhead and lifting items.
- Ability to perform CPR on a patient.
- Exposure to hazardous materials and bloodborne pathogens.

Statement of Purpose

The position of a Registered Nurse is one that supports the clinical and administrative mission of the business. This position is responsible for assessment, case management, and organization by using assessment skills and collaboration with nurse practitioner staff to provide the highest quality care to patients.

Minimum Qualifications

- Graduation from an accredited school of nursing.
- Current state licensure as a registered nurse.
- Current CPR certification.
- *Three-year experience in an outpatient setting*, including evidence of skills including but not limited to telephone triage, venipuncture, nebulizer treatments, and case management.
- Clinical experience in a similar business.
- Ability to practice independently, and as a valued team player.
- Knowledge of scope of practice (when collaboration with other clinicians is lawfully necessary).
- Ability to independently work with computer programs such as Microsoft Office; email, ExCel, word processing.

Duties and Responsibilities

Deliver evidence-based, safe care with oversight from nurse practitioner staff:

- Obtain complete medical history and immunization records.
- Perform telephone and in-person triage of illness, and make recommendations regarding self-care or referral for appointment.
- Perform comprehensive accurate multi-system patient assessments including; in-house rapid strep tests, mono tests, pregnancy tests, influenza tests, and urine exams.
- Provide office therapeutic procedures (e.g., asthma nebulizer, dressing changes, immunizations).
- Provide venipuncture and prepare laboratory samples for processing.
- Obtain, prepare, and ship biohazardous samples.
- Complete all requisitions and paperwork for ordering diagnostic testing.
- Report findings succinctly to staff.
- Collaborate with peers as needed.
- Educate patient/student regarding health/diagnosis (i.e., medication, side effects, self-care prevention, healthy life style choices, immunizations for travel).
- Distribute and educate patients in health topics including birth control, illness prevention, healthy lifestyle choices, illness management, travel requirements.
- Advocate for student/patient in obtaining needed services.
- Contact insurance companies when questions arise for coverage of patient care.
- Evaluate effectiveness of treatment regimen and/or alter plan to ensure desired outcome.

- Document the entire process detailed above.
- Maintain strict confidentiality of all patient information.
- Maintain up-to-date practice standards by attending continuing education.

Administrative:
- Comply with federal OSHA regulations.
- Complete annual training bloodborne pathogens/OSHA.
- Monitor temperature controls of vaccination refrigerator.
- Monitor expiration dates/oxygen levels/emergency equipment as needed.
- Comply with state of connecticut regulations.
- Maintain documentation standards.
- Conduct quality assurance/quality improvement reviews and assessments as assigned.
- Review peer's documentation.
- Monitor and suggest improvements in current policy and procedures.
- Develop and update policy and procedures as assigned.

Clerical:
- Clean exam rooms between patients and at the end of the day.
- Ordering and stocking rooms.
- Stock exam rooms with daily supplies.
- Monitor inventory for adequate amounts and communicate needs.
- Sterilize equipment with autoclave as needed.
- Answer phones as needed.
- Schedule daily appointments as needed.
- Reschedule missed appointments.
- Operate office equipment—faxes, copiers.

Physical Demands
- Physical activities will include sitting/extensive standing/walking/squatting and rare heavy lifting.
- Using a computer keyboard to type.
- Reaching overhead and lifting items.
- Ability to perform CPR on a patient.
- Exposure to hazardous materials and blood borne pathogens.

Secretary Job Description

Minimum Qualifications

- High school diploma.
- Two years secretarial experience in a medical office or any combination of education, training, or experience that provides the required knowledge, skills, and abilities.
- Ability to work efficiently without constant/direct supervision.
- Typing skills.
- Knowledge and experience with computers including the Office Suite (i.e., Word, ExCel, PowerPoint) and email.
- Knowledge of use of multiline phone system.
- Ability to use pleasant phone voice.
- Knowledge and implementation of proper phone etiquette.
- Knowledge and implementation of proper English language.
- Ability to maintain professional composure in an extremely sensitive and confidential environment.
- Ability to present clean and professional appearance.

Duties and Responsibilities

Reception Duties:

- Opening and locking the practice each weekday (see procedure).
- Greeting each individual either in person or on the phone.
- Providing assistance and directions to patients.
- Cleaning and straightening the waiting room nightly.

Secretarial:

- *Answering phone* on a multiline phone.
  - ☐ Taking accurate messages with pertinent and confidential information.
  - ☐ Distributing messages to staff confidentially.
  - ☐ Using judgment to interrupting clinicians when necessary.
- *Scheduling appointments* per the caller's prerogative.
  - ☐ Scheduling all of the appointments for each of the clinicians.
  - ☐ Using sensitivity in assessing the severity and urgency of every call
  - ☐ Arranging an appropriative visit for the patient complaint
  - ☐ Remembering patients who are in frequently and which clinician sees them
  - ☐ Knowing special requirements for returning patients and care/rooms needed for services offered (e.g., for GYN care, which requires special scheduling and room assignment).
- *Database entry* capturing the statistics for the utilization of the practice.

- *Ordering supplies* for both office needs and diagnostic supplies and maintaining office equipment including; fax, copiers, printers, computers, shredding service, radio, and, documentation paperwork.
- *Handling all mail* includes opening, sorting and distributing all U.S. Post Office, UPS supplies.
- *Handling all deliveries* includes refrigerating immunization deliveries and, handling biohazard deliveries and pickups.
- *Coordinating the filing of regulatory paperwork* with state and federal authorities.
- *Coordinating staff payroll paperwork* which includes compiling timesheets for staff, per diem staff and student workers for director review.
- *Accounting:*
  - ☐ *Collecting fees* tor the services provided (copays) either by overseeing petty cash, VISA charges, checks and writing receipts for all transactions.
  - ☐ *Securing payment* of all vendor invoices.
- *Medical Records Coordination:* Required Responsibilities
  - ☐ *Creating a medical record* for every patient at the time of enrollment in the practice.
  - ☐ *Processing the record* for completion and eligibility for enrollment per insurance requirements.
  - ☐ *Maintaining the record* for the career of the patient. Destroying records per state requirements.
  - ☐ *Pulling and refilling the records for each daily visit,* each phone call and, each lab result.
  - ☐ *Employee Records;* all records for employees who receive immunizations at the practice must be kept for 30 years.

7.2

Nurse Practitioner Evaluation

		1	2	3	4	5
	Duties and Responsibilities:					
	obtain complete medical history					
	perform comprehensive assessments					
	diagnose using and document differential list					
	implement evidence-based care					
	implement cost-effective care					
	use of office diagnostics					
	refer to physician/specialist as needed					
	evaluate plan and alter as needed					
	document patient education					
	document necessary follow-up					
	document legibly					
	maintain patient confidentiality					
	maintain CEU for current practice					
	comply with federal, state, practice regulations					
	maintain documentation standards					
	conduct QA/QI					
	conduct peer review					
	maintain professional appearance and demeanor					
	maintain licensures and certifications					
	Team Member Characteristics:					
	collaboration-with MD/peers/team/supervisors					
	organization-charting/meeting deadlines/OT					
	patient centered care					
	accountability-attendance/scheduling					
	professionalism					

Annual Goals: Evaluation points:

Z.10

Registered Nurse Evaluation

		1	2	3	4	5
	Duties and Responsibilities:					
	obtain complete medical history					
	perform comprehensive assessments					
	provide therapeutic procedures					
	report succinctly to staff					
	provide thorough patient education					
	use of office diagnostics					
	refer to NP/physician as needed					
	evaluate plan and alter as needed					
	document patient education					
	document necessary follow-up					
	document legibly					
	maintain patient confidentiality					
	maintain CEU for current practice					
	comply with federal, state, practice regulations					
	maintain documentation standards					
	conduct QA/QI					
	conduct peer review					
	maintain professional appearance and demeanor					
	maintain licensures					
	Team Member Characteristics:					
	collaboration-with MD/peers/team/supervisors					
	organization-charting/meeting deadlines/OT					
	patient centered care					
	accountability-attendance/scheduling					
	professionalism					

Annual Goals: Evaluation points:

After finding the right setting, negotiations begin. These negotiations precede the presentation of a written contract or agreement and should specify benefits, salary, and workplace requirements agreed to during the negotiating process. With the expansion of NP skills and increased acceptance of the NP role, an NP should be able to find an appropriate practice or niche.

Once a position has been secured, the first few days of employment include reviewing policy for the practice, as well as the work expectations articulated in the job description and evaluated in an annual review. This allows clear communication of expectations and goals can be set to meet those expectations from the start.

Finally, the points to consider when accepting a collaborative practice agreement were discussed. These points are articulated in the legislative requirement of each state's practice act.

Reflective Thinking Exercises

1. In your mind, create a model of your dream job in clinical practice. What service does it provide, and to whom? What philosophy does the company adopt? What aspects of employment make this your dream job?
2. Investigate the local job market. Can you find settings that match the parameters you established in Question 1?
3. Imagine you landed your dream job and negotiations for the employment contract begin in one hour. List all the points you consider nonnegotiable and those you can use as leverage to get the contract you desire.
4. The points listed as nonnegotiable in Question 3 MUST be provided in your contract.
5. Review the job description for the NP in Figure 7.6. Are these skills you possess? Can you think of other ways to demonstrate your proficiency upon annual review?

References

Alexander, N. (2009). Personal interview June 18, 2009 (M. O'Brien, Interviewer).

Chen, C., McNeese-Smith, D., Cowna, M., Upenieks, V., & Afifi, A. (2009, May–June). Evaluation of a nurse practitioner-led management model in reducing drug utilization and cost. *Nursing Economics, 27(3)*. p. 160 (9). Expanded Academic ASAP. Gale. Trinity College. 3 July 2009.

Goolsby, M. (2005, September). 2004 AANP national nurse practitioner sample survey, part I: an overview. *Journal of the American Academy of Nurse Practitioners, 17(9)*, 337–341. Retrieved July 5, 2009 from CINAHL with Full text database.

Hansen, R. (2009) Workplace Values Assessment: Do You Know the Work Values You Most Want in a Job and an Employer—and Does Your Current Employment Reflect Those Values? A Quintessential Careers Quiz Retrieved July 5, 2009 from http://www.quintcareers.com/workplace_values.html

Horrocks, S., Anderson, E., and Salisbury, C. (2002). Systematic review of whether nurse practitioners working in primary care can provide equivalent care to doctors. *British Medical Journal, 324*, 819–823.

Kaplan, L. and Brown, M. (2009, February). State and local APN salary data: the best evidence for negotiations. *The Journal for Nurse Practitioners, 5(2),* 91–97.

Kleinpell, R., and Perez, D. (2006, May). Negotiation strategies for ACNP practice. *The Nurse Practitioner, 31(5),* 6–11.

Mundinger, M., Kane, R., Lenz, E., Totten, A., Tsai, W., Cleary P., (2000). Primary care outcomes in patients treated by nurse practitioners or physicians: A randomized trial. *JAMA: The Journal of American Medical Association, 283*(1), 59–68.

Newland, J. (2006, May). 2006 Nurse practitioner salary & practice survey. *Nurse Practitioner, 31*(5), 39. Retrieved July 5, 2009 from CINAHL with Full text database.

Pearson, L. J. (2009). THE PEARSON REPORT, A National Overview of Nurse

Practitioner Legislartion and Health Care Issues. *The American Journal for Nursing Practitioners,* 8–82.

Pulcini, J., Vampola, D., & Levine, J. (2005). Survey: Nurse practitioner practice characteristics, salary, and benefits survey, 2003. *NPACE., 9(*1), 49–58.

Shaneberger, K. (2008, October). Staff evaluations: more than a formality. *OR Manager, 24*(10), 24. Retrieved August 30, 2009, from CINAHL with Full Text database

Sharp, K. (2006, March). Salary survey results from the northeast Tennessee nurse practitioner association. *The Tennessee Nurse, 69 (1),* 1. Retrieved July 5, 2009 from CINAHL with Full text database.

Entrepreneurial Models for Facilitating Best Practice: Specific Interventions for Maximizing Outcomes

8

Learning Objectives

1. Describe entrepreneurialism and how it applies to innovative methods of health care.

2. Describe how nurse practitioners (NPs) can be leading entrepreneurs in health care.

3. Differentiate among various models of care delivery that involve NPs.

4. Describe the process of outcome management in health care.

5. Analyze strategies to maximize patient outcomes, leverage resources, and improve patient satisfaction.

6. Develop an outcome management process to assess patient satisfaction.

7. Define standards in terms of obtaining practice agency accreditation.

Key Words: entrepreneurialism, models of care delivery, outcome management, practice accreditation, patient satisfaction

By using leadership, professional, managerial, and clinical skills, the NP can make specific contributions to and collaborate with colleagues in any practice area. The impact of NP entrepreneurialism in healthcare delivery is illustrated by:

- Developing a consumer base using one's practice,
- Securing referrals from the consumer base to potential clients,

- Creating a culture that encourages people to follow up on advice and remain connected with the practice,
- Establishing integrity in the marketplace by putting one's services on a pedestal of the highest quality, and
- Keeping competitive so positive cash flow can be generated and staff morale and enthusiasm maintained.

This chapter describes a variety of settings, including hospital, ambulatory care, community health, detention/prison, colleges, palliative care, complementary therapy/holistic, case management, acute care, and psychiatric/mental health. Results of interviews with experienced NPs describe:

- Feelings about models of care directing the practice,
- Use of reflective practice techniques,
- Methods of obtaining physician collaboration/supervision,
- Management of patient satisfaction,
- Use of cost saving methods,
- Use of diagnostics available on-site,
- Assessment of patients with screening tools,
- Management of on-call protocols, and
- Participation in emergency/disaster coverage in their practice/community.

In addition, NP perceptions of what masters students need to learn from a graduate Advanced Practice Role course are identified. Measuring patient outcomes, leveraging resources, and improving patient satisfaction are also discussed.

Entrepreneurialism

In health care, as in other professions, an entrepreneur must have courage, assertiveness, and vision, as well as be open to new and possibly risky options (Elange, Hunter, & Winchell, 2007). More than ever, each healthcare provider must have business savvy and the ability to manage business finances, participate in consumer marketing, maintain professional competency, display courage by thinking "outside of the box," and be able to take risks. Entrepreneurs use all these skills to develop a business, of which they are usually the sole proprietor. The Registered Nurse Response Network (RNRN) is a national organization that can be contacted for assistance in starting one's own business (http://www.nnba.net).

Before starting a business, answer the following questions. They are helpful in reviewing one's ideas.

- What kind of business operating model would best support an effective and cost-efficient agency?
- Does one feel comfortable and prepared to make decisions that may affect another person's livelihood?
- How best can a competitive healthcare agency be created given the current marketplace?

Every setting needs people with excellent communication skills. Agencies in which team members communicate directly with one another seem to be most effective in generating best outcomes. Saphiere (2005) and Brent (1990) provide excellent strategies for the NP to implement to generate change and growth in an organization. This entrepreneurial "spirit" is more specifically articulated in Cordock, *Business Upgrade: 21 Days to Reignite the Entrepreneurial Spirit in You and Your Team* (2007) and in Serota and Serota, *Starting from Scratch: Developing Your Own Practice Site* (2001).

Danna and Porche (2009) describe four approaches an NP can use to strategize as an entrepreneur:

- Aim to be a low-cost provider. This advocates a Wal-Mart type of business model applied to health care. Offer basic care to a large segment of the marketplace with less expensive visit charges, accessibility to the bus/metro, free parking, and no extra frills, such as a play area for children, television, a wide array of magazines, aquarium or other decorative distractions, and refreshments. This stresses profits based on the number of encounters instead of high cost.
- Offer services with some differentiation. Develop a reputation for being "special" in some way, such as always seeing patients on time, having laboratory services on site, and following up with patients by email or phone.
- Be known for having the best price. This is self-explanatory; it is also hard to do and still maintain quality. After performing a marketplace assessment, determine what other providers are charging for similar services and try to undercut your competitors' services through greater efficiency.
- Target your services to a specific population that wants a specific type of healthcare practice. This is similar to being niche focused. Generally, it means an upscale service that caters to people who do not worry about cost or what insurance will pay. They expect to "pay for what they get"; price is not a deciding factor. An example might be an agency in which the NP makes home visits and provides primary care. OR, perhaps, a practice focusing on patients who have undergone gender reassignment and have special healthcare needs (Sobralske, 2005).

Danna and Porche (2008) also list specific strategies an NP can use to establish partnerships with competitors:

- Strategic Alliances—This is when two agencies join together to accomplish the same mission and goals. An example would be a primary care practice and a diagnostic laboratory partnering to provide more convenient services.
- Merger and Acquisition—A merger occurs when two equal agencies create one new organization, such as when two small dermatology practices create one large practice. An acquisition is when one agency takes over a smaller or lower cost-generating agency, such as a world-acclaimed multiple provider Rheumatology Center acquiring a small one physician-based practice.
- Outsourcing—Often, healthcare agencies outsource their laundry, housekeeping, and perhaps billing to individuals/organizations specializing in

these areas. This allows the healthcare agency to concentrate fully on patient care and delegate to others functions outside of direct patient care. With this arrangement, the agency does not need to employ a specialist in-house to do these tasks. An entrepreneurial NPs could advertise a variety of services, such as Vaccination Update, Travel Clinic, Complementary Modes of Health Care, or Sports Physicals and Management of Sports-Induced Musculoskeletal Injuries. In addition, they could market these services to the consumer and other healthcare providers who may want to refer their patients.

Nurse practitioners should examine their own skill sets, agency resources, and staff abilities to determine if outsourcing is feasible, cost effective, and efficient. If little self-skill or knowledge is seen in an area, if sufficient financial resources are available to pay others, or if there is a lack of trained and/or educated staff, outsourcing may be the "best" decision. Outsourcing can be temporary (e.g., until the practice "gets its feet on the ground") or for whatever time duration makes sense. Mackey, McNiel, and Klingensmith (2004) define outsourcing as buying the services from vendors that can provide them in a high-quality and cost-efficient fashion. The services include:

- Information technology
- Business planning
- Billing and collection service
- Laboratory and radiology
- Accounting, marketing
- Staffing, payroll services
- Laundry
- Legal services

Some NPs believe staffing positions can be filled through outsourcing as well, particularly temporary staff positions, as the business could eliminate the cost of benefits for these employees, which generally average 25 to 30% of salary. However, outsourced staff has definite disadvantages as well. Such staff members may earn a higher salary, provide less consistency for patients, and possibly have less loyalty to the agency. In addition, team morale might decline as some of the staff is transient.

Intrapreneurs are individuals who, like entrepreneurs, are creative, like to try new things, do not worry needlessly, and enjoy taking risks. The difference is whose resources are being used and what risks the individual is taking. If the person works in an organization with an entrepreneurial style, the individual is an intrapreneur. In this case, the resources and risks are the responsibility of the organization and not the individual. The goal of the intrapreneur is to revitalize the organization and implement innovative initiatives. Nurse practitioners could use the entrepreneurial approach in creating his or her own business or choose to obtain experience as an intrapreneur in someone else's business, thereby learning to improve outcomes as well as one's salary and beneits package. Then, NPs could branch out after with less personal risk.

Strategies for Maximizing Patient Outcomes, Leveraging Resources, and Improving Patient Satisfaction

To obtain valued feedback, we interviewed nine seasoned NPs. The participants interviewed had between 4 and 25 years of NP experience, and the majority worked with adults aged 18 years and older. No one worked primarily in pediatrics, and only two worked in a family practice. All were women between 30 and 60 years of age. Questions were developed after a literature review revealed little information on specific topics. In addition, the authors' experiences have shown that most NPs were not savvy about these topics even though the information was important for NPs to know. The first topic was the use of a care model. Nurse practitioners use a nursing framework, along with the medical model, but some do not seem to realize this. The interviewees all thought in a similar fashion, using the same pattern of thought fairly consistently, as they analyzed the patient data after determining a differential diagnosis and establishing a care management plan. The questions are given below, with an analysis of the responses.

Questions and Answers

Question #1—*What model of care (e.g., a nursing model, medical model, or combination of both) do you follow?*

Answer:

Some used a combination of their nursing experience and the medical model, but they did not describe exactly how they came up with the plan for an individual patient. Rather, they just follow their "gut." One said that NPs have to think about how they get reimbursed from insurance companies, so they "have to" use their own model of care, coupled with the medical model of diagnosis. Several use *Orem's Self-Care Model* (Hartweg, 1991) and one NP in cardiology uses *Rosenstock's Health Belief Model* (Bradford, 1997), which specifically focuses on self-efficacy. Another NP uses a combination of models, including the *Trans-theoretical Model of Change* (Burbank, & Riebe, 2002), *Orem's Self-Care Model* (Hartweg, 1991), and *Erikson's Theory of Psychosocial Development* (Erikson, 1963), depending on the patient's problem(s). All follow some type of holistic approach, but they definitely have to use and document medical terminology or they will not receive appropriate reimbursement. Several NPs could not articulate which framework they used, but agreed they do think more about the patient as an individual and how they respond to treatments, adapt to change, and could potentially care for themselves, but do not necessarily use a specific model/framework. This is crucial in differentiating an NP philosophy of care centering on patient outcomes.

Question #2—*What is your perception of reflective practice as an NP? (When asked "what is meant by reflective practice?," the authors described it as continually evaluating one's own practice to inform oneself about approaches to reflection, such as critiquing self, developing and monitoring professional practice and, thereby, improving the quality of patient care).*

Answer:

I believe reflective practice is very important since it allows for personal and professional growth as a practitioner, which helps to improve care quality. As a new NP, reflective practice is very important since it helps you to learn about new and different approaches to situations and would be very beneficial to do consistently. I feel that obtaining more knowledge and skills from individuals who have been practicing longer has really helped me to be a better practitioner.

I continually reflect on my practice. The technology continues to change with my practice so I have to keep up with the new changes. Also, there are multiple clinical trials involving the care of heart failure patients, so I have to be sure to be educated about new guidelines. I continually educate myself on the new treatments in order to best care for my patients.

Reflective practice is important in order to be "present" for the patient and my own ongoing development and growth in reflection is necessary for excellence in practice.

I make it a practice to attend at least two conferences/year and network with a group of NPs to discuss patient management issues.

Every 6 months we are required to complete a self-evaluation tool for the Hospital Human Resources Department, and I also regularly [4–6 times/ year] meet with other APRNS to discuss our practice, development, and other professional issues.

I am constantly reviewing guidelines, doing on-line continuing education, attending conferences and professional meetings, and discussing cases with colleagues. I also review how I am interacting with patients and handling difficult situations. I know I can improve my communication techniques and try to do this using self-reflection.

Responses indicate there is a mixed understanding of reflective practice. Some NPs feel it involves only keeping up with new advances, skills, and technology; some see it as a method of self-critique; and still others see the use of self and being "present" with patients as very much a part of reflective practice.

Question #3—*How did you obtain collaborative agreement or supervision with a physician, if necessary, in your state?*

Answer:
"I have a physician I can call 24/7 if I need assistance; otherwise I practice independently." This was the predominant answer to this question by the NPs.

The NPs are responsible for stress testing [cardiologist is readily available during stress tests for collaboration], anticoagulation clinic, in-patient consults and follow-up visits, and out-patient visits. NPs do not see new cardiology consults in the hospital without the collaborating physician, so the APRN does the new consult's assessment and then reports to the physician. The MD sees the patient and writes a progress note, which includes the impression and recommendation. The APRN dictates the consult which is then cosigned by the MD. The APRN is not involved with new consults in the office. The APRN does follow-up visits in the hospital and office and these visits do not need to be cosigned by the MD.

I asked a physician and signed a collaborative agreement that we both agreed on, and we meet to discuss patients monthly.

A collaborative agreement with a physician(s) for most NPs in private practice, clinics, and specialty practices is necessary. Many NPs were not aware of the components of the collaborative agreement or how their employer negotiated this arrangement.

Question #4—*How do you measure patient outcomes and satisfaction?*

Answer:
Following office visits, all progress notes in the cardiology office are electronically forwarded to the primary care providers. This has greatly improved communication with these providers. APRNs also forward office visit write-ups to the cardiologists, so they have knowledge about the patient's progress.

We use the PROMISE Survey which is a Post-death Family Satisfaction Tool to evaluate our practice as palliative and hospice care providers.

I always do follow-up phone calls for my patients. I also emphasize how I want them to call or email me if they are not happy with the results of their visit.

I always try to give the patient [if appropriate] some control in the health-care decisions, such as giving him/her a choice on what exercise they would prefer or what stress-reducing practice would be best for them.

Mostly just monitor patient satisfaction verbally with good communication, education, and troubleshooting with the patient or family. No idea how this is done formally in my practice setting.

Patient outcomes are maximized through my efforts at integrating evidence-based strategies. I measure patient outcomes throughout their treatment.

I keep up with current practices and technology in order to maximize patient outcomes and provider satisfaction. Evidence-based practice keeps providers satisfied with the treatment that I am providing.

I follow up with a phone call or email after an office visit with my patients.

It seems all NPs are interested in receiving feedback, maintaining quality improvement, and improving patient outcomes. They all pair their outcomes to patient satisfaction. Only one is hospital based, one is in long-term care, and the rest are in out-patient settings, but none are doing chart review or outcome evaluation, such as the Healthcare Effectiveness Data and Information Set (HEDIS) that is used by 90% of American health plans to measure performance on service and care (National Committee for Quality Assurance [NCQA], 2009). A suggestion would be for all practices to initiate outcome evaluation processes, such as HEDIS, so NPs can become more involved in outcome evaluation.

Question #5—*Have you used any cost-saving techniques or found new ways of increasing resources in your practice?*

Answer:
Answers to the original question, "Do you leverage any of your resources with partners?," revealed that it is not widely incorporated. Leveraging is a way to supplement resources by sharing with partners. In some ways, it reflects a bartering concept. Nurse practitioners from a primary care clinic could collaborate with NPs from a women's health agency to assist both businesses in maximizing resources. For example, the primary care practice can use the women's health practice's wet mount and pap smear equipment, while sharing venipuncture supplies with the women's health practice. This leveraging of resources assists both agencies in providing more cost-effective service to patients.

> *Just recently, the stress testing was assigned to APRNs instead of MDs, so the MDs will have more time for office visits. This is extremely cost effective. The Anticoagulation Clinic was started by the APRNs, and it is revenue generating. We are very careful to avoid unnecessary duplication of diagnostics which, of course, is cost effective.*

> *The APRNs in the office developed an orientation program for APRNs, which has saved money and increased NP satisfaction with role considerably.*

> *We are a palliative care service in a hospital setting, so we now accept direct admissions. This has decreased cost and increased patient satisfaction.*

> *Since I am in dermatology, I do a lot of preventive teaching and that in itself saves the patient money.*

> *I try to prescribe generic drugs whenever possible. I also follow my heart failure patients very closely in order to keep them out of the hospital. I focus on cost-effective care for each of my patients, but I do not have any one idea that decreases costs for the practice.*

Moving practice to own home office has helped in decreasing my costs.

We went green in the office, and this has decreased costs. We also no longer use Rapid Strep or Rapid Flu screening on everyone with a sore throat or fever. We also stopped doing routine urine testing unless appropriate. We have extended our evening hours for our patients who work and also receive more urgent care visits, and these two changes have increased our revenue.

A number of good cost-saving recommendations were mentioned. In discussing this topic, several NPs said they are going to start thinking more about this. Others are considering a change and want to go out on their own or practice with one physician. The interview did stimulate some new thoughts and made some of the NPs think about doing something different and becoming more collaborative. Each NP has individually implemented cost-saving measures, but this could be dramatically increased by collaborating on a larger scale.

Question #6—*What type of diagnostics and screening tools do you have access to in your practice? Or, do you outsource the diagnostic work?*

Answer:
We have a lab station from a local hospital in our building so, in our office, we just do EKGs, spirometry, nebulizers, pulse oximetry, urine dips, rapid flu, and strep.

We perform regular stress tests, MIBI stress test, ECGs, Holter monitoring, ECHOs, PPM and ICD checks, Coumadin draws. All other lab work is sent to a laboratory.

The office staff do EKGs and blood work which is sent to the hospital laboratory. All INRs are drawn at the anticoagulation clinic as point-of-care testing.

We send our specimens out to a lab.

We are part of a hospital with complete lab services.

Finger sticks, mono, blood sugar, cholesterol, influenza, strep, and pregnancy tests are the only tests done in this clinic.

What about screening tools? List the three most frequently used tools.

The screening tools were specific to the type of specialty practice. Only a few NPs listed any other general tools, such as the CAGE, dyspnea, chest pain/discomfort, or depression screenings.

- Skin Typing for Skin Cancer Risk
- Dermatology Life Quality Index Tool
- Mini Mental/ Clock Drawing Screening Assessment
- Geriatric Depression Scale
- Noncancer Prognostic Criteria for Terminal Care
- Pain Assessment
- Beck Depression Inventory
- Speilberger State/Trait Anxiety Inventory
- Dissociative Experience Scale
- Borg's Scale of Perceived Exertion when doing Stress Tests
- Minnesota Living with Heart Failure Questionnaire
- We have an ROS and PE template designed for our cardiology patients which helps with standardization of findings and quality improvement
- Pulse oximetry, KOH and pH test strips, urine dipstick

The NPs offered no comments about outsourcing diagnostics, but those with more of a specialty focus were understandably more screening focused than those who work in more general practices and are bound by the restrictive 15-minute time frame for a visit. Of course, the psych NPs were more apt to use the mental health screening tools, but just about everyone identified the Beck Depression Scale as one of their most frequently used screening tools.

Question #7—*What is your on-call protocol, if you have one?*

Answer:
Cell phone and will get back to them in 24 hours. If out of town, have colleague cover.

NA

Hospital ED physicians handle the palliative care service calls.

Only the physicians provide 24/7 on-call.

I was on-call 24/7 unless on vacation, and my physician boss took call. I was not reimbursed for this.

There is no call for APRNs—there is a Cardiologist and Cardiology Fellow on 24/7.

We have one of our providers on-call 24/7 and share weekend call with another primary practice, so I only do call about 6 hours/week—we do not get paid for on-call but if we do extra on-call to cover someone, our office hours are compensated with time off.

Clearly, on-call is managed in many different ways. NPs earn little pay for this work, but more were saying that only the partners of the practice were responsible for off-duty calls. All but one NP said the physicians were not paid for their on-call work either, and it was evenly distributed among them.

Question #8—*What type of emergency/disaster coverage do you provide for your practice/network/community?*

Answer:
We are part of the hospital, so we use the hospital's ED and emergency system.

Patients are instructed to call 911 and/or go the local ED.

I am on the Disaster Team for the local hospital and the American Red Cross and our patients are covered for emergencies by our on-call protocol.

We are part of the hospital Disaster Team and serve the hospital and community.

Do not know.

None

We see patients who have skin emergencies by fitting them into our schedule, and our 24/7 on call protocol assists them to seek help otherwise. The physicians are linked with the local hospitals for Disaster Management.

Unless affiliated with a hospital, most NPs did not know much about their practice's link with the community in terms of providing Disaster/Emergency services.

Question #9—*Do you use any entrepreneurial interventions in your practice that could be helpful to other NPs? Do you have any advice on how to succeed as an NP?*

Answer:
Become specialized in your field and get all the extra courses/education/supervision you can about that area. Then, let your colleagues know what your specialty is; offer to do referrals and speak at conferences on the topic; publish articles; become certified in this area if you can; join listserves for this specialty; and join professional organizations in this area.

We use "Standing Stone," a software program to track patients being followed by an anticoagulation clinic. We are hoping to develop a software program for our heart failure patients.

I have multiple flow sheets for my patients in order to best follow their care.

We do daily rounding of our patients throughout the hospital and focus on their palliative care needs.

There is evidence that practice generates ideas for improvement in patient care.

The final question asked of these experienced NPs was their idea on what else NPs should learn to better fulfill the "Role" aspect of being an NP.

Question #10—*List five priority topics that should be included in an Advanced Nurse Practice Role Course [assume the following are included, so do not list: scope of practice, certification process and issues, rationale for educational preparation, and licensure process and issues].*

Answer:
Participants identified many of the same topics, including:

- Legal issues,
- Type of continuing education needed for board recertification,
- Research and quality improvement assessment,
- Program development,
- Outcome evaluation,
- Communication skills (motivational interviewing),
- Development of reflective practice techniques,
- Importance of lifelong learning,
- Day-to-day typical day activities of NP,
- New roles, such as hospitalist, and new procedures that NPs can do,
- Need to network and get connected to these new roles and processes,
- Business information must be part of everyday practice,
- Need for supervision/collaboration—what this means,
- Emphasize the autonomy of NP and need to not portray the helper or physician extender role,
- Negotiation tactics, salary, and promotion,
- What to expect with transition of student to NP role,
- Cost-effective approaches to care,
- Collaboration with everyone,
- Importance of thorough documentation, and
- Leadership training.

These interviews, although conducted with a small sample, validated that more education is needed about regulatory agencies and business practices. All the NPs felt that reflective practice was key to growth and tried to be cost effective in managing patients. The NPs had little in common regarding methods for cost savings, participating in emergency/disaster processes, use of screening tools, performing diagnostics in their practice setting, collaborative agreements, and practice models. Their recommendations for what should be included in a NP role course are reflective of what the inexperienced NPs in Chapter 1 identified. This confirms that the varied role of the NP encompasses leadership, management, professionalism, and clinical skills.

Sites of Entrepreneurialism for Nurse Practitioners

Community Health Centers

Working at Community Health Centers (CHCs) provides excellent opportunities for NPs to interact entrepreneurially with vulnerable populations and to generally care for rural, inner city, and homeless individuals. (These practice settings also result in a percentage of forgiveness for student loans. One can access the National Association of Community Health Centers at http://www.nachc.org. for more information on the loan forgiveness plan.) Often, a CHC system has multiple specialty clinics, several primary care satellites, and an urgent care center. During the school year, the CHC may also staff the city's school-based health clinics. Nurse practitioners need to be culturally aware, competent, and creative in managing the care of many of these patients, many of whom are seen only once for episodic care and tend to go from one clinic to another and from state to state. This episodic nature of care makes it difficult to monitor outcomes, particularly when electronic documentation is not available. But as CHCs become more accessible to patients, a stronger relationship between patient and provider and greater continuity is being established. This type of practice site has difficulty getting resources, will often collaborate with another clinic, and sometimes does not have basic equipment. Nurse practitioners can work autonomously in these clinics and have their own caseload of 400 to 450 patients.

Detention Centers

Detention Centers house teenagers who are alleged to have committed some criminal action. They tend to stay approximately three months. The staff consists of an NP, guards, the Detention Center Director, a secretary, a psychologist, and a housekeeper. While incarcerated, the teenagers receive primary health care, health promotion education, and health screening and vaccinations. Common problems are typical teenage ailments, such as headache, stomach ache, cough, and pharyngitis, but some have chronic illnesses, psychological problems, and acute health problems, while others have substance abuse and mental health disorders, pregnancy issues, and sexually transmitted infections. The majority of these adolescents need full dental, vision, and primary health care, as most have never received preventive health care, primary care, or dental prophylaxis. The NP needs to develop a collaborative relationship with each member of the center's staff, teaching the guards basic health treatments and how to communicate observations. Because there is usually no other nursing staff, the guards may need to be the NP's "eyes and ears." Emergency protocols need implementation for frequent problems (e.g., suicide attempts, severe respiratory infections, difficulty breathing, abdominal pain or any acute pain, fractures, burns, rashes that cause severe discomfort, anxiety, depression, head injuries, or any trauma), so that staff knows when to call 911 and when to call the NP who often takes calls 24/7. A policy book with clearly articulated procedures should be accessible, so the guards know how to proceed if the NP is not available. Frequent orientations of staff should be scheduled. The NP often implements many health promotion programs for the teens, but these programs need to be culturally appropriate and at the correct literacy level. Nurse practitioners working in this setting are successful when they can facilitate self-care and responsibility for health in the adolescents. These programs may be a mechanism by which detainees will acquire lifelong "good" health habits. Often, this setting is an ideal practice area funded by outside grants for health promotion and disease prevention programs.

College Health Clinics

College health offers the NP opportunities to work with young adults from 17 to 25 years of age. Most college health clinics care only for enrolled students; larger colleges care for students, faculty, and staff. Many models of care are being used in this clinical area, such as the overnight infirmary, the NP-run primary care clinic, and the physician-run primary care clinic. Faith-based colleges may limit access to contraception and abortion counseling and referral services, which is difficult as many college students need these services. More and more college health clinics are becoming primary care centers, managing student's health care needs, giving psychological counseling, providing emergency health services, and offering health promotion programs. These clinics are run generally with a staff of NPs and RNs, plus a secretary. Other clinics are NP run, with staffs consisting of ANPs, FNPs, and Psych NPs, an NP Director, a collaborating physician, a secretary, and an insurance manager. These clinics provide primary care to all enrolled students and coordinate care among the provider from the student's home, the clinic NP, and the subspecialist if a referral is needed. Students may present with common health problems, such as pharyngitis, mononucleosis, ear pain, headache, chest pain, and abdominal complaints; chronic illnesses, such as diabetes, asthma, cancer, Crohn disease, and lupus erythematosus; and acute problems, such as fractures, head injuries, pregnancy, sexually transmitted infections, hypothermia, dehydration, and anaphylaxis. In addition, these students need health promotion education and disease prevention care.

Palliative Care and Hospice

Nurse practitioners who work in palliative care and hospice are generally board certified as family nurse practitioners, pediatric nurse practitioners, gerontology nurse practitioners, or adult nurse practitioners; they may also have additional specialty certification in palliative care. As more providers use a palliative care model for individuals with end-stage chronic illness, the role of the NP in palliative care has expanded to include more consultations with primary care providers, referrals from hospitalists, and increased provision of advanced practice care. The focus of palliative care is holistic and comfort rather than curing. This care is now initiated earlier in the end stage of a disease. Quaglietti, Blum, and Ellis (2004) share their ideas about palliative care in advanced practice and highlight some helpful strategies. To enhance one's knowledge on palliative and end-of-life care, access the End-of-Life Nursing Consortium (ELNEC) program or

attend the graduate/advanced practice three-day course (http://www.aacn.nche
.edu/elnec/curriculum.htm).

Acute Care Nurse Practitioners

Kleinpell and Hravnak (2005) suggest some effective strategies for Acute Care
NPs to generate positive patient outcomes using a critical care model. Based on
nursing knowledge and experience, it has proven to be effective. In fact, they recommend Acute Care NPs identify problem areas, develop interventions, and
monitor effectiveness for evidence that these interventions are "better" than
what has been considered the "only tried-and-true way." Bahouth and Kopan
(2009) developed an Acute Care NP orientation program that used a model applicable for any setting. The National Organization of Nurse Practitioner Faculty
published the Acute Care NP Competencies, which are helpful to review when
thinking about practice models in critical care (http://www.nonpf.com/ACNP
Compsfinal20041.pdf).

Another frequent aspect of care challenging Acute and Primary Care NPs is
managing pain. Pain management is a growing industry, and NPs have the talent and skills to address the problems potentially causing the pain. This differs
from what seems to be "the mainstream method" of pain control, which is turn-
ing off the pain receptors temporarily with medication.

Psych Nurse Practitioners

Psych NPs work in a variety of settings, including hospitals, clinics, and private
practices. Many specialize in specific areas, such as bereavement, trauma, eat-
ing disorders, substance abuse, emergency departments, and fertility, or are
liaisons in primary care, acute care, or women's health. Some work with fibro-
myalgia patients, specialize in pharmacodynamics, or work with patients in hospice. Many use a holistic approach to care and deal with a variety of mental
health problems, including anxiety, depression, and thought disorders, and are
involved in intense psychotherapy with their patients (Wheeler, 2008). The
NONPF Psych NP Competencies can be accessed at http://www.nonpf.org/final
comps03.pdf.

Holistic Nurse Practitioners

Many NPs embrace complementary and alternative methods of care. Some combine these aspects of health management with more conservative medical model
interventions, while others follow completely holistic and complementary methods practices. These services are generally run as a boutique business, where the
consumer pays all costs directly. No insurance is involved. This acceptance of alternative methods highlights another difference between NPs and physician care.

Case Management

Case management can be divided into many areas of specialization, each with
its own approach and job description (Tahan & Huber, 2006). Nurse practitioners have traditionally been involved in case management practice and patient
outcome research often with high-risk patients (Daniels & Ramey, 2006; Huber
& Craig, 2007; and Umbrell, 2006) or patients with chronic illness. But, NPs are

now expanding their expertise to include new areas, including wound care, genetic screening, and geriatrics.

Wound Care

Within their scope of practice, NPs can implement the guidelines for wound care (MacLellan, Gardner, & Gardner, 2002) and provide expert care and case management. The same applies to high-risk patients in a tertiary care environment. Outcomes indicate that this NP practice model is efficacious.

Genetic Screening

Nurse practitioners also need to address the public's increasing awareness of the advantages and disadvantages of genetic screening. In some models of care, NPs teach and offer seminars explaining how one's genetic make-up relates to specific diseases. They have shown entrepreneurial spirit by also addressing the issue of how some people have a tendency to acquire specific diseases (Westwood, Pickering, Latter, & Lucassen, 2006). Zallen (2008) covers multiple issues in her book, *To Test or Not to Test: A Guide to Genetic Screening and Risk,* including:

- Diagnostics and yield for those who undergo testing for illness,
- Categories of people at high risk,
- Variables that mitigate screening,
- Decision process concerning testing, and
- Advantages of increasing knowledge about one's genes.

Geriatrics

Nurse practitioner expertise is also needed with the most complex and highest risk geriatric patients, who represent approximately 20% of the population and who account for about 86% of healthcare dollars, 67% of which are hospital based. Many patients hospitalized or in long-term care are being monitored by NPs. The limits of Medicare and insurance reimbursement make this a difficult practice area to manage. To succeed, this entrepreneurial opportunity needs a carefully planned NP business model. However, NPs should consider the high volume of potential patients who will need temporary and, sometimes, more extensive acute care management. They should strategize ways to provide high-quality care in suites with home-like atmospheres. Patients and their families could then become more involved with the patient's care, avoid or minimize the complications of immobility, and even manage nutritional needs. This model of care, built around Orem's Self-Care Model (Orem, 1980), would have the following mission:

- Be patient/family–centered,
- Provide patients with supervised care for activities of daily living and direct access to all the medical facilities needed, such as occupational, physical, and medical care, and
- Facilitate independence and self-responsibility for patient health.

The *vision* for this care model is a structured environment in which patients who are planning on returning to their own or a loved one's home could gain independence and improve their health status while family and loved ones learn how to administer appropriate care. All nutritional, pharmacological, and appropriate nursing interventions would be taught to the family members and the patient. The *goal* would be to discharge the patient as soon as self-care could be rendered. Specific *objectives,* with a target date or timeframe for completion, would be developed by the patient, family, and healthcare team. The NP would serve as coordinator (see Table 8–1). Thus, nurse practitioners can assist patients to change behaviors and, ultimately, improve healthcare outcomes (Miller & Rollnick, 1991; Rollnick, Heather, & Bell, 1992; and Jansink, Braspenning, van-der Weijden, & Niessen et al, 2009).

Strategic Planning

A small business owner/entrepreneur needs to use intuition and networking skills in the marketplace to learn what competitors are doing. Having a new business is chaotic. To be successful, the owner and employees need to measure patient and family satisfaction continuously. This demonstrates respect for consumer feedback and allows the adaptation of some or all of these ideas to promote maximum growth. At the same time, owners should stick to their general missions and visions (Moseley, 2009).

All NPs have been educated based on the NONPF Nurse Practitioner Competency Domains (2006), so practice owners should remember the NP staff has knowledge and experience in the following areas:

- Management of patient health/illness status.
- NP-patient relationship.
- Teaching-coaching function.
- Professional role.
- Managing and negotiating healthcare delivery systems.
- Monitoring and ensuring the quality of healthcare practice, and.
- Culturally sensitive care.

8.1 Components of Strategic Planning

Mission = agency or organization's purpose.

Vision = the ideal plan for the organization. Areas of growth and goals toward which the organization or agency is moving.

Goals = the overarching global goals that the agency/organization is striving to accomplish.

Objectives = the specific, planned actions, with a targeted timeframe for how the overall goals will be accomplished.

Many NPs have also had exposure to marketing, strategic planning, goal formation, evaluation techniques, and program planning and evaluation. They can easily transfer this knowledge if their role requires it. All 75 subcompetencies can be accessed at http://www.nonpf.com/NONPF2005/CoreCompsFINAL06.pdf.

Many specialty practices, such as pulmonary, cardiovascular, and oncology, provide comprehensive care from diagnosis through the end of life. They can manage effective patient outcomes, as the patient lives with chronic illness. These practices see patients on an out-patient basis, but the NP or physician also follows them during hospitalizations. Many NPs take call (i.e., are responsible for answering all patient phone calls after 5 PM and before 9 AM, as well as calls regarding the practice's patients from providers working in long-term care or hospitals), work with the hospitalist as a specialty consultant, and do palliative and hospice consultancies for other nonservice inpatients.

Some NPs in rural health or other practice models make effective use of telemedicine (Martin, 2000). This includes the exchange of detailed images of rashes, dental problems, and musculoskeletal deformities and videostreams that enable live interaction between the NP and the collaborative physician. Thus, telemedicine enhances this collaboration between the provider and a specialist or a visiting nurse and a NP/physician. Reed (2005) shares some examples of using telemedicine with a variety of NP practice models.

Outcome Management

With the escalating cost of health care, NPs have more opportunities to provide care and assist with improving patient outcomes. Most hospitals and large healthcare agencies have a department of Quality Improvement charged with monitoring patient outcomes. Small practice settings should also strive to conduct quality improvement audits. An excellent model that will help NPs review ideas for developing a quality improvement system is provided by the Institute for Health Care Delivery Research in Intermountain Health Care (www.ihc.com/xp/ihc/physician/research/institute/) In fact, each healthcare agency should monitor patient care in some fashion and not just assume every provider is documenting comprehensively and following patient care guidelines. Kane (2006) recommends that all outcome measurement be organized for analysis for the following reasons:

- Identification of the best practitioners/NPs/physician assistants/physicians. (This is important for individuals looking for the "right" provider, as well as for insurance companies that need to find the most effective care providers while maintaining cost effectiveness.)
- Establishment of accountability. (This process proves that the care is of adequate quality.)
- Improvement of the knowledge base. (If data are collected properly, they can validate evidence even though it is not derived from a randomized control trial.)

Patient-centered care requires patient input. Patient satisfaction is easy to measure and analyze using *Survey Monkey* or other tools, as long as the literacy level of the tool matches that of the population being evaluated. In addition, the type of tool should address the needs of the population under assessment. Patients should not be asked if they are "happy with the diagnosis," because patients are not able to judge the correctness of the care provided, and many may have received a poor prognosis. Visit http://www.SurveyMonkey.com for information and view the following example used at a College Health Primary Care Clinic (see Table 8.2). The tool questionnaire can be modified to support any type of patient care setting.

A conceptual model by which outcome assessment is planned is necessary. For example, the provider's hypothesis, or how they perceive herpes should be managed, needs to be tested. For example, is suppression therapy management, which would yield fewer clinic visits and provide greater comfort for the patient, more satisfactory to the patient than episodic management? Another hypothetical example would be whether to offer moderate level asthmatics a reduced fee for a spacer device for their inhaler. This would ultimately improve their breathing, decrease wheezing, increase energy, and decrease clinic visits. When assessing healthcare outcomes, NPs need a hypothesis or conceptual framework based on their clinical experience and intuition about how interventions given to specific types of patients affect specific outcomes. One might ask: "Wouldn't it be better for the practice to make the Asthmatic and Herpes 1 and 2 patients come to the clinic more frequently, thereby providing more revenue for the provider?" Probably not, because satisfied patients will recommend the practice to their friends and family—and patients will more likely be satisfied if they are managed with fewer visits. As satisfied patients recommend the practice, revenue will improve as the practice grows. Any and all areas of practice that intrigue or appeal to NPs can be analyzed for outcomes.

Further, NPs should realize that multiple variables influence patient outcomes, including general health status, age, genetic make-up, and compliance with treatment plan(s). This information needs to be documented, preferably on easy-to-read checklists. Berwick (1989) notes the importance of comprehensively recording all of the care and results, even if no negative finding arises. If a "negative" thing happens, you must be able to locate records of the treatments provided.

Another important point is that a large enough sample is needed to validate outcomes. Thus, collect data over several years and/or collaborate with other physicians and NPs to generate a large enough aggregate to evaluate. In addition, collaboration with others caring for similar patients means that more data can be collected over a shorter period of time, and the data analysis can occur quicker. This provides an excellent opportunity to network with other NPs with similar practices or roles.

Using Donabedian's (1966) original framework for quality of care, identify the following indicators so quality improvement can be monitored:

- Structure indicators (the training the providers received and the equipment at the practice site).
- Process indicators (whether the correct action was taken for a patient situation and if the action was performed correctly).
- Outcome indicators (the results of the process indicator actions).

8.2　Patient Satisfaction Tool

1. I am

   ☐ Male　　☐ Female　　☐ would prefer not to say

2. How would you identify yourself?

   ☐ African American　　☐ White American　　☐ International
   ☐ Hispanic American　　☐ Asian American　　☐ Other (please specify)

3. Would you describe yourself as:

   ☐ Heterosexual　　☐ Bisexual　　☐ Questioning
   ☐ Transsexual　　☐ Gay or Lesbian

4. When scheduling your appointment, were you seen?

   ☐ The same day I inquired　　☐ The day you wanted
   ☐ The following day　　☐ Other (please specify)

5. I found it easy to make an appointment

   ☐ Yes　　　☐ No

6. The receptionist treated me with courtesy and professionally

   ☐ Yes　　　☐ No

7. How long did you wait in the waiting room to be seen?

   ☐ Less than five minutes　　☐ 11–20 minutes
   ☐ 5–10 minutes　　☐ Greater than 20 minutes

8. FOR EACH STATEMENT BELOW, CHECK THE BOX THAT BEST INDICATES HOW
   SATISFIED YOU WERE AT THIS VISIT:

	Very Satisfied	Satisfied	Unsatisfied	Very Unsatisfied	I have no opinion
The Nurse Practitioner spent enough time with me.	☐	☐	☐	☐	☐
The Nurse Practitioner treated me with courtesy and respect.	☐	☐	☐	☐	☐
The degree to which the Nurse Practitioner respected your privacy and protected your confidentiality.	☐	☐	☐	☐	☐
The Nurse Practitioner gave me the opportunity to ask questions.	☐	☐	☐	☐	☐

	Very Satisfied	Satisfied	Unsatisfied	Very Unsatisfied	I have no opinion
The amount of information the Nurse Practitioner gave you about your medical condition.	☐	☐	☐	☐	☐
The relief from worries about your medical condition that the Nurse Practitioner provided.	☐	☐	☐	☐	☐
The amount of information the Nurse Practitioner gave you about preventive practices.	☐	☐	☐	☐	☐

9. If necessary, would you consider a return visit to the Health Center?

   ☐ Yes   ☐ No

10. Do you know that a Nurse Practitioner is on-call after hours?

    ☐ Yes   ☐ No

11. Do you know that the Health Center has a health information web site?

    ☐ Yes   ☐ No

12. Are there any additional services that you would like the Health Center to provide?

    ☐ Yes (please describe) _____

    _____

    _____

    ☐ No

13. What type of insurance do you have?

    _____

14. Have you seen any of the Health Education programs in the community?

    ☐ Yes   ☐ No

Practice Accreditation

Accreditation is a process of evaluation that results in accountability and quality services. Just as educational institutions must prove the quality of education provided, practices can obtain accreditation to prove the quality of care provided. Practice accreditation is available for multiprovider practices, providers of certain subspecialties, and some provision models. Private, single-provider practices generally do not seek accreditation.

Accreditation by the appropriate authority signals excellence in care and quality outcomes. As an analogy, imagine shopping for meat for dinner. A NY strip will provide a nice meal, but purchasing "certified Angus" ensures the best quality available. If having a procedure at an ambulatory surgical center, recommendations from friends or providers is helpful, but accreditation by the Accreditation Association for Ambulatory Health Care (AAAHC) provides knowledge about the level of care provided and the competence of the staff. Accreditation is a "seal of approval" indicating that the practice has established guidelines, performance standards, and expected outcomes in key clinical, financial, and service areas. Accreditation reports about each practice are publically available, so they allow patients to compare different providers offering the same services. Patients are empowered to make an informed decision. The inspection or survey of the business examines more than 60 areas of operations. In these areas, the business is held accountable to meeting established standards. Generally the following six categories are reviewed:

- Quality management and improvement in clinical outcomes
- Member rights and responsibilities
- Utilization standards, including decision-making standards and clinical protocols
- Preventive health interventions
- Credentialing of staff
- Medical records policies and systems

Another aspect of the inspection is a comparison between the practice and the nationally standardized clinical and financial outcomes measured by the Health Plan Employer Data and Information Set (HEDIS). More than 50 measures are addressed in HEDIS, including the management of cancer, heart disease, smoking, and diabetes. A standardized member satisfaction survey is also incorporated (Neuman & Ptak, 2003). The original accreditation standards were written for medical healthcare services, but standards are now available in multiple areas and specialties, such as:

- *The Joint Commission*—offers accreditation in Ambulatory Care, Behavioral Health Care, Critical Access Hospitals, Home Care, Hospitals, Laboratory Services, Long Term Care, and Office-Based Surgery, as well as International Accreditation (http://www.jointcommission.org).
- *The Accreditation Association for Ambulatory Health Care* (AAAHC)—offers accreditation in Ambulatory Health Care Organizations, Managed Care Organizations, and Office-Based Surgery Centers (http://www.aaahc.org).
- *The Accreditation Commission for Health Care, Inc.* (ACHC)—offers accreditation in Home Health, Infusion Nursing, Hospice, Sleep Lab, Home/ Durable Medical Equipment Services, Clinical Respiratory Care, Medical Supply Provider, Complex Rehabilitation and Assistive Technology Supplier, Fitter Services, Pharmacy Services, Infusion, Pharmacy, Ambulatory Infusion Center, Specialty Pharmacy, Non-Certified/Private Duty Program, Private Duty Nursing, and Private Duty Aide (http://www.achc.org).

- *Utilization Review Accreditation Commission* (URAC)—offers accreditation in Case Management, Claims Processing, Consumer Education and Support, Core Accreditation Comprehensive Wellness, Credentials Verification Organization, Credentialing Support Certification, Disease Management, Drug Therapy Management, Health Call Center, Health Content and Personal Health Management Providers Accreditation, Health Network, Health Plan, Health Provider Credentialing, Health Utilization Management, Health Web Site, HIPAA Privacy, HIPAA Security, Independent Review Organization, Mail Service Pharmacy, Medicare Advantage Deeming Program, Pharmacy Benefit Management, Specialty Pharmacy, Workers' Compensation Utilization Management, Workers' Compensation Pharmacy, and Vendor Certification (http://www.urac.org).
- *The Community Health Accreditation Program, Inc.* (CHAP)—offers accreditation in home health care and hospice (http://www.chapinc.org).
- *Electronic Healthcare Network Accreditation Commission* (EHNAC)—offers accreditation in Service providers for Electronic Health Records, e-Prescribing, Financial Services, Health Information Exchange, Health-Care Network, and Outsourced Services (http://www.Ehnac.org).
- HealthCare Quality Association on Accreditation (HQAA)—offers accreditation in DME (http://www.hqaa.org).
- Healthcare Facilities Accreditation Program (HFAP)—offers accreditation to all hospitals, ambulatory care/surgical facilities, mental health facilities, physical rehabilitation facilities, clinical laboratories, critical access hospitals, and stroke centers (http://www.hfap.org).
- Commission on Accreditation Healthcare Management Education (CAHME)—offers accreditation to agencies hosting education in any field of healthcare (http://www.cahme.org).

Conclusions

An NP with solid leadership skills has the ability to provide optimum and cost-effective care to patients and their families. With creativity and confidence, an NP can use entrepreneurial skills to offer new or unfamiliar services to patients. Nurse practitioners perform a special function because they combine nursing models of care with the medical model. The result is a holistic approach to patient mind and body health.

Nurse practitioners in hospital settings are involved in many outcome assessments, including patient satisfaction measurements. In comparison, NPs in outpatient care delivery areas are more frequently involved in preventing episodic events that require hospitalization and ensuring sound fiscal management, which also facilitates patient compliance. However, NPs in every setting are under pressure to fulfill benchmarks, including patient satisfaction, and are targeting their care to demonstrate use of evidence-based guidelines. Thus, NPs need to expand their knowledge in various areas of care, such as pain management, palliative care, and genetic screening. At the same time, they must focus on their leadership, management, and professional roles. Results from interviews with experienced NPs confirm that additional education is needed, so NPs will not serve solely as clinical technicians who follow guidelines and achieve patient benchmarks. Finally, practices should be aware of the dynamic and challenging methods for receiving accreditation, even if the agency involved is not mandated to be accredited.

We cannot leave our nursing roots behind and concentrate only on completing patient care in 20 minutes. To maximize outcomes, NPs need to embrace their rich nursing experience and lead in transforming health care so that it encompasses patient's accountability and participation in health care.

Reflective Thinking Exercises

1. Browse the entrepreneurial Web site, Entrepreneurs (http://www.entrepreneurs.about.com). Read a few of the links about business plan development, sales and marketing, or other business ideas. Then read Warren Buffet's explanation of *sustainable competitive advantage* (http://entrepreneurs.about.com/od/beyondstartup/a/whatwarrenwants.htm) and answer the following question in 30 seconds: What is your business best at or what do you want it to ultimately be best at?
2. Given your experience and readings on measuring patient outcomes, develop a framework for monitoring patients with hypertension, asthma, or hyperlipidemia in a primary care practice. Consult the Guidelines for the Seventh Report of the Joint National Committee on Prevention, Detection, Evaluation, and Treatment of High Blood Pressure (JNC 7), Diagnosis and Management of Asthma, and Expert Panel on Detection, Evaluation, and Treatment of High Blood Cholesterol in Adults (Adult Treatment Panel III, or the JNC (http://www.nhlbi.nih.gov/guidelines/index.htm).
3. Develop a mission statement, vision, two or three goals, and objectives for a targeted timeframe of 12 months for your "ideal" healthcare agency or organization. Review the mission, vision, and goal statements from other agencies. Remember to be creative, yet competitive with the marketplace. Think BIG!
4. Develop a patient satisfaction tool such as shown in Table 8–1 that encompasses your patient population's demographic variables and care needs. Obtain peer feedback on the tool, and edit the revisions. Be sure to use appropriate terminology for non-healthcare professionals to understand. Review health literacy, which is the ability to understand health information so that appropriate decisions can be made. Use the U. S. Department of Health and Human Services Office of Disease Prevention and Health Promotion Health Communication Activities on health literacy improvement as a guide (http://www.health.gov/communication/literacy/default.htm). Conduct a pilot survey on five non-healthcare professional people whom you know but do not have as patients. Adjust the tool based on the feedback they provide.

References

Accreditation Association for Ambulatory Health Care. (2009). Accreditation. Retrieved July 22, 2009 from http://www.aaahc.org/eweb/StartPage.aspx.

Accreditation Laws and Regulations by State. (n.d.). Retrieved July 22, 2009, from Accreditation Association for Ambulatory Health Care—AAAHC.org: http://www.aaahcnewyork.org/lawsbystate.htm.

Bahouth, M. & Kopan, K. (2009). *APN Leadership Development—Part II—Educational Needs and Practice Development for Acute Care Nurse Practitioners.* Retrieved on June 22, 2009 from. http://www.aacn.org/wd/nti_cd/data/papers/main/43331.pdf.

Berwick, D. (1989). Continuous improvement as an ideal in health care. *New England Journal of Medicine, 320*(1), 53–56.

Bradford, R. (1997). *Children, families and chronic disease: Psychological models and methods of care.* New York: Routledge

Brent, N. (1990). Setting up your own business, facing the future as an entrepreneur. *AORN Journal 51*(1), 205, 208, 210–213.

Burbank, P. & Riebe, D. (2002). *Promoting exercise and behavior change in older adults: Interventions with the transtheoretical model.* New York: Springer Publishing.

Cordock, R. (2007). *Business upgrade: 21 days to reignite the entrepreneurial spirit in you and your team.* Chichester, England: John Wiley & Sons, Ltd.

Daniels, S. & Ramey, M. (2005). *The leaders guide to hospital case management.* Sudbury, MA: Jones and Bartlett Publishers.

Danna, D. & Porche, D. (2008). Entrepreneurial strategy. *The Journal for Nurse Practitioners. 9,* 573–575.

Donabedian, A. (1966). Evaluating the quality of medical care. *Milbank Memorial Fund Quarterly, XLIV*(3), 166 – 206.

Elange, B., Hunter, G., & Winchell, M. (2007). Barriers to nurse entrepreneurship: a study of the process model of entrepreneurship. *Journal of American Academy of Nurse Practitioners. 19*(4), 198–204.

End of Life Nursing Consortium (ELNEC) Graduate Modules Program. Retrieved March 4, 2009 from http://www.aacn.nche.edu/elnec/curriculum.htm.

Health Plan Employer Data & Information Set. (2009). *HEIDIS and Quality Measurement.* Retrieved July 22, 2009 from http://www.ncqa.org/tabid/59/Default.aspx.

Erikson, E. (1963). *Erikson's theory of psychosocial development.* New York: W.W. Norton & Co.

Hartweg, D. (1991). *Self care deficit theory of care.* Newbury Park, CA: Sage Publications Inc.

Huber, D. & Craig, K. (2007). Acuity and case management. *Professional Case Management, 12*(3), 132–146.

Institute for Health Care Delivery Research in Intermountain Health Care. Retrieved. May 13, 2009 from www.ihc.com/xp/ihc/physician/research/institute/

Jansink, R., Braspenning, J., van der Weijden, T., Niessen, L., Elwyn, G. & Grol, R. (2009). Nurse-led motivational interviewing to change the lifestyle of patients with type 2 diabetes (MILD-project): protocol for a cluster, randomized, controlled trial on implementing lifestyle recommendations, *BMC Health Services Research,* 9:19, http://www.biomedcentral.com/1472-6963/9/19.

Kane, R. Ed., (2006). *Understanding health care outcomes research.* 2nd.ed. Sudbury, MA: Jones and Bartlett Publishers.

Kleinpell, R. & Hravnak, M. (2005). Strategies for Success in the Acute Care Nurse Practitioner Role. *Critical Care Nursing Clinics of North America, 17*(2), 177–181.

Mackey, T., McNiel, N., & Klingensmith, K. (2004). Outsourcing issues for nurse practitioner practices. *Nursing Economics, 22*(1), 21 – 26, 32.

MacLellan, L. Gardner, G. & Gardner, A. (2002). Designing the future in wound care: The role of the nurse practitioner. *Australian Journal of Wound Management, 10*(3) 97, 101–3, 105–106.

Martin, K. (2000). Nurse practitioners: A comparison of rural-urban practice patterns and willingness to serve in underserved areas. *Journal of the American Academy of Nurse Practitioners. 12,* 491 – 496.

Miller, W. R., & Rollnick, S. (1991). *Motivational interviewing: Preparing people for change.* New York: Guilford Press.

Moseley, G. (2009). *Managing health care business strategy.* Sudbury, MA: Jones and Bartlett Publishing.

National Association of Community Health Centers. *Loan Forgiveness.* Retrieved April 12, 2009 from http://www.nachc.org

National Committee for Quality Assurance. (2009). *HEIDIS & Quality Measurement.* Retrieved August 2, 2009 from http://www.ncqa.org/tabid/59/default.aspx.

National Organization of Nurse Practitioner Faculty. *Acute Care NP Competencies.* Retrieved May 12, 2009 from http://www.nonpf.com/ACNPCompsfinal20041.pdf.

National Organization of Nurse Practitioner Faculty. (2006). NP Competency Domains. Retrieved May 13, 2009 from http://www.nonpf.com/NONPF2005/CoreCompsFINAL06.pdf.

National Organization of Nurse Practitioner Faculty. *Psychiatric NP Competencies.* Retrieved May 12, 2009 from http://www.nonpf.org/finalcomps03.pdf.

Neuman, K., & Ptak, M. (2003). Managing managed care through accreditation standards. *Social Work, 48*(3), 384–391. Retrieved August 16, 2009, from CINAHL with Full Text database.

Orem, D. (1980). *Nursing: Concepts of practice.* New York, NY: McGraw-Hill.

Quaglietti S; Blum L; Ellis V. (2004). The role of the adult nurse practitioner in palliative are. *Journal of Hospice & Palliative Nursing, 6* (4): 209 – 214.

Reed, K. (2005). Telemedicine: Benefits to advanced practice nursing and the communities they serve, *Journal of the American Academy of Nurse Practitioners, 17*(5), 176–180

Rollnick, S., Heather, N., & Bell, A. (1992). Negotiating behavior change in medical settings: The development of brief motivational interviewing. *Journal of Mental Health, 1,* 25–37.

Saphiere, H. (2005). *Communication highwire.* London: Intercultural Press.

Serota, J. & Serota, F. (2001). Starting from scratch: Developing your own practice site. *Journal of Pediatric Health Care, 15*(4), 215–217.

Sobralske, M. (2005). Primary care needs of patients who have undergone gender reassignment. *Journal of the American Academy of Nurse Practitioners. 17*(4), 133 – 138.

Tahan, H. & Huer, D. (2006). The CCMC's national study of case manager job descriptions. *Lippincott's Case Management, 11*(3), 127–144.

The Registered Nurse Response Network (RNRN). *Starting one's own business.* Retrieved March 3, 2009 from http://www.nnba.net.

Umbrell, C. (2006). Trauma case management: A role for the advanced practice nurse. *Journal of Trauma Nursing, 13*(2), 70–73.

U.S. Department of Health & Human Services. Agency for Healthcare Research and Quality. Retrieved on July 12, 2009 from www.hhs.gov.

Westwood, G., Pickering R., Latter, S., Lucassen, A., Little, P. & Temple, I . (2006) Feasibility and acceptability of providing nurse counselor genetics clinics in primary care. *Journal of Advanced Nursing 53*(5), 591–604

Wheeler, K. (2008). *Psychotherapy for the Advanced Practice Psychiatric Nurse,* St. Louis: Mosby Elsevier.

Zallen, D. (2008). *To test or not to test: A guide to genetic screening and risk.* Newark, NJ: Rutgers University Press.

Conclusions and Implications

9

Learning Objectives

1. Describe the possibilities for continued expansion of the nurse practitioner (NP) role, with emphasis on clinician, leader, manager, and professional functions.

2. Describe evidence-based practice.

3. Apply an evidence-based research framework to the analysis of a clinical problem or population.

4. Analyze the level of evidence in several studies relevant to your clinical problem or population.

5. Create ways to participate in health policy initiatives.

6. Describe methods of networking locally, regionally, nationally, and internationally with individual NPs or organizations.

7. Outline the process for starting one's own NP business.

Key Words: independent practice, NP role, future trends, evidence based practice, health care policy

The future is wide open for NPs to develop their role and "own" a piece of health care. Buerhaus, Staiger, and Auerbach (2009) project a high demand for advanced practice nursing and NPs, particularly in medically underserved rural and inner city communities. This trend is also apparent in primary care centers, hospitals, and some specialty out-patient practices. As NPs use entrepreneurial skills, demonstrate leadership and management savvy, and participate in multiple professional organizations and local provider networks, their role will continue to advance.

Still, NPs face, and must overcome, the following challenges:

▓ Unequal Medicare reimbursement policy for equivalent care rendered by NPs when compared with physicians,

▓ Required physician collaborative agreements in many states, and

▓ Failure to perceive the NP as an autonomous provider.

Each NP must communicate to the consumer what NPs do, how they are different from other healthcare providers, and ways in which the role of the NP will continue to expand. Rashotte (2005) emphasizes that troubled economic times have positively affected the NP role in shaping health care for the future. NPs will also benefit from newly developed doctoral programs that further prepare them for an expanding role and give them the status of an advanced degree to match other healthcare professionals.

The chapter discusses how NPs can use evidence-based practice to improve their services and patient outcomes. Ideas for becoming involved in health policy development and taking on responsibility in a professional organization are also shared.

This chapter offers suggestions for widening NP connections from "practice site only" to include local colleagues and then national and international providers. It also summarizes how to start your own NP business, as a way to encourage reflection on existing or new ventures. Finally, some trends regarding the evolution of the NP are also discussed.

Evidence-Based Practice

Certainly the role of the NP as a clinician, manager, leader, and professional can be refined by evidence-based practice (EBP), which Melnyk and Fineout-Overholt (2005) define as using knowledge from literature reviews and results from individual research studies, along with evidence from experts, the products of reasoning, and patient preferences. Nurse practitioners cannot practice the way "they think is best" or "how it has always been done," but rather must practice based on evidence of effectiveness. A practicing NP must embody all four functions of the NP role if engaged in EBP, either independently or with a group of providers. As clinicians, NPs are well versed in the clinical management of patients with a variety of problems. As managers, NPs can collect data from their own practices and begin to determine if current practice needs improvement or if recommendations from others should be incorporated in providing care for specific populations. They can also determine if any emerging patterns show improved outcomes based on patient response. This can be studied to determine if the changes can also be generalized to other patients. Evaluating what has been done and interpreting new outcomes is the foundation of EBP. Kovner, Fine, and D'Aquila (2009) share examples of evidence-based management at medical centers that assist NPs in managing their healthcare practices. As leaders, NPs can think of creative ways to change practices and use the new information to affect other providers' patients as well as their own small group. As professionals, NPs can disseminate new knowledge, thereby replicating the new "evidence" in other practices. The providers can be interdisciplinary and can include ancillary personnel as well.

Melnyk and Fineout-Overholt, (2005) and Craig and Smyth (2007) state that few nurses have the time and skills to engage in evidence-based research. However, if NPs could use the Population/Problem, Intervention, Comparison, Outcome, and Timeframe (PICOT) format and divide care into steps or phases, they could more easily incorporate EBP into daily practice. By using Melnyk and Fineout-Overholt's framework, EBP can become a consistent part of a practice. The result would be improved patient outcomes.

In evaluating a study, the level of evidence is most important. Melnyk and Fineout-Overholt (2005) suggest the following framework to use when analyzing evidence levels:

- Level I = systematic reviews of randomized trials
- Level II = randomized control trials
- Level III = case controlled analytical studies or nonrandomized control trials
- Level IV = studies based totally on opinion and not on evidence (i.e., anecdotal reports)

The goal is to validate findings with Level I and II studies, which would lend credence to applying the results to the delivery of care.

The literature has many examples of nurses' perceptions of evidence-based practice (Mantzoukas, 2009; Koehn, M. & Lehman, K. 2008) and of actual evidenced-based practice studies (Hutchinson & Johnston, 2008; Harper, 2007). Nurse practitioners can easily perform a database search electronically using their hospital or university library to obtain multiple studies in their area of interest. If their area of interest is very new and no studies have been published, the NP has an opportunity to forge ahead in developing an evidence-based study. To begin, one needs to:

- Conduct studies (using Level I or II study designs)
- Publish findings
- Disseminate findings to colleagues, so new data can be replicated to see if it can be generalized to larger populations

This, in essence, is building the evidence for improved patient outcomes.

Some nurses do not want to be involved in studies or collaborative projects to evaluate patient outcomes and improve care. The challenge demands time, and current patient scheduling models provide little time to work on independent projects. What kind of care delivery model would enable NPs to spend the time allocated for one patient visit (approximately 15 to 30 minutes per day) on an evidence-based research project? Is it possible to negotiate for this time in an employment contract once an NP has been at a practice for at least six months? Or, what about a compromise, perhaps one hour a week set aside for conducting an EBP study? Some critics believe NPs will schedule this one hour at the end of a day so they can go home early. Others complain that one hour a day is insufficient for such a large endeavor; the hour will be lost just arranging materials. Still others do not consider best practices as necessary and are interested only in seeing patients.

However, even an hour can provide the NP with an opportunity to research and improve care to patients, which should be every NP's goal. Nurse practitioners who say, "I cannot think about EBP when I know a patient is waiting for me," need to understand that EBP helps maximize patient outcomes. Others say, "I could be calling for labs, getting an MRI scheduled, seeing another patient who really needs to be seen." These excuses point to an inefficient practice in which the right person is doing the wrong job. The NP should not be calling for MRI scheduling; this should be delegated to someone else. Some NPs really do not enjoy this kind of research, but they need to realize that their practice will become stagnant without engaging in EBP. They say, "Once I get home, I do not get paid for doing the research and writing, so why should I do it?" "Why would someone ever do something like EBP on their own time?" is the question commonly asked. What about a model of care allowing the collaborative physician or NP Director to see patients a certain number of hours/week? By pairing with each scheduled NP, there could be time to work on an EBP project each week. Each NP could be scheduled for some desk time for EBP. With some thorough outcome measurement, this time could generate more cost-effective patient outcomes. To encourage EBP, recertification could require proof of implementation of EBP in practice or of each NP's participation in EBP studies. The bigger picture of healthcare requires implementation of EBP across practice sites. It can result in business opportunities that could affect costs and improve quality. If a practice is stagnant it is out of date.

Increased Nurse Practitioner Participation in Healthcare Policy

Nurse practitioners need more awareness of how politics and economics affect practice and system-wide initiatives affecting care. They need the skills to participate in institutional, local, state, federal, and international health policy discussions. For example, NPs are in an excellent position to influence consumers about healthcare reform, insurance/government/state reimbursement, regulations affecting healthcare legislation, palliative care, mental health initiatives, long-term care, and a variety of other health issues. By becoming politically active and recruiting like-minded people with more political savvy, perhaps our healthcare delivery system could be reframed to improve patient access. In addition, the NP role would become more respected and fairly reimbursed.

A copy of the Public Policy Agenda, which includes legislation and regulatory issues impacting NP practice, can be downloaded from www.Acnpweb.org. The *American Journal for Nurse Practitioners* publishes the Pearson Report annually. This is a state-by-state national evaluation of NP legislation and other healthcare issues affecting NP practice. In addition to clinical conferences, NPs need to participate in Health Policy and Leadership Summits/Conferences to discuss and analyze issues affecting practice. Nurse practitioners need to build coalitions with patients and colleagues to advocate for causes, as well as to empower them to fight for other workforce issues. Many Web sites can assist NPs in educating themselves about health policy, including:

- Commonwealth Fund http://www.commonwealthfund.org
- Henry J. Kaiser Family foundation http://www.kff.org
- Mathematica Policy Research http://www.mathematica-mpr.com/health
- The Urban Institute http://www.urban.org

The Evolving Role of the Nurse Practitioner

Nurse practitioners are beginning to concentrate on patient-centered, as opposed to provider-focused, health care. Consider how reflective thinking can help the role of the NP role evolve. According to Ruth-Sahd (2003), reflective thinking can lead to the acquisition of new knowledge, particularly if one considers ways to improve practice results through EBP. NPs who are not currently incorporating reflective thinking in their practice can easily be taught, as discussed by Kuiper & Pesut (2004). This self-reflection is good for practitioners as well as patients in their everyday lives. Nurse practitioners can design programs and support groups to promote good health practices for their patients, while simultaneously acting as role models of reflective practice. Minelli and Breckton (2009) provides some creative ideas on public health education, and Goodson (2009) gives examples of program development, along with an evaluation framework that can help increase reflective thinking skills. Patients can gain great insight into their own behaviors and health patterns by using reflective techniques.

A challenging situation for NPs is how to handle a noncompliant patient. Releasing a patient from a practice is a provider-centered action. As a concept, compliance implies that someone in authority presents a mandate that others are required to follow. If patients are noncompliant and, therefore, "fired" by a provider, patient-centered care is not being practiced. If this situation develops the patient would be incapable of following the management program. It is not a good healthcare system when clinicians work harder to achieve patient health than the patients do. Remember to incorporate the patient in the planning process to arrive at achievable actions and outcomes.

Future Trends for Nurse Practitioners

More outcome studies and cost comparison reviews of healthcare providers and NPs are necessary to provide more data showing that NPs are providing excellent and high-quality care, resulting in outcomes comparable with other providers. Research that documents cost-efficient and quality patient care will strengthen the NP's position in terms of equal reimbursement from all payers and improve the NP's image across the nation. Mills (2009) cites studies illustrating that the NPs' scope of practice is approximately 80% of a physician's. As a result, the author states, "for medical problems outside that 80%, the patient needs to see a physician" (p. 3). O'Grady (2009) contends that NPs should receive full reimbursement for their work with Medicare patients, rather than just 85%, because "providers should be paid the same rate for the same services, and NPs can provide high-quality care at a lower rate than physicians" (p. 8).

Nurse practitioners also need to access and work with healthcare and professional organization boards to lower barriers. Eadie (2009) identifies the following three themes as crucial for consistent evaluation and reevaluation in order for a successful not-for-profit organization to prosper and grow:

- Is the organization significantly diversified and moving in a direction that will provide long-term growth? (strategic plans, vision, and target dates)
- What structure does the organization have now? Does the leadership seem transparent? (specific goals of current leader need defining, mission, programs, organizational structure, budget, and policies)
- Is the organization doing well financially and with consumers? (outcome evaluation, fiscal stability, revenue plan)

Healthcare organizations with Trustee Boards should follow the abovementioned guide. Board members are expected to participate by ensuring appropriate accountability, communication, and transparent authority on the part of themselves and the Chief Executive Officer (CEO). Eadie provides a Model Committee Structure template for not-for-profit groups to use in his book, *Extraordinary Board Leadership: The Keys to High-Impact Governing.*

Just as electronic documentation is used in all areas of health care today, advanced technology is also necessary to learn about the most recent guidelines and medications. Resources such as the *Monthly Prescribing Reference* and the *Nurse Practitioner Prescribing Reference,* allow direct access to information for accurate and easily obtainable information about prescribing all drugs. The references also provide contact information on the last page for most pharmacological companies in the United States (www.empr.com).

By 2010, trends show that more NPs will be in independent practice. There will also be more doctoral prepared NPs, as more NPs earn the MSN–DNP degree and baccalaureate nursing graduates move to the doctoral program instead of a master's degree in NP education. Graduates from these programs obtain more knowledge and experience concerning the business of running a practice, health information technology, electronic health information, economics, and financing (Alpert, Fjone & Candela, 2002; Wallace, Grossman, & Lange, 2009). The DNP experience serves as an "internship" for baccalaureate students. However, some of the DNP-NP graduates may need a residency if they choose to work in a specialty area without previous experience. New partnerships will need to be developed between academia and clinical sites to provide educational sites for these new graduates. Nurse practitioners returning to academia for a DNP program may need some partnering with their employing healthcare agency to fulfill capstone requirements and still work full time. Perhaps some partnering can be creatively worked out to assist new nonexperienced NP graduates in securing paid internships, while experienced and employed NPs receive tuition assistance with course work.

Nurse practitioners will be performing more complex procedures (Mayhew, 2009) if employed in specialty areas, such as gastrointestinal, dermatology, cardiovascular, and neurology. Since reimbursement is less than that given to a physician, the cost of healthcare for some patients may be reduced. However, NPs need to acknowledge the necessity of working with physician teams, so that if a patient has an abnormal response, an emergency, a complication, or needs a more invasive technique during a "common procedure," an expert physician will be available.

Healthcare delivery needs to change, so that new models of NP-driven primary care and NP–MD team specialty care can emerge. Perhaps, group appointments with diabetics, asthmatics, the morbidly obese, and others who require intensive follow-up can be arranged to increase efficiency and provide support for those needing behavior changes. These group appointments may be billable and reimbursed by payers. At the same time, they generate savings for patients and allow providers to see more patients. More focus needs to be placed on patients to assume increased responsibility to lifestyle changes necessary for improved health. Telehealth methodology can be used in areas where it will increase cost effectiveness and decrease time lost by patients and providers. Nurse practitioner consultants, independent NPs, NP-RN partners, and NP-MD teams will be formed to manage primary care as, for example, in the Health Home Model. Nurse practitioners have expertise regarding motivational techniques for patients to use to change lifestyles and promote improved health behaviors. In addition to providing the medical component of primary care, NPs can make a difference by helping patients make health style changes. Nurse practitioners have long been recognized for their holistic healthcare delivery and comprehensive health teaching skills. With new payer systems that highlight patient responsibility and self-accountability to obtain full financial coverage, the idea of teaching health promotion alongside primary care delivery is part of an NP's approach. The NP has the advanced clinical assessment skills, as well as the diagnostic reasoning ability, to independently diagnose and prescribe for medical management of patients. This differs from the registered nurse, who primarily participates only in screening and implementation of a plan. Only the MD or NP role can diagnose and, therefore, serve the primary care needs of all populations. Educators of NPs need to use more experiential strategies in their teaching and help NPs gain competency, acquire assessment and diagnostic skills for patient challenges, and have more experience with the tools and knowledge needed to find data, guidelines, and protocols. As healthcare becomes more complex, it is crucial to understand the concept of lifelong learning. Rounds and Rappaport (2008) explore many teaching-learning strategies, such as hybrid on-line interactive methodologies that use problem-based learning and case scenarios. Simulations with simulated patients give students experience in accessing "patients" and their data (Ebbert & Connors, 2004). Many products, such as SimClinic/SimHospital and Microsim, allow students the opportunity to use diagnostic reasoning and manage a patient with immediate feedback. This kind of pedagogy, in contrast with didactic lectures, is the way of the future. With the growing shortage of NP faculty, NPs in practice have more opportunities to do adjunct teaching or guest lectures for educational programs.

Networking with Nurse Practitioners

Nurse practitioners would benefit from exchanges with NPs in other parts of the country and throughout the world to compare advanced practice education, legislation, scope of practice, and patient management outcomes. Collaboration between our graduate NP students and those from other countries, such as the UK and Australia, would also be of interest. Students could compare notes on how they have progressed through their ANP programs using reflective practice techniques, which are popular in Europe, or discuss knowledge and skills taught universally to NPs. The literature offers little about NP practice in other countries although more is published in Australia and the UK than in other countries.

In addition, networking would enhance cultural awareness. According to Benkert, Tanner, Guthrie, Oakley, and Pohl (2005), the growing diversity of the U.S. population points to the obvious need for NPs and all healthcare providers to be culturally sensitive. The Institute of Medicine (2002) recommends that healthcare educators include cultural responsiveness as a future goal for all healthcare providers. This "fits" well with the NP's interest in reflective practice. Smith (1988) defines cultural competence as an ongoing process of care that involves awareness of self and others, developing relatedness with patients, and competent use of interpersonal skills and knowledge. Networking with NPs in other countries could aid in understanding different cultures.

As a case in point, interesting ideas about providing healthcare to the people of Australia are published in the NEWS column of the *Australian Nursing Journal,* which is available free-of-charge at http://www.highbeam.com/Australian+Nursing+Journal/publications.aspx. The literature shows that Australian general practitioner physicians are supportive and respectful of the service NPs provide. These Australian NPs could be contacted to discuss their healthcare delivery experiences and collaborate with Americans regarding current challenges. Another example is the International Council of Nurses, which has annual conferences and has a section, The International Nurse Practitioner/Advanced Practice Nursing Network, that can be accessed at http://icn-apnetwork.org/.

Nurse practitioners and NP faculty should also be members of professional organizations, such as the American Academy of Nurse Practitioners, the American College of Nurse Practitioners, the American Association of Critical Care Nurses, the National Association of Pediatric Nurse Practitioners, and the Women's Health Nurse Practitioner Association. Nurse practitioner faculty need to be members of the National Organization of Nurse Practitioner Faculty. All NPs might consider joining other organizations, such as Sigma Theta Tau International, the American Nurses Association, and specialty multidisciplinary organizations. They should participate professionally in one or more of these organizations and join list-serves, blogs, and committees to assist in expanding networking and achieving the goals of these organizations. Networking with NPs outside of those seen every day in work settings would benefit the profession.

Creating an Independent Business: A Summary

An NP who wants to begin an independent practice should first perform a marketing survey to determine a solid business location. This means investigating competitive medical practices and the demographics of the population one wants to serve. Some information can be obtained from the local hospital and public health departments. Connections with both of these health care agencies will also improve networking. The hospital may offer space for your practice or know of a place that might be suitable.

Then, choose an appropriate business structure. With input from your legal adviser and business consultant, establish your strategic plan, mission, and vision statements. By this time, you should have shared your vision with colleagues and others in health care. Perhaps one of them will want to join the new practice or perhaps a partner or colleagues will agree to part time or per diem employment to help you defray costs until the practice expands and can finance a full time associate.

This new business associate may be able to bring patients from their current practice if they did not sign a noncompete clause. However, with providers on specific insurance panels, patients often follow their providers. More than enough patients need primary and specialty care to support more than one practice.

Nurse practitioners may need a collaborative agreement or some type of supervision with a physician to open an NP care practice. This agreement provides access to immediate medical support, chart review, and/or prescriptive authority. In addition, the practice might want to outsource or hire experts in marketing and billing. In particular, billing, coding, and reimbursement requires specialized knowledge of so many details, as set forth by Medicare/Medicaid and private insurers, that outsourcing may be a cost-efficient and less worrisome approach.

Try new techniques that do not require major expenditures and provide positive outcomes. Think high quality and low cost at every juncture of opening and expanding the practice, but remember that the highest frequency etiologies correlate with malpractice suits (Buppert, 2009, p. 321). These complaints include:

- Breast changes and lumps in supraclavicular and axillary areas
- Chest and shoulder pain in an individual with history of more than 20 packs of cigarettes a year
- Chest pain in an adult
- Lower abdominal pain

The related diagnoses are breast cancer, lung cancer, myocardial infarction, appendicitis, and colorectal cancer.

Finally, manage finances with the lowest overhead possible and keep expenditures down, including your own salary, until revenue increases. Be positive, use reflective practice techniques, think YES you can do what you want (Zanders 2000).

Conclusions

This book addresses the need for a comprehensive resource to assist NPs in developing or revising healthcare delivery practice settings and fostering new and more autonomous roles. This information is critical, as more NPs are managing primary care settings, an increasing number of NPs are collaborating with physicians as hospitalists and in specialty practices, and the educational requirements mandate that as of 2015, APNs must earn a clinical doctorate. In addition, as the Institute of Medicine states, almost 100,000 preventable patient deaths occur annually in the United States. Nurse practitioners can assist in decreasing this number. With improved primary care, patients should have less acute, episodic Emergency Department visits and hospitalizations, as well as improved health outcomes.

This text has answered the question so many friends and patients ask NPs, "What is the difference between an NP and a physician?" The answer is clear.

NPs offer a different, often improved, kind of care. Studies have repeatedly shown that NPs provide competent quality health care with health outcomes and patient satisfaction equal to those achieved by physicians in primary care with 80% of presenting complaints. Nurse practitioners provide the care that patients want. For the other 20%, NPs need healthcare colleagues with whom to collaborate, network, and arrange patient referrals. But NPs are different for other reasons, as clinical care is only 25% of an NP's advanced practice role. Nurse practitioners are also leaders in improving healthcare policy, researching to improve patient outcomes, and advocating for patients. They manage patient care, pharmaceutical use, and healthcare expenditure as part of their routine functions. In addition, NPs are conscious of patient barriers to executing the care plan and assist in obtaining resources to realize success. Finally, NPs are professionally accepted by patients. Patients will say, "the NP treats me like a person and gets to know me not just my disease." The hallmark of NP practice is viewing patients holistically, as unique individuals with all types of influences on their health, including financial, family, psychological, interpersonal, employment, stress, and biological. Before prescribing medication for pain or depression, an NP takes a history that reveals the etiology, which may not be based on any cause a pill can alleviate. NPs MUST NOT become the "physician extender" in the physician practice medical model and convert our multifactorial teachings to a 6 to 10 minute meet, treat, and street mentality. Resist the temptation to earn more by "making numbers," as this may be the death knell of healthcare.

This book has also answered the question, "Why should I go back to get a doctoral degree?" To be effective as a provider, many tools and skills must be learned in the areas of business, policy, statistics, evidence-based practice, billing/coding, and compliance. Additional education in these areas, over and above the clinical care taught in a master's program, is necessary to succeed and to have the profession evolve.

Reflective Thinking Exercises

1. Read *Your First NP Position: Advice from Those Who've Been There* (http://nurse-practitioners.advanceweb.com/Editorial/Content/Editorial.aspx?CC=200814). After reading the various NP perspectives, develop your own plan for obtaining a first or new NP position. In addition, establish a timeframe for implementing your plan.
2. Research hints for finding employment by using the American Academy of Nurse Practitioners (AANP) Career link www.aanpcareerlink.com. Develop your résumé and cover letter. Ask a colleague to edit them before you send them out.
3. Imagine you are an NP in 2020, who is preparing for daily virtual rounds at the Older Adult Assisted Living Agency that you opened approximately one year previously. Prepare an outline of your "typical" day and an action plan for proceeding from start to finish. Be sure to include time and energy spent on community service and academic support.

4. Use the PICOT system to assess a clinical problem of your choice. As you analyze the literature, be sure to evaluate the study in terms of the level of evidence it provides.
5. Join a list-serve for NPs in your area. Network with these NPs at monthly meetings and dinners by email, blogging, or in person. Get on the mailing list for at least two NP journals that are mailed or sent electronically to enrollees. Examples of these are *ADVANCE for Nurse Practitioners, Clinical Provider, The American Journal for Nurse Practitioners,* or *Nurse Practitioner World News.*

References

Alpert, P., Fjone, A. & Candela, L. (2002). Nurse practitioner: reflecting on the future. *Nursing Administration Quarterly, 26*(5), 79–89.

American College of Nurse Practitioners (2009). *Public Policy Agenda.* Retrieved April 3, 2009 from www.Acnpweb.org

Australian Nursing Journal. (2009). Nurse practitioner clinic gets overwhelming support. NEWS column of the *Australian Nursing Journal 16*(7), 5. Retrieved June 29, 2009 from http://www.highbeam.com/Australian+Nursing+Journal/publications.aspx.

Benkert, R., Tanner, C., Guthrie, B. Oakley, D., & Pohl, J. (2005). Cultural competence of nurse practitioner students: A consortium's experience. *Journal of Nursing Education, 44*(5): 225–233.

Buerhaus, P., Staiger, D., & Auerbach, D. (2009). *The future of the nursing workforce in the United States: Data, trends, and implications.* Sudbury, MA: Jones and Bartlett Publishers.

Buppert, C. (2009). Know the red flag chief complaints. *The Journal for Nurse Practitioners, 5,* 321–322.

Craig, J. & Smyth, R. (2007). *The evidence-based practice manual for nurses.* 2nd ed., Edinburgh, Scotland: Churchill Livingston Elsevier.

Eadie, D. (2009). *Extraordinary board leadership: keys to high-impact governing.* 2nd ed. Sudbury, MA: Jones and Bartlett Publishers.

Ebbert, D. & Connors, H. (2004). Standardized patient experiences: Evaluation of clinical performance and nurse practitioner student satisfaction. *Nursing Education Perspectives. 25*(1), 12–15.

Goodson, P. (2009). *Theory in health promotion research and practice: thinking outside the box.* Sudbury, MA: Jones & Bartlett.

Harper, J. (2007). Emergency nurses' knowledge of evidence-based ischemic stroke care: A pilot study. *Journal of Emergency Nursing. 33*(3): 202–207.

Hutchinson, A. & Johnston, L. (2008). An observational stud of health professionals' use of evidence to inform the development of clinical management tools. *Journal of Clinical Nursing, 17*(16): 2203–2211.

Institute of Medicine. (2008). *Knowing what works in healthcare: A roadmap for the nation.* Washington, DC: The National Academic Press.

International Council of Nurses. *The International Nurse Practitioner/Advanced Practice Nursing Network.* Retrieved May 12, 2009 from http://icn-apnetwork.org/.

Koehn, M. & Lehman, K. (2008). Nurses' perceptions of evidence based nursing practice. *Journal of Advanced Nursing, 62* (2): 209–215.

Kovner, A., Fine, D., & D'Aquila, R. (2009). *Evidence based management in healthcare.* Chicago, IL: Health Administration Press.

Kuiper, R. & Pesut, D. (2004). Promoting cognitive and metacognitive reflective reasoning skills in nursing practice: Self regulated learning theory. *Journal of Advanced Nursing, 45*(4), 381–391.

Mantzoukas, S. (2009). The research evidence published in high impact nursing journals between 200 and 2006: A quantitative content analysis. *International Journal of Nursing Studies, 46*(4), 479–89

Mayhew, M. (2009). Off-label prescribing. *The Journal for Nurse Practitioners, 2,* 122–123.

Melnyk, B. & Fineout-Overholt, E. (2005). *Evidence based practice in nursing and healthcare.* Philadelphia, PA: Lippincott, Williams & Wilkins.

Mills, C. (2009). Why NPs need full practice and prescriptive authority. *Nurse Practitioners World News, 14*(5/6), 3, 13.

Minelli, M. & Breckton, D. (2009). *Community health education: Settings, roles, and skills.* 5th ed., Sudbury, MA: Jones & Bartlett.

Monthly Prescribing Reference and/or *Nurse Practitioner Prescribing Reference.* Retrieved May 3, 2009 from www.empr.com.

O'Grady, E. (2009). Cost effectiveness vs. comparable worth. *Nurse Practitioners World News, 14*(5/6), 8–9.

Rashotte, J. (2005). Knowing the nurse practitioner: Dominant discourses shaping our horizons. *Nursing Philosophy, 6,* 51–62.

Rounds, L. & Rappaport, B. (2008). The successful use of problem-based Learning in an online nurse practitioner course. *Nursing Education Perspectives. 29*(1), 12–16.

Ruth-Sahd, L. (2003). Reflective practice: A critical analysis of data based studies and implications for nursing education. *Journal of Nursing Education, 42*(11), 488–497.

Smith, L. (1998). Concept analysis: Cultural competence. *Journal of Cultural Diversity, 5*(1), 4–10.

Wallace, M., Grossman, S. & Lange, J. (2009). The Clinical Nurse Leader (CNL) in *The clinical nurse leader & doctorate of nursing practice: Essentials of program development and implementation into clinical practice.* Edited by Fitzpatrick, J. & Wallace, M. New York: Springer Publishers.

Zander, R. & Zander, B. (2000). *Using the art of possibility: Transforming professional and personal life.* Cambridge, MA: Harvard Business Book Press.

Templates, Documents, Policy, Procedures, and Plans

Administrative Policies

Organizational Framework Policies

Blank Policy Form
Mission Statement
Governance Policy
Governance Meeting Documentation Form
Organizational Chart
Staff Meeting Policy
Staff Meeting Documentation Form
Official Documents of Clinic Policy
Policy and Procedures Policy

Patient Rights, Responsibilities, and Eligibility

Eligibility to Receive Services Policy
Notice of Available Services Policy
Patient Bill of Rights
Patient Responsibilities
Patient Complaints and Grievance Policy

Medical Records Information

Medical Records Policy
Chart Order Policy
Visit Documentation Form
Release of Information Policy
Release of Information Authorization
Referral Form
Problem-Oriented Medical Record Form
Patient Health History Form
Disposal of Medical Records Policy

Staffing/Provider Information

Appointment to Medical/Clinical Staff Policy
Orientation Policy

Administrative Policies: Organizational Framework Policies

Blank Policy Form

_____ Policy

Purpose:	
Policy:	It shall be the policy of XXXX
Equipment:	
Procedure:	

Implemented:

Revised:

Reviewed:

Mission Statement

The Mission of XXXX is to provide evidence-based, patient-centered health care and to promote health and wellness. The consumers of the practice are (define practice clientele here)

Evidence-based, patient centered health care is the foundation of healthcare services provided at XXXX. Treatment plans will include care based on current research showing efficacy with patient input to assure acceptance and compliance.

Wellness is not simply the absence of illness. In the practice of XXXX, wellness means exhibiting personal behaviors that enable one to enjoy optimal health by making healthy lifestyle choices acknowledging any health-related deficiencies. Wellness incorporates more than biological health; it also includes the psychological, emotional, spiritual, social and biological components of the human being.

The components of wellness acknowledged by our service include a nutritious diet, physical fitness, safety, sleep, weight control, and the absence of substance abuse/dependence. Other important foundations are healthy relationships, effective stress management, self-control and effective communication of feelings and needs.

XXXX staff is committed to teaching and enabling patients to care for their bodies, minds, and spirits in an intentional and preventive manner. This will help each patient maximize his or her health and achieve their highest potential.

XXXX focuses on accessible clinical care and/or education of patients, quality on-site care and/or referring to trusted specialist treatment in the community, and advocacy to remove barriers to appropriate care.

Lastly, XXXX encourages self management of illness and care through education of personal case management.

Governance Policy

Purpose:	To provide structure for the reporting of operational business items and responsibilities of XXXX to the governance board of the business
Policy:	It shall be the policy of XXXX that YYYY will be responsible for the day-to-day operations of XXXX and will report pertinent information to the governance board.
Equipment:	Meeting documentation
Procedure:	YYYY will report on a (timeline) basis during the fiscal year to the governance board and to (i.e. supervising/collaborating physician (staff meeting). The report will include but is not limited to the functional operations. Report topics discussed in these meetings should include;

- Clinical/service operations
- Utilization
- Patient satisfaction
- Staffing concerns
- Fiscal concerns
- Policy and procedure changes
- Public health concerns affecting practice
- Marketing efforts

Minutes of the Governing Board meeting will be kept in a binder.

The Governance Board and supervising/collaborating physician will receive and review the Policy and Procedure Manual annually.

Implemented:

Revised:

Reviewed:

XXXX — Governance Meeting Documentation Form

Date: _____

In attendance:

<u>Agenda</u>

▦ Operational points:

▦ Patient Satisfaction:

▦ Utilization:

▦ Staff:

▦ Policy/Procedure Changes:

▦ Management:

▦ Budget:

▦ Finance/Reimbursement:

▦ Public Health Issues:

Organizational Chart

OWNER LEVEL: Chief Executive/Operating/Financial/Board of Directors
Clinical Services Director/Office Manager

Adjunct Staff	Clinical Staff	Administrative Staff
Nutritionist	Nurse Practitioners	Receptionist
Social Worker	Nurses	Health Insurance Specialist
Physician	Medical Assistants	Billing/Coding Specialist
Substance Abuse Counselor		
Physical Therapist		
Message Therapist		

(Delete extraneous roles and draw arrows to show who reports to whom.)

Staff Meeting Policy

Purpose:	To provide open communication with all staff members about the operations of XXXX in an effort to ensure maximum efficiency.
Policy:	It shall be the policy of XXXX that YYYY will be responsible for the day-to-day operations of XXXX and will report pertinent information to the staff.
Equipment:	Staff Meeting Documentation
Procedure:	YYYY will conduct staff meetings on a regular (insert time frame). The meeting will include updates about: ▪ Patients of concern ▪ Clinical operations/ service operations ▪ Utilization ▪ Patient satisfaction ▪ Staffing concerns ▪ Fiscal concerns ▪ Policy procedure changes ▪ Public health concerns effecting practice ▪ Marketing efforts Every staff member will receive a copy (electronic) of the meeting's minutes and will be held responsible for implementation of the information as of the date of delivery even if identified as not present at the meeting.

Implemented:

Revised:

Reviewed:

Staff Meeting Documentation Form

Date: _____

In attendance:

Agenda

- Patients of concern:

- Patient satisfaction:

- Utilization:

- Staff information:

- Operational points:

- Policy/procedure changes:

- Management:

- Fiscal points:

- Public health Issues:

Official Documents of Clinical Policy

Purpose:	To identify whereabouts of official documents concerning XXXX in order to provide efficient access when needed.
Policy:	It shall be the policy of XXXX to maintain orderly storage of official documents of operation as described below.
Equipment:	Various binders and/or electronic filing systems.
Procedure:	▨ The COO of XXXX or designee will maintain and update annual personnel files of all employees, including licensure and certification information. ▨ The COO of XXXX or designee will maintain original copies of all contracts. ▨ XXXX will maintain records of equipment maintenance and building repair. ▨ Patient medical records will be maintained in accordance with the policy on medical records. ▨ Pharmacy and sample logs will be archived by XXXX ▨ XXXX will maintain an electronic folio or notebook of all official documents and operating licenses. ▨ OSHA training requirement records of employees will be maintained by XXXX including medical waste transit papers. ▨ Fire inspection documentation will be maintained by XXXX. ▨ Electrical inspection documentation will be maintained by XXXX.

Implemented:

Revised:

Reviewed:

Policy and Procedures Policy

Purpose:	To ensure that ALL staff members are knowledgeable and current in expectations for operations and procedures by having written expectations in the form of policies and procedures. To provide a reference for operational questions.
Policy:	It shall be the policy of XXXX that written policies shall guide the operations of XXXX. ▓ XXXX shall formulate policies and procedures to control and coordinate the operation of XXXX. No policy or procedure shall be so construed as to violate or infringe in any way upon state and or federal law or the power and authority of the controlling board of the organization. ▓ XXXX shall issue revisions to the policies and procedures manual as appropriate, supervise the annual review of staff members, and receive recommendations on policies and procedures for the inclusion in or deletion from the manual. ▓ Annually, all staff members will read, sign, and date the declaration page at the front of manual upon review. ▓ All staff members are encouraged to tender suggestions for the editing, inclusion, and or deletion of policies as they deem appropriate as it relates to their role within the organization,
Equipment:	Binder to hold policies and/or electronic folder. Annual signatory/declaration page.
Procedure:	All staff must review the policy and procedure manual annually and sign the declaration page to show proof of review.

Implemented:

Revised:

Reviewed:

Administrative Policies: Patient Rights, Responsibilities, and Eligibility

Eligibility to Receive Services Policy

Purpose:	To articulate the parameters that need to be met to be eligible to become a patient of the business/practice.
Policy:	It shall be the policy of XXX that patients who meet the following criteria are eligible to receive services at XXXX: ▨ A ▨ B ▨ C (List here all of the parameters of your practice. If it is underserved, fee for service, Medicaid, a certain specialty like cardiology etc. Be as comprehensive as possible for the instance where it may be necessary to use this document as evidence to remove someone from your practice.)
Equipment:	Orientation of scheduling staff.
Procedure:	Patients will be asked upon scheduling an appointment and when registering for services if the above criteria have been met. Those who do not meet the criteria above will be referred to a local emergency room or walk-in center for care.

Implemented:

Revised:

Reviewed:

Notice of Available Services Policy

Purpose	To list for the public services available through the practice,
Policy	It shall be the policy of XXXX that available services shall be made known to the community in a variety of ways: ▦ Each year XXXX will publish a flier to be distributed in newspaper and other print media. ▦ Brochures, pamphlets, and other suitable written materials shall be printed and made available to all patients in the waiting room. ▦ XXXX will maintain a Web page publicizing services offered. ▦ Local radio and TV will be utilized to publicize services available.
Equipment	Brochures pamphlets, giveaways, computer (Web page).
Procedure	The Office Manager shall maintain a brochure and be responsible for the maintenance of the practice's Web page with the assistance of a marketing firm when available.

Implemented:

Revised:

Reviewed:

Patient Bill of Rights

XXXX supports the rights of patients and encourages the responsibility of patients by publicizing this document of Patient Rights and Responsibilities. XXXX believes observance of these rights contributes to more effective care with a greater satisfaction for both patients and healthcare professionals.

Information Disclosure: The patient has the right to:

Know who comprises the staff, including their educational and experiential credentials.

Request the staff member of their choice.

Expect that within the capacity of the clinic, staff will respond to each request for services, including evaluation and/or referral using easily understood information.

Participation in Treatment Decisions: The patient has the right to:

Fully engage in healthcare planning and decisions being made regarding the healthcare plan.

Complete information, to the degree known, concerning your diagnosis, treatment, and prognosis in terms that can be reasonably understood. When medically inadvisable to give the information directly, it will be made available to an appropriate person on the patient's behalf.

Receive information necessary to give informed consent prior to any procedure or treatment. Except in emergencies, this information should include the specific procedure or treatment, significant risks, probable duration, and available medical alternatives.

Refuse treatment to the extent permitted by law and to receive information about the medical consequences of refusal.

Expect reasonable continuity of care, including knowing in advance which doctor or nurse is available and being made aware of care required following the visit.

Receive an explanation of any fees.

Confidentiality of Health Information: The patient has the right to

Expect that all communications and records will be treated as confidential and protected, unless less than 18 years old. Then, guardians may be notified in certain circumstances.

Have access to their own medical record either by a copy or to view with a staff member.

Respect and Nondiscrimination: The patient has the right to

Respect and consideration.

Appropriate privacy during examinations, treatments, discussions, and consultations.

Know the staff expects to be treated with as much respect and consideration as they afford the patient.

Complaints: The patient has the right to

Request from a staff member, a copy of the procedures to register a complaint regarding care.

Make a complaint to the State Licensing Board if not satisfied with the decision of the business.

Adapted from The Advisory Commission on Consumer Protection and Quality in the Health Care Industry (2007, http://www.hcqualitycommission.gov/final/append_a.html)

Patient Responsibilities

Patients are afforded rights and along with those rights, patients at XXXX have the following responsibilities:

1. Providing accurate and truthful information about health history, including all medication information.

2. Asking questions if information is not understood, including the explanation of diagnosis, treatment, and prognosis, as well as any educational instructions.

3. Providing the necessary personal information to complete the health record.

4. Paying any charges as a result of care.

5. Seeking medical attention promptly and during regular hours if not an emergency.

6. Reporting significant change in symptoms or failure to improve.

7. Keeping scheduled appointments or canceling in a timely manner.

8. Providing useful feedback about our services and policies.

9. Knowing the names, purposes, and effects of medications prescribed.

Patient Complaints and Grievance Policy

Purpose:	To provide a means for patients to voice their suggestions, complaints, and grievances to appropriate levels of authority to ensure a satisfactory response.
Policy:	It shall be the policy of XXXX that ▓ Complaints are taken seriously. ▓ Every effort shall be made to listen carefully to the complaints of patients. ▓ Patients shall be informed of the results of any suggestions or complaints that they bring forward. Each complaint will be recorded in writing and forwarded to XXXX.
Equipment:	
Procedure:	▓ Any complainant will be encouraged by a staff member to put their complaint in writing in any format available to them. ▓ The written complaint will be forwarded to XXXX, and it will be addressed at the next scheduled governance meeting. ▓ A written response will be returned to the complainant after a complete evaluation and a best course of action is established.

Implemented:

Revised:

Reviewed:

Administrative Policies: Medical Records Information

Medical Records Policy

Purpose:	To maintain a medical record system from which patient information can be collected, processed, maintained, stored, retrieved, and distributed promptly.
Policy:	The following constitutes the the policy of XXXX regarding medical records: 1. Clinical information relevant to patient care is to be available to authorized personnel only and only during operational hours of the clinic unless electronic access is available. Authorized personnel include administrative staff and clinicians. 2. A system of identification and filing shall be employed that ensures the prompt location of patient records. 3. An individual medical record is to be established for every patient receiving care. The record is owned and maintained by the business. 4. Medical records shall not be removed from the practice without permission of XXXX. 5. Except when otherwise required by law, any record that contains clinical, social, financial, or other data on a patient is to be treated as strictly confidential and protected from loss, tampering, alterations, destruction, and unauthorized or inadvertent disclosures. 6. When appropriate, a signed "consent for care form" is to be obtained and included in the record. 7. The content and format of the medical record, including the sequence of information, shall be uniform. 8. Records shall document patient's treatment and progress accurately. 9. Entries in records shall be completed and authenticated by the signature of the clinician rendering care. 10. All record entries shall be legible and comprehensible. 11. Written consent shall be obtained from the patient before medical information is released in any form. Copies of medical records may be given directly to a requesting patient after written consent is obtained. A full-time staff member shall review contents of all information to be released. 12. Allergies shall be noted in red on the problem list. 13. All records shall contain a problem list and a completed allergy sticker to provide a quick summary of ongoing care. 14. Telephone calls of significant medical content shall be documented in the medical record. 15. All medical records shall be kept secure in a locked file and away from possible damage. 16. All staff will utilize S.O.A.P format. Entries shall include: date, chief complaint, history of present illness, physical findings, diagnosis or clinical impression, therapies and education, disposition, recommendations, and instructions and signature of the practitioner. 17. Nothing listed above should supersede the state regulation of medical records.
Equipment:	Release of Information Authorization, Problem List, Progress Note
Procedure:	Patients will sign a written release of information for any medical records. The release will be filed in the correspondence section of the medical record and a notation will be placed on the problem list. Records can only be released to the patient, not to any third party.

Implemented:

Revised:

Reviewed:

Chart Order Policy

Purpose:	To ensure the maintenance and uniformity of each chart.
Policy:	The policy of XXXX is that charts will be maintained as follows: ▓ Right side of the chart: All progress notes shall be numbered and filed by fastening at top and shall be read from the bottom (oldest note) to the top (newest note). Subsequent visits shall be documented in chronological order, numbered consecutively, and placed on top of right side. The patient's name will be identified on each note page. ▓ Left side of the chart: Problem list, with documented allergies and history is on top. Insurance information/demographic page is next down. Diagnostic results (lab/X-ray) chronologically, bottom to top is next. Health history form next. Correspondence records and consultation notes received from other providers are put on the bottom of the left side in the order received. Chart tab includes last name, first name, date of birth, and home address.
Equipment:	End tab charts with enclosure tabs on left and right sides, Progress note form, problem record, and allergy notation.
Procedure:	Each chart will be created identically as described above.

Implemented:

Revised:

Reviewed:

Visit Documentation Form

XXXX Address Town, State ZIP PH: Fax:

Name: _____ **Date/Time:** _____

<u>*S:*</u> **C/C:**

   HPI/ROS:

Current Meds/OTCs:

Med Allergies:

<u>Medical Hx:</u> PastMedHx: FamMHx:

<u>Social Hx:</u> *Sleep:*   *Diet:*   *Relationships:*

Smoker: (No)(Yes) #____/day___:yrs *ETOH:* (No)(Yes) #/wk: ____ *Drug use:* (No)(Yes) ____

<u>*O:*</u>   Encouraged cessation/moderation

HT: _____ WT: _____ T: _____ Pulse: _____ Resp: _____ BP: _____ (♀ L MP: _____)

		WNL	Variant-describe
GENERAL:	WDWN, Alert, cooperative ♀ ♂ in NAD:	( )	
SKIN:	Warm and dry, intact, without lesions or infection	( )	
HEENT:	<u>Eyes:</u> PERRLA,EOM x 6, cornea clear, no papilledema, Sclera and conjunctiva clear, anicteric, without d/c	( )	
	<u>Ears:</u> canals clear, TMs: no bulging, nl reflex, nl landmarks	( )	
	<u>Nose:</u> mucous membranes wnl, no exudate, sinus not tender	( )	
	<u>Oropharynx/Postpharynx:</u> Mucous membranes wnl, no erythema, lesions, or exudate; tonsils not enlarged	( )	
	<u>Neck:</u> FROM, supple, no adenopathy, no thyromegaly	( )	
HEART:	RRR, S1 S2 without murmur, peripheral pulses equal bilat	( )	
LUNGS:	clear, gd aeration, no crackles, wheeze, or rhonchi	( )	
ABDOMEN:	audible BS, soft, nontender, no masses or HSM	( )	
	no CVA tenderness	( )	
MUSCULOSKELETAL:	FROM all extrems, no bruising, no joint tenderness, swelling or erythema, gd tone and strength = bilaterally	( )	
NEURO:	A&O x 3, Cranial nerves intact, Rhomberg WNL	( )	

(continued)

Visit Documentation Form (*continued*)

		WNL	Variant-describe
RECTAL:	Skin clear, no lesions, no masses or hemorrhoids	( )	
GU:	Male: Penis: __ circumcised, no lesions, no d/c	( )	
	Scrotum: no masses, no hernias, testicles ↓↓ bilat	( )	
GYN:	Female:		
	Breasts: no axillary nodes or skin retractions noted	( )	
	no palpable abnl masses, lesions or expressible d/c		
	External genitalia: nl hair distribution, no lesions	( )	
	BUS/Vulva: no tenderness, no redness, no d/c, no lesions	( )	
	Vagina: pink, rugated, no lesions, no d/c	( )	
	Cervix: pink, nontender, no CMT, no d/c, nonfriable	( )	
	Uterus: firm, no masses, nontender	( )	
	Adnexa: no masses, nontender	( )	

testing in office:

Urine HCG : _____ Rapid Mono: _____ Rapid Strep: _____ Rapid Flu: _____

Urine Dip: pH· _____ color: _____ leukocytes: _____ Sp. Grav: _____ blood: _____ nitrites: _____

ketones: _____ urobili: _____ bili: _____ protein: _____ glucose: _____

Wet Prep. pH: _____ whiff: _____ Clue cells: _____ WBC's: _____ RBC's: _____

trich: _____ yeast hyphae: _____

A/P:

Diagnostics:

Rx:

Education/follow up instructions/ Handout(s) given and discussed:_____

(Y) (N) Patient has given me permission to leave a voicemail/email message about this visit.

Examiner's Signature:_____ Date:_____ Contact Phone:_____

Interim/Phone Notes:

Authorization for Use or Disclosure of Protected Health Information

Release of Information Policy

Purpose:	To provide guidelines to ensure consistent actions when releasing personal health information (PHI) .
Policy:	It shall be the policy of XXXX that a written signature on our Release of Information form is required before any information is given to any person or office.
Equipment:	Release of Information form.
Procedure:	Any patient requesting information from the medical record of the practice must obtain, complete, and provide the practice our Release of Information with written signature. It is the preference of the practice that the released PHI be given to the patient directly to do whatever is desired.

Implemented:

Revised:

Reviewed:

Release of Information Authorization

(Required by the Health Insurance Portability and Accountability Act – 45 CFR Parts 160 and 164)

I consent to the use and/or disclosure of my protected health information described below:

To _____

_____

From _____

_____

This release covers all treatment and visits for the dates:

_____ to _____

( ) I consent to release of my complete health record
    (Including records pertaining to mental health care, communicable diseases, HIV or AIDS, and treatment psychiatric issues including alcohol/drug abuse).

OR

( ) I consent to release of my complete health record with the exception of the following:
    ( ) Mental health records
    ( ) Communicable diseases (including HIV and AIDS)
    ( ) Alcohol/drug abuse treatment
    ( ) Other (please specify): _____

This authorization shall be in force and effect until _____.

I understand that I have the right to revoke this authorization, in writing, at any time. I understand that a revocation is not effective for any information already released.

_____   _____
Signature of Patient/Personal Representative   Date

_____
Print name of patient (or) personal representative //relationship to patient

Referral Form

XXXX * Address * Town, State Zip Tel: * Fax:

Patient's Name: _____

Date: _____ DOB: _____ Contact Phone: _____

Reason for referral: _____

_____

_____

Best day/time for pt:

Referring Clinician _____

- -

Referred to _____ (name of specialist)/
(specialty)

_____ (address)

_____

_____ (tele/fax)

_____ Appt date and time

Dear Consultant/Referral Source:
Please complete and return this form or follow-up letter as soon as your consultation is complete. As a reminder this communiqué is for the purpose of continuity of care and under HIPAA a release/signature is not required to return this to us (referring office).

Findings/treatment:

Follow up recommendation:

Thank you very much for your consultation and care of our patient.

Problem-Oriented Medical Record

XXXX * Address * Town, State Zip Tel: * Fax:

NAME: _____   DOB: _____

(Last)   (First)   (Initial)

Date	Diagnosis:	Date	Medications: RFs

Last mammogram:	Last occult test:	Last flu shot:	Last pneumovax:
Last pap smear:	Last colonoscopy:	Last cholesterol screening:	Last tetanus booster:

ALLERGIES: **Page ____ of _____**

Patient Health History Form

PART A – Demographic Information

PLEASE PRINT

Name: _____   ❑ Male   ❑ Female
      (LAST)   (FIRST)   (M.I.)

Birth Date: ___ /___ /___ Birth Place: _____ Cell Phone: (___) _____

Permanent Home Address: _____ Home Phone: (___) _____

City: _____ State: _____ Zip: _____

Email address to contact you: _____

Employer: _____

Employer's address: _____

IN CASE OF EMERGENCY NOTIFY

Full name: _____ Relationship: _____
       (Last)   (First)

Business phone: _____ Cell/Home phone: _____

consent for care and confidentiality acknowledgement

I hereby authorize XXXX staff to provide medical treatment and services. This authorization will remain in effect as long as I am a patient of the practice. In the case of a minor (under 18 years of age), a parent or legal guardian's signature below permits health care in the absence of the guardian.

I consent to the use or disclosure of my protected health information by XXXX to any person or organization for the purposes of carrying out treatment, obtaining payment, or conducting certain healthcare operations. Protected health information used or disclosed by XXXX may include HIV/AIDS related information, psychiatric and other mental health information, and drug and alcohol treatment information, as long as such information is used or disclosed in accordance with state and federal law, which may require specific written authorization. I understand that information regarding how XXXX will use and disclose my information can be found in XXXX's Notice of Privacy Practices. I understand that this consent is effective for as long as XXXX maintains my protected health information.

By signing below, I understand and acknowledge the following:
- I have received a copy of the Privacy Practices and
- I understand this consent is in effect upon signing.

_____ Date: _____
Signature

Patient Health History Form (*continued*)

PART B – Medical History

List all **allergies** you have (meds, foods, metals, latex, environ, etc.) _____

list type of reaction do you have?_____

List all medicines taken regularly (including ones you purchase without Rx). Please include dosage and timing. _____

Have you ever had surgery, been a patient in a hospital overnight, or had a major illness? (**Yes**) (**No**) If yes, explain _____

REVIEW OF SYSTEMS

Have you had/have any of the following (please mark each item). Explain **YES** answers in the space provided.

Yes	No		Yes	No		Yes	No	
☐	☐	Recent weight gain/loss >25 lbs.	☐	☐	Palpitations	☐	☐	Easy bruising
☐	☐	Night sweats/hot flashes	☐	☐	Heart Murmur	☐	☐	Anemia/low iron
☐	☐	Acne	☐	☐	Thrombophlebitis/blood clots	☐	☐	Blood clotting disorder
☐	☐	Atopy/Eczema/other skin problems	☐	☐	Varicose veins	☐	☐	Blood transfusion
☐	☐	Migraines	☐	☐	Mitral valve prolapse	☐	☐	Sickle cell anemia or trait
☐	☐	Concussions	☐	☐	High cholesterol	☐	☐	Thalesemia
☐	☐	Severe head injury (TBI)	☐	☐	High blood pressure	☐	☐	Thyroid problems
☐	☐	Eye problems	☐	☐	Bladder, kidney, or urinary issue	☐	☐	Diabetes
☐	☐	Frequent ear infections	☐	☐	Ovarian cyst, fibroids, endometriosis	☐	☐	Chicken pox
☐	☐	Frequent nosebleeds	☐	☐	Abnormal pap smear	☐	☐	Mononucleosis
☐	☐	Frequent sinus infections	☐	☐	Nipple discharge	☐	☐	Whooping Cough
☐	☐	Snoring	☐	☐	Breast surgery	☐	☐	Rheumatic fever
☐	☐	Breathing problems/asthma	☐	☐	Arthritis	☐	☐	Meningitis
☐	☐	Chronic cough	☐	☐	Fractures or dislocations	☐	☐	MRSA skin infection
☐	☐	Fainting, blackouts, seizures	☐	☐	Painful joints	☐	☐	Malaria
☐	☐	Persistent numb or tingling	☐	☐	Back trouble	☐	☐	Sexually-transmitted infection
☐	☐	Insomnia	☐	☐	Stomach &/or liver problems	☐	☐	Do you smoke or chew tobacco?
☐	☐	Depression	☐	☐	Need special diet	☐	☐	Do you drink alcohol?

Explain **YES** answers:

To the best of my knowledge, the information on this history form is complete and correct.

Signature _____ **Date** _____

Disposal of Medical Records Policy

Purpose:	To describe the procedure for the disposal of medical records to ensure compliance with state and federal laws.
Policy:	It is the policy of XXXX medical records and reports are to be kept in XXXX per YYY state regulation. The Office Manager will oversee the destroying of medical records, which will be done as needed. Medical records shall be kept in a locked storage container until a company contracted for disposal arrives for removal.
Equipment:	Contract with company for confidential destroying of records with Business associate agreement in place. Locked bin.
Procedure:	Staff will place confidential records in a locked storage container for disposal. Paperwork generated through the normal workday which needs to be disposed of confidentially can also be placed in the storage container for confidential disposal.

Implemented:

Revised:

Reviewed:

Administrative Policies: Staffing/Provider Information

Appointment to Medical/Clinical Staff Policy

Purpose:	To provide instruction as to how the medical staff of XXXX is appointed.
Policy:	It is the policy of XXXX that medical staff shall be appointed by the COO. Reappointment shall be done on an annual basis.
Equipment:	Letter of Appointment.
Procedure:	Initially, XXXX medical/clinical staff appointments are confirmed by a letter of offer from the COO or owner of XXXX. Each year, after annual review, a letter is generated from XXXX. This letter is sent to the employee and serves as annual reappointment notification.

Implemented:

Revised:

Reviewed:

Orientation Policy

Purpose:	To identify the necessary components for a complete orientation for new employees of XXXX.
Policy:	It is the policy of XXXX that orientation for new employees shall take place before the commencement of patient care. Orientation is mandatory for all new employees to become familiar with personnel policies and procedures. Orientation includes but is not limited to benefits, pensions, sick time, vacation days, and the following: ▪ Orienting to physical layout of XXXX ▪ Review Policy and Procedure Manual ▪ Review Fire Drill Policy ▪ Review Disaster Plan ▪ Review Universal Precautions Policy ▪ Review Infection Control Policy ▪ Review Exposure Control Plan ▪ Review In-House Lab Testing ▪ Review site specific paperwork (i.e., lab and X-ray requests) ▪ Review referral process ▪ Review scheduling of patients ▪ Review patient charts ▪ Review key use ▪ Review opening and closing procedures ▪ Review emergency box and lock ▪ Review clinical work and call schedule ▪ Review use of time sheets ▪ Review parking and pass ▪ Review personnel file to include: CV, references, licenses, Certs, CPR cert, HBV, PPD, evaluations annually
Equipment:	Keys, Policy and Procedure Manual
Procedure:	Staff members will sign an orientation check list at the conclusion of their orientation, and they will sign the P/P Manual declaration page.

Credentialing Upon Hire Policy

Purpose:	To provide consistent guidelines for the credentialing of each clinician employee of XXXX upon hire.

Policy:	It is the policy of XXXX that each employee of XXXX will adhere to the following requirements as a condition of employment and provide documentation of adherence:
	
	▓ Provide list of all states where professional licensure has occurred.
	▓ Provide list of all institutions of higher education attended.
	▓ Provide permission to confirm veracity of presented credentials.
	▓ Provide evidence of Hepatitis B series completion or declination.
	▓ Complete HIPAA Training.
	▓ Complete OSHA training.
	▓ Address varicella, tetanus, and pertussis status.
	▓ Complete a Tuberculin (Mantoux) test.
	▓ Provide current CPR certification.
	▓ Provide current licensure per state regulation.
	   ☐ RN: RN license
	   ☐ APRN:RN and APRN License
	   ☐ MD: Medical Doctor license
	▓ Provide current independently sought malpractice insurance.
	▓ Provide current National Certification by an Accrediting Agency.
	▓ Provide current State Consumer Protection (DEA) licensure.
	▓ Provide current Federal DEA licensure where applicable.
	▓ Provide NPI number where applicable.

Equipment:	Personnel files checklist, credentialing permission
Procedure:	Office Manager will review credential files during the hiring and orientation process.

Implemented:

Revised:

Reviewed:

Annual Credentialing Policy

Purpose:	To provide consistent guidelines for the credentialing of each clinician employee at the time of the annual review.

Policy:	It is the policy of XXX that each employee will adhere to the following requirements as a condition of employment and provide documentation of adherence.
	
	 ▓ Tuberculin (Mantoux) test.
	 ▓ Completion of annual OSHA bloodborne training.
	 ▓ Provide current CPR certification.
	 ▓ Provide current state licensure per state regulation.
	   ☐ RN: RN license
	   ☐ APN:RN and Nurse Practitioner License
	   ☐ MD: Doctor of Medicine license
	 ▓ Provide current independently bought malpractice insurance.
	 ▓ Provide current National (Board) Certification by an Accrediting Agency.
	 ▓ Provide current State Consumer Protection (DEA) licensure.
	 ▓ Provide current Federal DEA licensure information where applicable.
	 ▓ Provide completed Collaboration Agreement.
	 ▓ Evidence of 3 continuing education attendance.

Equipment:	Personnel files checklist
Procedure:	Annually the Office Manager will review personnel files during the annual review and inform each employee of items required for the year.

Implemented:

Revised:

Reviewed:

Personnel File Checklist

Name:		Review year:	
ADMINISTRATION			
Application	have need N/A	**MANDATED TRAINING UPON HIRE**	
Resume/CV	have need N/A	OSHA training	Done
Standards of Documentation	have need N/A	Confidentiality Training	Done
Confidentiality Agreement	have need N/A	HIPAA	Done
Medical Records Policy	have need N/A	Hepatitis B	have need N/A
ID Badge	have need N/A	Varicella	have need N/A
PAC Code	have need N/A	MMR	have need N/A
Computer Access	have need N/A	Pertusis/Tetanus	have need N/A
Mailbox	have need N/A		
Keys Agreement	have need N/A		
Orientation Sign-Off	have need N/A		
Offer Letter	have need N/A		
CLINICAL PRACTICE REQUIREMENTS			
Collaborative Practice Agreement	have need N/A	exp	Exp
RN License	have need N/A	exp	Exp
APRN License	have need N/A	exp	Exp
Certification	have need N/A	exp	Exp
Federal DEA License	have need N/A	exp	Exp
State DEA License	have need N/A	exp	Exp
UPIN	have need N/A	exp	Exp
NPI	have need N/A	exp	Exp
Malpractice Insurance	have need N/A	exp	Exp
CPR Certification	have need N/A	exp	exp
PPD Annually	have need N/A	exp	exp
OSHA Training Annually	have need N/A	exp	exp
Continuing Ed Classes/Payment	1		
	2		
	3		
Physician Chart Review	done	done	done
Annual Self Evaluation	done	done	done
Annual Evaluation	done	done	done
Staff Appointment	yr	yr	yr

Staff Performance Review Policy

Purpose:	Staff performance is reviewed annually to assure clinical quality and to set performance goals for the employee.
Policy:	It is the policy of XXX that each year the COO or Office Manager will conduct staff performance reviews.
Equipment:	Self-Evaluation Guide, Annual Evaluation Guide
Procedure:	The COO or Office Manager dispenses and collects annual self-evaluations from each employee. Using this as a guide, management will conduct annual staff performance reviews.

Implemented:

Revised:

Reviewed:

Staff Performance Review Form

Based on expectations listed in the job description, grade each performance parameter on the Likert scale each (provide examples on back to support grading).

Performance Review of: _____ Date: _____

Job Skills: 1 = exceeds, 2 = meets, 3 = partially meets, 4 = needs oversight to meet, 5 = fails to meet

Deliver high-quality, evidence-based health care

Comprehensive assessments	1	2	3	4	5
Use of diagnostic ordering	1	2	3	4	5
Use of pharmacotherapeutics	1	2	3	4	5
Use of patient education	1	2	3	4	5
Comprehensive documentation	1	2	3	4	5
Legibility of documentation	1	2	3	4	5
Comprehensive follow up of care	1	2	3	4	5
Constructive use of collaboration	1	2	3	4	5
Constructive use of referrals	1	2	3	4	5
Provides patient advocacy as needed	1	2	3	4	5

Delivers care in a professional manner

Maintains confidentiality	1	2	3	4	5
Maintains compliance with policies	1	2	3	4	5
Maintains good patient communication	1	2	3	4	5
Maintains expertise through CEUs	1	2	3	4	5
Maintains professional appearance	1	2	3	4	5
Maintains collegial relationship with staff	1	2	3	4	5

Job behaviors:

Provides patient-oriented care	1	2	3	4	5
Demonstrates commitment to patient satisfaction	1	2	3	4	5
Demonstrates commitment to achieving	1	2	3	4	5
Completes work on time	1	2	3	4	5
Is organized in the completion of job duties	1	2	3	4	5
Is accountable for care rendered	1	2	3	4	5
Is on time for work with limited absenteeism	1	2	3	4	5

Use this space for documenting examples to substantiate grades given.

_____ _____ _____
Staff member's signature   Supervisor's signature   date

Peer Review/Chart Audit Policy

Purpose:	To review clinical records for content and quality of care with feedback from peers not supervisors.
Policy:	It is the policy of XXXX that peer chart review will take place on a regular interval (insert interval).
Equipment:	Medical records, peer evaluation tool.
Procedure:	At each (interval) at a staff meeting, each clinician will remain and five medical records will be randomly reviewed for content and thoroughness. Minutes of the meeting shall serve as documentation of the peer review process.

Implemented:

Revised:

Reviewed:

Peer Review Form

Date: Practitioner Name:

DOCUMENTATION					
All documentation of visits will be in a S.O.A.P. format.					
Documentation must include date and time of visit.					
Name of patient on progress note					
Page number on note					
Legibility					
S: subjective data includes:					
Chief compliant					
History of present illness					
Review of systems					
Relevant/contributory past medical history					
Pertinent social history					
O: objective data includes:					
Pertinent vital signs					
General observation					
Head-to-toe findings documented					
A: assessment data includes:					
Diagnosis consistent with objective findings					
Diagnosis ** must be proven by diagnostics or use symptom Diagnosis, ICD 9/10					
P. Plan data includes:					
Diagnostics- appropriate/cost effective					
Therapeutics – appropriate/ cost effective					
Interventions – appropriate/ cost effective					
Actions taken are evidence based					
Education - pt ed given, implications and prognosis discussed/ return instructions.					
Problem List					
Visit entered onto list					
Medications recorded					
ACTIONS TAKEN					
Reviewed with practitioner					
Documentation updated					
Signature/initials of evaluator					

MD/APRN Collaborative Practice Agreement

Collaboration is a mutually agreed upon working clinical relationship between an Advanced Practice Registered Nurse (APRN) and a Physician who is educated, trained, or has relevant experience related to the work of such APRN.

I, (physician name), MD, and I (APRN name), APRN agree to enter into a collaborative agreement for the provision of health care at XXXX.

The APRN will provide services consistent with the Scope of Practice for the care of acute and/or chronic illnesses and health maintenance. This includes but is not limited to ordering, performing, and/or interpreting any laboratory test, diagnostic procedure, or medical therapeutics necessary and consistent with applicable training of the APRN.

The APRN will prescribe pharmacotherapeutics, including controlled substances, schedule II through V medications, for the acute and chronic physical conditions requiring their use as related to current practice standards of care. The APRN must have an independent DEA (state and federal) and an NPI number.

Consultation and referral shall be on a case-by-case basis as warranted by patient condition, level of expertise, and clinical judgment of the APRN. Circumstances that require consultation with the MD or a specialist are agreed upon and listed on the bottom of this agreement. Physician oversight will be by observation when consulting the physician and the structured review of patient care via ten (10) clinical charts which will be randomly chosen, reviewed, and discussed each (insert time frame).

Clinical care will be assessed by evaluation patient outcomes and measured by clinical response and/or laboratory data, as per standard chart review.

Coverage for patients during nonoffice hours and vacations will be arranged and mutually agreed upon and written into the contractual arrangements known to all parties.

Disclosure of Physician-APRN collaboration will be either by verbal or written declaration to the patient. The APRN shall educate patients and families about his or her role as a nurse practitioner in the workplace through brochures, signage, or pamphlets.

Each party to this agreement will provide his or her own malpractice insurance coverage to be not less than 500,000 per incident and 1,500,000 per aggregate.

Signed

_____   _____
, MD   , APRN

Date:

Administrative Policies: Infection Control Information

Infection Control Policy

Purpose:	To provide guidelines for the prevention of exposure to blood and body fluids.
Policy:	It is the policy of XXXX that every employee utilize Universal Precautions at all times with all patients. Universal Precautions includes using Personal Protective Equipment (PPE). PPE will be made available to all staff members.
	Proper hand washing techniques are to be followed by all staff members.
	Dressings and disposable supplies, including syringes and needles are to be discarded according to OSHA guidelines in red bag waste receptacles.
Equipment:	PPE: Gloves, masks, gowns, red bag waste receptacles.
Procedure:	Universal Precautions will be in effect at all times with PPE when providing patient care.
	PPE will be provided to each staff member at no personal cost.
	Any patient with a diagnosis inferring communicable disease or who is immunosuppressed and at risk for infection will be kept isolated from the general population as soon as the issue is discovered.
	See Blood Borne Pathogen Exposure Control Plan.

Implemented:

Revised:

Reviewed:

Cleaning and Decontaminating Spills of Blood or Body Fluids Policy

Purpose:	To provide guidance and ensure safety while cleaning potentially hazardous materials.
Policy:	All spills of blood or other body fluids will be cleaned and the area decontaminated promptly.
Equipment:	"Body Fluid Clean-Up Kit", "Infection Control Kit" (bacteriacidal/viricidal) _____ Cleansers
Procedure:	Obtain the Clean-Up kit located in the _____. Gloves must be worn when cleaning up blood or body fluids contaminated with a visible body fluid. Dirty linen should be handled as contaminated and placed in a nonporous bag for transport to a laundry facility. Articles contaminated with more than 100 cc of blood or body fluids should be bagged and placed in the red bag waste container in each exam room. _____ Cleanser can be used to clean up smaller spills on surfaces.

Implemented:

Revised:

Reviewed:

Handwashing Policy

Purpose:	To ensure that staff members wash their hands as a means of preventing the spread of infection.
Policy:	It is the policy of XXXX that all staff members wash their hands under the following conditions: ▓ When coming on duty. ▓ Whenever hands are obviously soiled. ▓ Before patient contact. ▓ Before preparing or handling medication. ▓ After patient contact. ▓ After handling contaminated items or equipment. ▓ After contact with blood, urine, feces, oral secretions, vomit, bodily fluids, or broken skin. ▓ After personal body functions such as toilet use, blowing one's nose, applying make-up, and before and after eating or drinking. ▓ Upon completion of duty.
Equipment:	Running water, soap, paper towels, or liquid alcohol-based gel.
Procedure:	1. Turn on faucet and wait for water to reach desired temperature. 2. Wet hands and wrists thoroughly. Spread soap over the entire area of hands and wrists. 3. Rub hands together vigorously to create suds. Work lather over hands and wrists. Rub one lathered hand against the other (friction removes surface organisms). Scrub for at least 20 seconds. 4. Rinse hands thoroughly under running water. 5. Dry hands well with paper towels. Turn off the water by using a paper towel to cover the handle of the faucet. 6. Discard the paper towels in waste container.

Implemented:

Revised:

Reviewed:

Medical Waste Policy

Purpose:	To provide guidelines for the identification and disposal of medical waste.
Policy:	XXXX will contract with _____ (a medical waste provider) for the proper disposal of all medical waste. The following will be considered medical waste according to the guidelines published by the U.S. Office of the Environmental Protection Agency: Human blood, body fluids and blood products Sharps (needles, syringes, scalpels) Cultures and stocks Pathological wastes Animal waste Isolation wastes Spill/cleanup materials
Equipment:	Sharp container boxes, red bag waste receptacles
Procedure:	Each patient area will contain a sharps disposal container and/or a red bag waste receptacle. These will be emptied by staff when appropriate and placed in a collection box until pick up. The calendar for expected pick up dates will be posted. Universal Precautions will be maintained at all times, especially when handling medical waste. Documentation of the medical waste pick up should be provided by the pick-up company and should be kept for 7 years.

Implemented:

Revised:

Reviewed:

Business Cleaning Policy

Purpose:	To maintain an efficient and accurate accounting of the cleaning process of XXX. XXX must be kept clean at all times to avoid problems with our license or operations and delivery of health care in the clinic.
Policy:	It is the policy of XXXX that cleaning be done thoroughly as follows: 1. Floors will be swept daily. 2. Floors will be buffed YYY (at regular intervals). 3. Carpets will be vacuumed daily. 4. Carpets will be shampooed YYY (at regular intervals). 5. Waiting room runners will be replaced YYY (at regular intervals). 6. All trash cans in each room and work area will be emptied daily. 7. Every sink cleaned daily. 8. Toilets cleaned daily. 9. Bathroom counters cleaned daily. 10. Bathroom floors washed twice weekly. 11. Waiting room surfaces cleaned with antibacterial product. 12. Waiting room windows and backdoor windows cleaned YYY (at regular intervals). 13. Waiting room furniture vacuumed/cleaned monthly. 14. Exam tables and exam room counters will be cleaned at least at the end of each day with an antibacterial-antiMRSA product or more often as the condition requires. Sign-off sheet must be completed to document cleaning. 15. Red bag (OSHA) and sharps containers will be changed as needed by XXXX staff. 16. Desk tops and phone receivers will be cleaned daily. All doors must be kept closed and secured at ALL times to insure confidentiality of contents of XXXX. Nothing can ever be stored under a sink.
Equipment:	Antibacterial cleaning products, vacuum.
Procedure:	As package directions indicate by cleaning staff.

Implemented:

Revised:

Reviewed:

Administrative Policies: Emergency-Related Information

Mandatory Reporting Policy

Purpose:	To provide information to authorities about medical conditions divulged that may have required reporting or have insurance implications.
Policy:	All lawful and appropriate reporting forms will be completed by the clinician seeing the patient and forwarded to authorities according to confidentiality laws. If in the act of delivering clinical services, information is obtained concerning an accident, potential abuse of a minor, or a reportable disease, pertinent clinical information will be forwarded to the authorities.
Equipment:	Appropriate report forms.
Procedure:	Consult with Office Manager. Motor Vehicle Crashes: Release of medical information must be signed by patient. Forms are completed and sent to attorneys as instructed by patient. Disability: Release of medical information must be signed by the patient. Forms are completed and sent to attorneys. Suspected Abuse: Appropriate contact with social service agencies and/or police. Reportable Diseases: Forms are obtained, completed, and returned to state public health department. A copy of any report completed and given to patient should be kept in the chart for documentation purposes.

Implemented:

Revised:

Reviewed:

Emergency Equipment Policy

Purpose:	To establish regular checks for the maintenance and function of emergency equipment.
Policy:	It is the policy of XXXX that all emergency equipment will be checked on a regular basis and recorded in the OSHA log. Eye Wash Station – weekly Oxygen Tank – monthly Fire Extinguisher – monthly Emergency Box- quarterly EKG Machine/AED – as manufacturer recommends
Equipment:	Oxygen tank, emergency box. eye wash station, fire extinguisher, EKG/AED.
Procedure:	See the individual policies for the above equipment.

Implemented:

Revised:

Reviewed:

Clinical Practice Policies: Operational Guidelines and Policies

Clinical Guidelines Policy

Purpose:	To establish the existence of a resource used to guide the clinical practice of the business.
Policy:	It shall be the policy of **XXXX** that care rendered will follow the guidelines of the *text Clinicial Guidelines of Family Practice,* by **XXXX** unless variance in the care rendered is supported in documentation within the medical record.
Equipment:	*Clinical Guidelines of Family Practice.*
Procedure:	Staff will be familiar at the minimum guidelines for care outlined in the text *Clinical Guidelines of Family Practice.* If care varies from that suggested, documentation in the medical record should explain why the variance was necessary.

Implemented:

Revised:

Reviewed:

Emergency Equipment/Medication Box Policy

Purpose:	To ensure that the Emergency Equipment/Medication Box is kept clean, supplies are in date, and in good repair.
Policy:	It is the policy of XXXX that one regular staff member will be assigned the quarterly task of lock checking and completing inventory of the emergency medicine box and documenting the procedure.
Equipment:	Emergency medicine box, inventory list, replaceable locks, OSHA log.
Procedure:	1. Once a quarter the emergency box will be checked. 2. Remove the plastic lock. 3. Inventory each item and check expiration date. 4. Report to XXXX if items need replacing. 5. Document the check was done by date and initials in the OSHA log.

Implemented:

Revised:

Reviewed:

Emergency Equipment/Medication Box Checklist

quantity & expiration date noted

Biohazard Bag (2)				
Vinyl Gloves (6)				
Safety Glasses (1)				
Triangular Bandages (2)				
Rolled Gauze – Sterile (3)				
Rolled Gauze – Nonsterile (4)				
4×4 Sterile Gauze Pads (10)				
Adhesive Tape (1)				
1×3 Bandaids (10)				
Steri Strips – varied sizes				
Sphygmomanometer				
Stethoscope				
All-Purpose Shears				
Arm Splint – Foam and Aluminum				
Velcro Tourniquet				
Splinter Forceps				
Kelly Clamp (hemostat)				
Flashlight with working batteries				
Tongue Depressors(5)				
Large Bandaids (5)				
Antiseptic Swabs (10)				
Alcohol Swabs (10)				
Ammonia Inhalants – 1 box				
CPR Micromask				
Oxygen Tank				
Ambu Bag/Mask/Tubing				
Instant Glucose Gel (2)				
Adult Epi Pen (2)				
Burn Gel Packets				
Disposable Burn Dressings (2)				
Bloodborne Pathogens Disposal Kit				
Initials of person completing checklist				
Date				

Eye Wash Policy

Purpose:	To ensure that the eye wash station is kept clean, the pipes are cleared of residue, and the unit is in good repair.
Policy:	It is the policy of XXXX that one regular staff member will be assigned the weekly task of rinsing the eye wash station and documenting the procedure. The eyewash will be maintained in an area that has un-fettered access within 15 seconds.
Equipment:	Sink, eye wash, running tepid water flow, OSHA log.
Procedure:	1. Once a week the eye wash station will be rinsed. 2. Remove the covers over each nozzle. 3. Turn on the faucet. 4. Ensure the water bubbles up through the two eye nozzles at a height of at least 6 inches. 5. Allow the water to run through the nozzles for 15 minutes. 6. Turn off the water and recap each nozzle. 7. Document the check was done by date and initials in the OSHA log.

Implemented:

Revised:

Reviewed:

Oxygen Tank Policy

Purpose:	To ensure oxygen is available, and tank is functional.
Policy:	It is the policy of XXXX that one regular staff member will be assigned the monthly task of testing the oxygen tank. The tank will be turned on to ensure functioning and an adequate level of oxygen. The oxygen tank will be observed for level after each use.
Equipment:	Oxygen tank, oxygen tank regulator.
Procedure:	1. Take wrench off oxygen tank. 2. Place wrench over valve of regulator. 3. Turn to the left to start the flow of oxygen. 4. Observe the gauge and record the level of oxygen in the tank in the OSHA log. 5. Turn to the right to stop the flow of oxygen. 6. Turn nut on bottom of gauge to release oxygen from gauge. 7. Check that an adequate supply of nasal canula and re-breather masks are available. 8. Inform XXXX if tank requires filling or if labeled expiration date is approaching.

Implemented:

Revised:

Reviewed:

Fire Drills Policy

Purpose:	To review procedures to ensure a safe evacuation in the event of a fire.
Policy:	It is the policy of XXXX that a quarterly fire drill occur.
Equipment:	Fire drill documentation sheet.
Procedure:	▓ Call a mock fire drill. ▓ Observe staff procedures consistent with the Fire Policy including, evacuation of patients, locking of entrances that patients may enter unobserved during a fire, closing of doors and windows, and removal of oxygen tanks. ▓ Record drill on documentation sheet. ▓ Have all staff that participated in drill sign. ▓ File drill on OSHA log.

Implemented:

Revised:

Reviewed:

Fire Policy

Purpose:	To communicate guidelines on what to do in the event of a fire.
Policy:	It is the policy of XXXX that each room will have a posted evacuation route. All staff members will know the location of the fire boxes, extinguishers, exits, and the evacuation procedure below.
Equipment:	Evacuation routes, fire extinguishers
Procedure:	<ul><li>All personnel will evacuate in the event of a fire.</li><li>Do not try to fight a fire; pull the nearest fire pull box and/or call 911.</li><li>Evacuate all patients and families immediately.</li><li>Lock all nonexiting doors so patients cannot enter the building unnoticed.</li><li>Close all doors and windows, checking to be sure each room is empty.</li><li>Staff should evacuate with all oxygen tanks if possible.</li><li>Stay with patients in a safe place until fire personnel have deemed to building safe for reentry.</li></ul>

Implemented:

Revised:

Reviewed:

Fire Extinguisher Policy

Purpose:	To ensure the proper functioning of the fire extinguisher.
Policy:	It is the policy of XXXX that one assigned employee will check the fire extinguisher tag and level monthly. The proper use of a fire extinguisher "P.A.S.S." will be reviewed at one staff drill annually. P=pull pin, A=aim, S=squeeze, S=sweep the spray.
Equipment:	fire extinguisher, fire extinguisher tag.
Procedure:	▓ Observe gauge on top of extinguisher for level of fullness. ▓ Observe tag on fire extinguisher for current status. ▓ Record results on OSHA log. If tag or extinguisher needs replacing, inform XXXX.

Implemented:

Revised:

Reviewed:

Fire Drill Documentation

Time and date mock drill was called: _____

Check completion of events:

- Evacuation of patients completed safely. (Yes) (No)

- Locking of non-evacuation doors to stop unintended entry. (Yes) (No)

- Closing of hallway doors and windows. (Yes) (No)

- Removal or oxygen tanks. (Yes) (No)

Signatures of all participants:

Implemented:

Revised:

Reviewed:

Hours of Operation/Staffing Policy

Purpose:	To ensure patient and staff safety and quality of care.
Policy:	It is the policy of XXXX that whenever the business is open, two licensed professionals will be onsite. If only one licensed professional is available, no scheduled appointments will take place. Rather, patients will be triaged (on-site or on-call) to facilities in our community. Hours of operation for XXXX are: Monday–Friday: 8:30 A.M. – 5:30 PM Saturday: Noon – 4:00 PM On-Call Coverage: A staff member is on call whenever XXXX is not open for business. A brochure will distributed to all clientele detailing the on-call procedure.
Equipment:	Work schedule, on-call schedule.
Procedure:	A monthly clinical schedule will be posted at least six weeks in advance of the time frame covered by the schedule.

Implemented:

Revised:

Reviewed:

Contact Phone Policy

Purpose:	To make available important contact numbers and resources to staff members.
Policy:	It is the policy of XXXX that YYYY will create, update, and distribute to staff members a "Contact Telephone List"
Equipment:	Contact Telephone List.
Procedure:	The Office Manager will update and distribute "Contact Telephone List" every six months and as needed.

Implemented:

Revised:

Reviewed:

Contact Telephone List Form

Staff:

_____ , APRN	home:	cell:
_____ , APRN	home:	cell:
_____ , Receptionist	home:	cell:
_____ , Office Manager	home:	cell:
_____ , MD	home:	cell:

Local Resources:

Lab Results	(111) 111-1111	44 Main Street Anytown., NY
Counseling	(111) 111-1111	44 Main Street Anytown., NY:
Ambulance	(111) 111-1111	44 Main Street Anytown., NY

Poison Control   800-343-2722 (local) 111-111-1111

Walk-In Clinic   XXX (111) 111-1111   44 Main Street Anytown., NY
                      Hours: M-F 8am-8pm; Sat. 9am-5pm; Sun 10am-4pm.

Emergency Departments

XXXX Hospital

Main Hospital	111-111-1111
Main E.R Desk	111-1111
Triage Nurse	111-1111

Pharmacies:

Arrow	(111) 111-1111	44 Main Street Anytown., NY
CVS (**24 hours**)	(111) 111-1111	44 Main Street Anytown.,
Rite Aid	(111) 111-1111	44 Main Street Anytown., NY
Walgreen's	(111) 111-1111	44 Main Street Anytown., NY

Dental Emergency:

XXX, DMD	(111) 111-1111	44 Main Street Anytown., NY
Weekdays:	(111)-111-1111	
Emergencies:	(111)-111-1111 (Nights & weekends)	

On-Call Policy

Purpose:	To notify patients of XXXX of the on-call services available.
Policy:	It is the policy of XXXX to offer on-call service whereby a staff member is available for phone consultation after hours when XXXX is unavailable or not open for clinical services. Call duty will be shared among staff members. A schedule of call will be published monthly. All calls received while on duty will be documented on a progress note and filed in the patient's chart the next day.
Equipment:	Call schedule, progress note (interim note section).
Procedure:	The Office Manager will create and distribute an on-call schedule to staff members.

Implemented:

Revised:

Reviewed:

Discarding of Expired Pharmacological Therapeutics Policy

Purpose:	To·ensure the proper disposal of unused medications.
Policy:	To document of and dispose of expired and unused medications in a safe an appropriate manner.
Equipment:	Destruction inventory sign-out sheet.
Procedure:	XXXX maintains an inventory of all drugs used in the facility. Inventory sheets include the name of medication, lot number, quantity of medication, and each dose dispensed. Expired or unused medications will be removed from the medication area and stored in the bottom drawers of the refrigerator until disposal can be completed. When disposal occurs, a record of removal/destruction will be documented on the inventory sign-out sheet with the appropriate date/lot number/and items destroyed. A record of destruction must be signed by two staff members on the inventory sheet. The medications will be disposed of according to hazard level. Some being ruined by adding water and discarded in trash and some held until the next hazard waste pick up.

Implemented:

Revised:

Reviewed:

Prescription Pad Policy

Purpose:	To provide guidance as to the distribution, control, and safe keeping of prescription pads.
Policy:	It is the policy of XXXX that the inventory supply of blank prescription pads is to be maintained by the office manager in a locked cabinet. Nurse practitioners (APNs) who have obtained prescriptive authority shall have a supply of prescriptions with their name imprinted on them. They are responsible for assuring protection of the prescription pads. The pad will have both the APN and physician names on it. Pads not currently in use MUST be locked in the medication room.
Equipment:	Prescription pads, locked cabinets.
Procedure:	Storage of the unused pads will be in a locked cabinet in the medication area. When necessary the Office Manager will arrange to have more prescription pads made.

Implemented:

Revised:

Reviewed:

Fax Cover Sheet

DATE:

TIME:

TO:

FAX #:

FROM:

       XXX: _____ _____

       Phone:

       Fax:

RE:

PAGES (INCLUDING COVER): _____
If you do not receive all pages, please call the number above

CONFIDENTIALITY NOTICE:

This fax message, including any attachments, is for the <u>sole use of the intended recipient(s)</u> and may contain confidential and privileged information. Any unauthorized review, use, disclosure, or distribution is prohibited. If you are not the intended recipient, please contact the sender by phone number above and DESTROY all copies of the original message. Information contained in this fax should be treated as confidential and is intended to only be read by the recipient in the TO line above. Dissemination of this information in any other capacity violates patient's confidentiality.

Index

A

Abuse, mandatory reporting of, 148, 278

Accident reporting, 153

Accreditation, 13, 50–51, 207–209

Accreditation Association for Ambulatory Health Care, 50, 208

Accreditation Commission for Health Care, Inc., 208

Acquisitions, 189

Acute care nurse practitioners, 44, 201

Adaptation model, 79

Administrative policies and forms, 145, 148, 231–240

  blank policy form, 232

  for emergencies, 277–279

  governance meeting documentation, 235

  governance policy, 234

  for infection control, 271–276

  for medical records, 247–258

  mission statement, 233

  official documents of clinical policy, 239

  organizational chart, 236

  organizational framework, 231–240

  for patient rights, responsibilities, and eligibility, 241–246

  policy and procedure policy, 240

  staffing/provider, 259–269

  staff meeting documentation form, 238

  staff meeting policy, 237

Advanced nurse practitioners, 4, 11. *See also* Nurse practitioners

Advanced nursing practice, 49–50

Advanced practice nurses, 4, 5. *See also* Nurse practitioners demand for, 90, 213

Advanced practice registered nurses (APRN), 12. *See also* Nurse practitioners

ADVANCE for Nurse Practitioners, 4, 167

Advocacy, 62

Agency for Healthcare Research and Quality, 38, 79, 84–85, 86

American Academy of Family Practitioners, 31

American Academy of Nurse Practitioners, 62, 221

  certification from, 52, 53

  professional policies of, 11

  salary survey by, 90, 167

  Standards of Practice for Nurse Practitioners of, 79

American Academy of Pediatrics, 31

American Association of Colleges of Nursing, 13–14, 33, 36

American Association of Critical Care Nurses, 221

American Association of Nurse Attorneys, 5, 89, 104, 128

American College of Nurse Practitioners, 10–11, 62, 221

American College of Physicians, 31, 69

American Journal for Nurse Practitioners, 11, 54, 217

American Nurses Association, 5, 13–14, 62, 221

American Nurses Credentialing Center, 13, 51, 52, 53